W9-AEV-056

DISCARDED

ANNUAL REVIEW OF NURSING RESEARCH

Volume 13, 1995

EDITORS

Joyce J. Fitzpatrick, Ph.D.
Dean and Professor
Frances Payne Bolton School of Nursing
Case Western Reserve University
Cleveland, OH

Joanne S. Stevenson, Ph.D.
Professor
College of Nursing
The Ohio State University
Columbus, OH

ASSOCIATE EDITOR

Nikki S. Polis, Ph.D.
Researcher
Frances Payne Bolton School of Nursing
Case Western Reserve University
Cleveland, OH

ADVISORY BOARD

Violet Barkauskas, Ph.D.
School of Nursing
University of Michigan
Ann Arbor, MI

Marie Cowan, Ph.D.
School of Nursing
University of Washington
Seattle, WA

Claire Fagin, Ph.D.
School of Nursing
University of Pennsylvania
Philadelphia, PA

Suzanne Feetham, Ph.D.
National Institute for Nursing Research
National Institutes of Health
Bethesda, MD

Phyllis Giovannetti, Sc.D.
Faculty of Nursing
University of Alberta
Edmonton, Alberta, CA

Ada Sue Hinshaw, Ph.D.
School of Nursing
University of Michigan
Ann Arbor, MI

Kathleen McCormick, Ph.D.
Office of the Forum for Quality and Effectiveness in Health Care
Agency for Health Care Policy and Research
Rockville, MD

Jane Norbeck, D.N.Sc.
School of Nursing
University of California, San Francisco
San Francisco, CA

Christine Tanner, Ph.D.
School of Nursing
Oregon Health Sciences University
Portland, OR

Roma Lee Taunton, Ph.D.
School of Nursing
The University of Kansas
Kansas City, KS

Harriet Werley, Ph.D.
School of Nursing
University of Wisconsin-Milwaukee
Milwaukee, WI
Founding Editor
Annual Review of Nursing Research

ANNUAL REVIEW OF NURSING RESEARCH

Volume 13, 1995

Joyce J. Fitzpatrick, Ph.D.
Joanne S. Stevenson, Ph.D.
Editors

CARL A. RUDISILL LIBRARY
LENOIR-RHYNE COLLEGE

SPRINGER PUBLISHING COMPANY
New York

RT
81.5
.A55
V 13
Jed. 1996

Order ANNUAL REVIEW OF NURSING RESEARCH. Volume 13, 1995, prior to publication and receive a 10% discount. An order form can be found at the back of this volume.

Copyright © 1995 by Springer Publishing Company, Inc.
All rights reserved

No part of this publication may be reproduced, stored in a retrieval system, or transmitted in any form or by any means, electronic, mechanical, photocopying, recording, or otherwise, without the prior permission of Springer Publishing Company, Inc.

Springer Publishing Company, Inc.
536 Broadway
New York, NY 10012

95 96 97 98 99 / 5 4 3 2 1

ISBN-0-8261 8232-1
ISSN-0739-6686

CARL A. RUDISILL LIBRARY
LENOIR-RHYNE COLLEGE

ANNUAL REVIEW OF NURSING RESEARCH is indexed in *Cumulative Index to Nursing and Allied Health Literature* and *Index Medicus*.

Printed in the United States of America

Contents

Preface

This thirteenth volume of the *Annual Review of Nursing Research (ARNR)* series continues the tradition of selecting recognized scholars as authors to complete a critical review of the nursing research in a defined area. As the series has developed over the years, we collectively, authors, editors, advisory board members, reviewers, and readers, have been able to chart the expansion of our science.

In Part I, "Research on Nursing Practice," we have included nursing research related to key social and health issues. William L. Holzemer and Holly Skodol Wilson review research related to quality of life and the spectrum of human immunodeficiency virus (HIV) infection. Ada M. Lindsey describes research on the physical health of homeless adults. Susan J. Kelley presents a review of research on child sexual abuse and Heidi vonKoss Krowchuck reviews research on the neurobehavioral effects of childhood lead exposure.

Part II, "Research on Nursing Care Delivery," includes the following chapters: "Case Management," by Gerri S. Lamb; "Technology and Home Care," by Carol E. Smith; "Nursing Minimum Data Set," by Polly Ryan and Connie Delaney; and "Pediatric Hospice Nursing," by Ida M. Martinson. In this section, an effort was made to select current topics for review.

Part IV, "Research on the Profession of Nursing," includes two chapters: "The Professionalization of Nurse Practitioners," by Bonnie Bullough and "Feminism and Nursing," by Peggy Chinn. Part V includes a chapter by Sara Torres and Antonia M. Villarruel on health risk behaviors for Hispanic women.

Special acknowledgments are due to our scientific reviewers of manuscripts, our Advisory Board members, editorial staff, and support staff.

JOYCE J. FITZPATRICK
SENIOR EDITOR

Contributors

Bonnie Bullough, Ph.D.
Department of Nursing
University of Southern California
Los Angeles, CA

Peggy L. Chinn, Ph.D.
School of Nursing
University of Colorado Health Sciences Center
Denver, CO

Connie Delaney, Ph.D.
College of Nursing
The University of Iowa
Iowa City, IA

William L. Holzemer, Ph.D.
School of Nursing
University of California, San Francisco
San Francisco, CA

Susan J. Kelley, Ph.D.
School of Nursing
Georgia State University
Atlanta, GA

Heidi vonKoss Krowchuk, Ph.D.
School of Nursing
University of North Carolina at Greensboro
Greensboro, NC

Gerri S. Lamb, Ph.D.
Carondelet St. Mary's Hospital
Tucson, AZ

Ada M. Lindsey, Ph.D.
School of Nursing
University of California, Los Angeles
Los Angeles, CA

Ida M. Martinson, Ph.D.
School of Nursing
University of California, San Francisco
San Francisco, CA
and
Frances Payne Bolton School of Nursing
Case Western Reserve University
Cleveland, OH

Polly Ryan, Ph.D.
John L. Doyne Hospital and Clinics
Milwaukee, WI

Sara Torres, Ph.D.
College of Nursing
University of North Carolina at Charlotte
Charlotte, NC

Carol E. Smith, Ph.D.
School of Nursing
University of Kansas
Kansas City, KS

Antonia M. Villarruel, Ph.D.
School of Nursing
University of Michigan
Ann Arbor, MI

Patricia Hinton Walker, Ph.D.
School of Nursing
University of Rochester
Rochester, NY

Holly Skodol Wilson, Ph.D.
School of Nursing
University of California, San Francisco
San Francisco, CA

FORTHCOMING

ANNUAL REVIEW OF
NURSING RESEARCH, Volume 14

Tentative Contents

PART I

Research on Nursing Practice

Chapter 1

Quality of Life and the Spectrum of HIV Infection

William L. Holzemer
Holly Skodol Wilson
School of Nursing
University of California, San Francisco

CONTENTS

QUALITY OF LIFE AS AN OUTCOME MEASURE

Public discourse on quality of life (QOL) has made health care providers keenly aware of client choices in therapy decisions. Scholarly work on QOL has broadened conceptualizations of the outcomes of care, ultimately changing standards of care. Although the literature on QOL is expansive, little work has focused on defining and measuring the meaning and dimensions of QOL for persons with human immunodeficiency virus (HIV) infection. Little is known about the impact of age, gender, ethnic diversity, and stage of illness on perspectives of QOL in HIV-infected persons. Of particular importance is the need to understand the meaning and dimensions of QOL from patients' perspectives (Oleson, 1990).

In her content analysis of the QOL literature during a 10-year period, Kleinpell (1991) traced the history of efforts to measure QOL to three national studies measuring the overall well-being of populations. Continued interest in the concept had yielded more than 3,000 Index Medicus citations by 1991. Kleinpell concluded that the concept is associated with vague and abstract meanings, including "life satisfaction," "perceptions of well-being," "worth of life," "value of life," "self-esteem" "contentment," or "satisfaction with life." Others propose that QOL is based on conditions, such as the ability to enter into relationships with others and the capacity to reason and have emotions. Still others define QOL using criteria, such as income, housing, and physical functions. Most, however, define it as referring to attitudes, feelings of well-being, and perceptions. Goodinson and Singleton (1989), Kleinpell (1991), Muthny, Koch, and Stump (1990), and Spitzer (1987) have provided excellent overviews of QOL research for areas other than HIV/acquired immunodeficiency syndrome (AIDS).

When focusing on health-related QOL, Goodinson and Singleton (1989) concurred with the elusive multidimensionality of the concept, suggesting that QOL should be measured at different times during illness and should include information from patients. Measuring health-related QOL has served diverse purposes. Among the most commonly cited are (a) to justify or refute different forms of treatment (Glover, 1977; Greer, 1987); (b) to identify disease sequelae that may be mediated by palliative measures; (c) to evaluate cost-effectiveness of treatments; and (d) to identify treatments with potential to maximize the "quality-adjusted life years" (Siegrist & Junge, 1989).

Health-related QOL has become an important component in evaluating patient outcomes in progressive, debilitating, and terminal diseases. QOL has been studied in hypertensive disease (Rockey & Griep, 1980), chronic obstructive pulmonary disease (McSweeny et al., 1982), myocardial disease (Ott et al., 1983), and end-stage renal disease patients (Koch & Murphy, 1990). Research has been conducted on QOL among cancer patients (Morris, Suissa, Sherwood, Wright, & Greer, 1986; Padilla et al., 1983). Quality of death has also been studied (Wallston, Burger, Smith, & Baugher, 1988) as has QOL in children and adolescents with cancer (Hinds, 1990). Investigators agree that there is no "gold standard" for measuring QOL, but that it is a critical variable for investigation because lethality, mortality, and rehabilitation alone are insufficient (Kober, Küchler, Broelsch, Kremer, & Henne-Bruns, 1990). They further agree that health-related QOL is a dynamic concept that changes during the course of illness (Künsebeck, Korber, & Freyberger, 1990). Expanding the choice of end points beyond the traditional "hard" variables has had widespread support (Padilla et al., 1983; Troidl et al., 1987). Experts also urge that future research be "based on conceptual models" that clarify relationships among QOL domains throughout illness and attend to multiethnic issues (Aaronson, 1991; Marshall, 1990).

Few systematic attempts have examined ethnic differences in QOL in general or in HIV specifically. Experts agree that perceptions of QOL are embedded in cultural beliefs about what constitutes normalcy, health, and even physical appearance and functioning. Culture and ethnic background influence every aspect of the experience of both health and illness, including the meaning attached to physical symptoms; responses to symptoms, such as pain; and the selection of care. Because health care and disease ideology differ among cultures, assessments of QOL must be understood within the boundaries that maintain and reinforce life experiences (Marshall, 1990). This understanding cannot be gained through simple language translation. For example, many Hispanics are bilingual or multilingual but not necessarily acculturated within the dominant Anglo society (Marshall, 1990). Kleinman (1986) was critical of any attempts to evaluate QOL that did not account for the personal significance of an illness and its expression in cultural norms and social relationships.

Despite these areas of agreement, confusion surrounds the concepts of health status, QOL, and functional status. Debate continues on the merits of global versus disease-specific scales. Some QOL measures are clinician scored, and others employ patient self-reports (Spitzer, 1987). There are gaps in knowledge regarding cross-class and cross-cultural approaches to the assessment of QOL, in methods to assess the QOL for family systems, and in development of age-specific norms for assessing QOL across the life span (Aaronson, 1991). General agreement exists on three central points, however. First, health-related QOL is a multidimensional concept that includes functional status, psychological and social well-being, health perceptions, and disease- and treatment-related symptoms. Second, QOL assessment is essentially subjective, because the person whose life quality is in question is the primary source of information (Aaronson, 1991). And, third, research on QOL should be based on strong conceptual models, although relevant models have not yet been fully developed. Conceptual models are needed that address the multidimensionality of QOL, the interrelationship among QOL domains, both patient coping and support resources, and the effects of nursing and medical interventions (Jaloweic, 1990). Such models are particularly critical in cross-class, multiethnic populations to avoid overgeneralizing existing theory or research findings based solely on the perspectives of the majority culture. Awareness of the importance of QOL is reflected in the growing body of HIV/AIDS care literature that includes QOL measures.

Literature Review Process

Searches were conducted to identify studies that examined QOL and HIV/AIDS, and were available in the English language. The searches included all combinations of "quality of life," "AIDS," and "HIV" as exact subject, key words, and title words. Forty-one studies were selected from those published between 1989 through September 1993. The following categories were excluded: case studies, research reports based only on statistical projections with no actual data, and cost and resource use studies.

This literature review is organized in five sections, beginning with essential information on the changing HIV/AIDS epidemic. In the second section, definitions and measurement strategies for QOL in HIV infection are presented. The third section examines QOL across the spectrum of wellness to illness. In the fourth section, HIV-related signs and symptoms are linked to studies of QOL, and intervention studies using QOL measures are reported in the fifth section.

HIV/AIDS EPIDEMIC

As the AIDS pandemic enters its second decade, two emerging trends are profoundly affecting the ability to care for persons living with HIV infection. First, the fabric of HIV infection in the United States has changed (Vermund, 1991). Although the incidence of HIV infection is decreasing slightly among the white gay male population, it is increasing among people of color, women, and children (Centers for Disease Control [CDC], 1993). Second, providers are becoming more aware that HIV-positive persons are experiencing longer healthy, symptom-free phases as a result of more effective therapies. These trends have important implications for understanding QOL in persons with HIV infection.

The CDC has reported 315,390 confirmed AIDS diagnoses (CDC, 1993; Resource Booklet, 1993), 60% of which are in homosexual/bisexual populations. People of color are overrepresented in the 1992 HIV statistics. Hispanics account for 8% of the U.S. population and 16.5% of the adult AIDS diagnoses; African Americans comprise 12% of the population and 30% of the adult AIDS diagnoses. Of the reported cases of AIDS in women, African American women account for 52.9%, and Hispanic women account for 20.9%. The preponderance of persons living with AIDS worldwide are people of color—particularly women of color (Fullilove et al., 1990).

Newer treatment options have made possible early intervention for HIV infection and more aggressive management of HIV disease. Some authorities believe HIV disease has become a chronic illness (Moore, 1991). This view may be premature; however, treatment options, such as zidovudine, may be slowing disease progression. HIV-infected persons are living longer without clinical symptoms, and individuals with HIV disease are surviving longer (Lemp, Hirozawa, Araneta, Young, & Niera, 1991; Moore, Hidalgo, Sugland, & Chaisoon, 1991). Unfortunately, this extended symptom-free period might be correlated with increasing incidence of lymphomas in late-stage HIV illness (Bartlett, 1992). Shifting patterns in the HIV/AIDS epidemic have implications for the meaning, definitions, and measurement of QOL.

QUALITY OF LIFE AND HIV INFECTION: DEFINITION AND MEASUREMENT

Formidable questions surround measurement of QOL. Should a subjective or objective approach be adopted? Which dimensions should be included to assess the impact of disease or therapy? Is a global evaluation more useful than one relying on assessment of symptom distress? What form should the instrument take—visual analogue scales, Likert scales, or interviews (Yancik & Yates, 1986)? Apart from the difficulties of selecting appropriate dimensions of QOL and resolving the problems of measurement approaches, evaluating existing work in this area yields several methodological problems (Fava, 1990; Ganz, Bernhard, & Hurny, 1991; Katz, 1987).

Varricchio (1990), Foreman and Kleinpell (1990), and Slevin, Plant, Lynch, Drinkwater, and Gregory (1988) have discussed who should measure QOL: the patient, the physician, or the caregiver. Research literature indicates that assessments made by care providers do not correlate well with patient perceptions (Holzemer, Henry, Reilly, & Slaughter, 1994); however, there is some suggestion that the caregiver's assessment does indeed agree with the patient's (Curtis & Fernsler, 1989). It is possible that HIV/AIDS patients may be too confused or fatigued to complete

QOL scales. Oversimplified instruments, although easier and quicker to administer, may lack the sensitivity to distinguish the effectiveness of one intervention over another (Mor & Guadadnoli, 1988).

Goodinson and Singleton (1989) summarized their review of QOL assessment issues by offering the following criteria for instrument adequacy: (a) QOL measures should be obtained from subjects themselves; (b) information about QOL cannot be obtained from the subject in isolation from coping strategies, past experiences of illness, and other personality variables; (c) any QOL test should incorporate a weight of importance to the subject; (d) the test should cover a range of dimensions based on the conceptualization from which it was developed; and (e) the test should apply at different stages of illness. None of the scales reviewed met all of their requisite criteria.

In three studies, researchers employed qualitative methods to describe QOL for HIV-infected persons. Ragsdale, Kotarba, and Morrow (1992a) and Weitz (1989) focused on quality of life in late-stage HIV illness. Ragsdale et al. (1992a) interviewed 13 males and 1 female using a grounded theory approach to explore QOL issues in the HIV-positive individual. Weitz (1989) interviewed 23 males to learn how they managed the uncertainty of HIV infection in their lives. Both researchers discussed the process of how the HIV-positive person "controls" the illness. Ragsdale et al. (1992a) described six "management styles" used: loner, activist, victim, timekeeper, mystic, and medic. Weitz (1989) discussed control problems arising from uncertainty in the lives of respondents and reported their need to explain HIV-related events, such as health status before HIV testing, living with HIV-positive test results, and initial experience with opportunistic infections. Because these study samples are male and white dominated and because of the assumptions inherent in the study designs, it is inappropriate to generalize the need for control to other HIV-positive groups.

O'Brien and Pheifer (1993) reported on the physical and psychosocial nursing care needs of patients with HIV infection in a third qualitative study every 3 months over a three-year period. They interviewed and observed 138 HIV-positive gay/bisexual men at home and, when appropriate, in the hospital. The authors identified two physical needs (fatigue and weight loss) and six psychosocial needs (self-concept, loneliness, sexual integrity, home management, spiritual distress, and impaired communication) as shared among people living with HIV, and conceptualized QOL for HIV-infected persons as having both a physical and psychosocial component.

Research has begun on the measurement of QOL for persons with HIV infection. The nine scales reviewed here have been used with HIV/

AIDS samples in two or more studies, and focus primarily on QOL. Three of them—the Karnofsky Performance Scale (Karnofsky & Burchenal, 1949), Kaplan's Quality of Well-Being (Kaplan et al., 1989), and the Quality Audit Marker (Holzemer, Henry, Stewart, & Janson-Bjerklie, 1993)—are completed by a provider or researcher, whereas the other six scales are designed to be completed by the person with HIV/AIDS.

Several QOL-related scales have *not* been included in this review because they were not developed to measure QOL; however, they do measure selected components of QOL and may be appropriate for a QOL study. All have been used with HIV/AIDS subjects. These include Profile of Moods State (McNair, Lorr, & Droppelman, 1971), Beck Depression Scale (Beck, Ward, Mendelson, Mock, & Erbaugh, 1961), Brief Symptom Inventory (Derogatis & Melisaratos, 1983), Symptom Distress Scale (McCorkle & Young, 1978), and Sickness Impact Profile (Bergner, Bobbitt, Carter, & Gilson, 1981). Finally, six QOL-related scales that have been developed for HIV/AIDS research and reported only once in the literature are identified.

Visual (Linear) Analogue Scale. The Visual Analogue Scale (VAS) (Goodinson & Singleton, 1989) usually presents a 0- to 100-mm line denoting a continuum of experience, with anchor words or phrases marking the extremes. This method is sensitive, subjective, and quick to complete, but physical weakness may distort scores, and the use of fixed end points may produce the "ceiling effect" (Goodinson & Singleton, 1989). Another problem is that all experiences assessed are given equal weight despite the likelihood that different dimensions of life may be weighed differently by respondents. VAS scales have been used to measure QOL in four studies with HIV/AIDS subjects (Fawzy, Namir, Wolcott, Mitsuyasu, & Gottlieb, 1989; Henry et al., 1992; Nordic Medical Research Councils HIV Therapy Group, 1992; Presant, 1993).

Karnofsky Performance Status Scale. The Karnofsky Performance Status Scale (KPS) (Karnofsky & Burdenal, 1949) is a unidimensional measure of physical performance and level of assistance needed. First used with lung cancer patients to assess the impact of palliative treatments, the KPS scale is a scale from 0 to 100 with 11 classifications of functioning. A score of 100 indicates absence of disease, normal independent functioning, and the ability to work (Bowling, 1991). It has been used primarily as a global assessment of patient function by a professional providing direct care. Interrater reliability and validity have been established in non-HIV samples. Three studies have used the KPS scale to measure QOL in HIV-positive individuals treated with zidovudine (ZDV) versus a placebo (Fischl et al., 1987, 1990; Rabkin, Remien, Katoff, & Williams, 1993; Wu et al., 1990).

Quality of Life Index. The Quality of Life Index (Spitzer, Dobson, Hall, Chesterman, & Levi, 1981) measures five dimensions (activity, daily living, health, support, and outlook) using a 3-point Likert scale and assigns a single total score for QOL. Williams and Rabkin (1991) examined the content validity of the QOL Index in a sample of 29 HIV-positive asymptomatic males and 21 HIV at-risk males. Because there were no differences as expected between the known groups (HIV-positive and HIV-negative), caution is advised in selecting this scale. The index has been used in two studies with HIV subjects (Rabkin et al., 1993; Williams & Rabkin, 1991).

Quality of Well-Being Scale. The Quality of Well-Being Scale (Kaplan et al., 1989) assesses three constructs (mobility, physical activity, and social activity) and was used in two reported studies. The instrument is completed by the care provider and the scaling technique is referred to as "preference-weighted measures of symptoms and functioning" (p. S32). A total score is possible by combining the weighted scale scores. Wu et al. (1990) had difficulty using the Quality of Well-Being Scale because death was included in the weightings and the absence of differences between experimental and treatment groups was attributed to the inclusion of death.

Medical Outcomes Study: 20-Item Short Form. The Medical Outcomes Study (MOS) 20-Item Short Form (Stewart, Hays, & Ware, 1988) measures six health status concepts (scales): physical functioning (6 items), role functioning (2 items), social functioning (1 item), mental health (5 items), health perceptions (5 items), and pain (1 item). Participants can complete the scale in approximately 3 minutes (Stewart et al., 1988; Wachtel et al., 1992). The MOS-20 uses Likert scales. High MOS scores indicate high functioning and low symptomatology (Wu et al., 1993).

Wachtel et al. (1992) administered the 20-item MOS to a sample of 520 HIV-positive patients (90% male) receiving health services. The purpose of the study was to test the reliability and validity of the scale in a community-based sample. Participants rated the frequency of a selected list of nine AIDS-related symptoms. Coefficient alphas for the multiitem scales ranged from 0.82 to 0.87, similar to the Wu et al. (1991) findings. "Respondents with four or more symptoms reported significantly lower scores in all areas than did respondents with fewer symptoms for all variables" (p. 132).

Cleary et al. (1993) evaluated eight dimensions of health-related quality of life in persons with AIDS: life satisfaction, general health perception, physical functioning, emotional well-being and fatigue, disability, pain, memory problems, and symptoms. Emotional well-being and fatigue were measured with the 20-item short form MOS. The investigators conducted 189 face-to-face interviews in three primary care settings. Adequate validity and reliability estimates (Cronbach alphas over 0.80 for scales) were reported. "The strongest correlate of average health in the past month was the measure of fatigue. The next strongest correlates were limitations in intermediate ADLs and physical symptoms" (p. 575). This study presented an expanded conceptualization of quality of life for people living with AIDS and supported the use of both discrete symptoms and more "general measures of functioning when assessing patients' health" (p. 576).

Medical Outcomes Study: 30-Item Short Form (MOS-30) (Stewart et al., 1988). Wu et al. (1991) tested the validity and reliability of the MOS-30 in a sample of 73 participants with asymptomatic HIV infection and 44 with symptomatic disease, finding predicted differences between these two groups. The 30-item MOS required approximately 5 minutes for subjects to complete. Symptomatic patients scored significantly lower scores on the 11 scales. Asymptomatic patients had significantly better overall health, better physical and role function, and less pain than the symptomatic patients.

Burgess, Dayer, Calalan, Hawkins, and Gazzard (1993) examined the reliability and validity of the MOS-30 in a sample of 99 HIV-positive men ($n = 33$ asymptomatic; $n = 41$ symptomatic; $n = 35$ AIDS). Cronbach's alpha reliability estimates ranged from 0.78 to 0.91 for the subscales. Construct validity was supported for the MOS-30 through correlations with an investigator-developed QOL scale and by demonstration of decreasing QOL scores with disease progression.

Health Assessment Questionnaire. The Health Assessment Questionnaire (HAQ) (Lubeck & Fries, 1992, 1993) consists of six scales measuring components of QOL, partially adopted from the MOS-30 (Lubeck & Fries, 1992, 1993). Items are scaled on a 1 to 3 Likert rating. Reliability and validity of the HAQ self-report scale have been documented (Lubeck & Fries, 1992, 1993; Lubeck, Bennett, Mazonson, Fifer, & Fries, 1993). The researchers have reported missing data because the instrument appears to be too complicated for individuals with advanced HIV infection to complete.

The Quality Audit Marker. The Quality Audit Marker (QAM) (Holzemer et al., 1993) was designed to measure changes in the status of hospitalized AIDS patients (Holzemer et al., 1993). The 10-item HIV-QAM includes three scales: Self-Care (6 items), Ambulation (2 items), and Psychological Distress (2 items). Four- and 5-point Likert scales are used. A high score on the QAM indicates high functional status and low patient symptomatology (Janson-Bjerklie, Holzemer, & Henry, 1992).

The QAM is completed by a nurse investigator based on the nurse's judgment about the patient's status, determined by observation, interview with the patient and the patient's nurse, reviews of chart and kardex, and listening to intershift report. Estimated time to complete this instrument is less than 2 minutes.

In a study of 201 hospitalized AIDS patients with *Pneumocystis carinii* pneumonia (PCP), the QAM was used as an outcome measure of nursing activities or interventions (Holzemer et al., 1993). The internal consistency reliability of the 10-item QAM's three scales was high in this study. Cronbach's alpha for the Self-Care, Ambulation, and Psychological Distress scales were 0.89, 0.88, and 0.84, respectively. Adequate content, construct, concurrent, and predictive validity for patient mortality at 3 and 6 months have been reported (Holzemer et al., 1993).

HIV Overview of Problems-Evaluation System. The HIV Overview of Problems-Evaluation System (HOPES) (Ganz, Schag-Coscarelli, Kahn, Peterson, & Hirji, 1993; Schag-Coscarelli, Ganz, Kahn, & Peterson, 1992) includes five factors (physical, psychosocial, medical interaction, sexual, and significant other/partner) as well as a total score. It was validated on 318 HIV-infected persons across the disease spectrum.

Six instruments appear in only one study with HIV/AIDS samples, and they are listed here because future investigators may wish to examine them: *Derdiarian's Behavioral System* (Derdiarian & Schobel, 1990), *Quality of Life Index* (Ferrans & Powers, 1985), *Functional Independence Measure* (O'Dell, Crawford, Bohi, & Bonner, 1991), *Support Team Assessment Schedule* (Butters, Higginson, George, Smits, & McCarthy, 1992), *Quality-Adjusted Time Without Symptoms and Toxicity* (Gelber et al., 1992), and *The European Questionnaire for Research and Treatment of Cancer Core Quality-of-Life Questionnaire* (de Boer, van Dam, Sprangers, Frissen, & Lange, 1993).

Critique of Instruments

Review of the psychometric properties of measures of QOL used with HIV-positive persons offers strong evidence of the validity and reliability of the scales. Subscales on these measures include a combination of assessments of the physical, psychological, and social components of QOL. Although the scales have all been used with HIV-positive women as well as HIV-positive people of color, the samples have often been small, and further work is needed. Little qualitative, inductive work was reported as a basis for scale development addressing the QOL for people living with AIDS. Research must continue to explore the definitions, meanings, measurement, and importance of QOL for people with HIV/

AIDS. The state of the art in the measurement of QOL in HIV/AIDS disease has shown that existing measures work well with this group. However, concepts or dimensions of QOL perhaps unique to HIV/AIDS group have not been identified. The challenge for health care, especially nursing, is to enhance the QOL for clients and patients through effective interventions. Developing valid and reliable measures for QOL as an outcome variable will enhance our ability to test the effectiveness of nursing interventions.

QUALITY OF LIFE ACROSS THE HIV SPECTRUM

Eight studies examined QOL for HIV-positive persons by examining quality of life at a certain point in the spectrum of infection or by following infected individuals over time. Jewett and Hecht (1993) wrote, "people with HIV infection have different stage-specific health maintenance needs that form an important part of comprehensive care for people in all stages of infection" (p. 1144). Lubeck and Fries (1993), Ragsdale and Morrow (1990), and Fawzy et al. (1989) evaluated QOL in relatively healthy samples of HIV-positive individuals.

Lubeck and Fries (1993) reported on a repeated measures analysis of QOL for HIV-positive persons in an analysis of an ongoing database titled AIDS Time-Oriented Health Outcomes Study (ATHOS). ATHOS is a longitudinal, observational database of more than 3,000 HIV-infected patients seen by community-based physicians. Data were collected from charts and questionnaires. These researchers examined seven dimensions of quality of life (disability, general health, social functional, mental health, cognitive functioning, energy, and disease symptoms) for three subsets of HIV-positive individuals over 9 months. These constructs were measured with HAQ, developed and validated for the ATHOS project. Most of the items from the HAQ are from the MOS scales.

Samples in this analysis included $n = 99$, HIV-positive only and no symptoms; $n = 238$, HIV-positive with symptoms; and $n = 145$, HIV-positive with diagnosed AIDS. In this predominately male, gay/bisexual, white sample, "Patients with AIDS scored significantly worse on all quality-of-life dimensions when compared with asymptomatic individuals after 9 months" (p. 274). The authors concluded that this scale can be useful in detecting changes in health and psychosocial status throughout HIV illness, although these findings may not apply for those with advanced HIV infection or women and ethnic minorities.

Ragsdale and Morrow (1990) examined QOL cross-sectionally in a sample of 95 males divided into HIV-positive ($n = 24$), AIDS-related complex (ARC) ($n = 15$), and AIDS ($n = 56$) categories, a schema no longer recommended to classify severity of illness related to HIV infection. Ragsdale and Morrow (1990) used the Sickness Impact Profile (Bergner et al., 1981), which measures 12 dimensions (sleep and rest, emotion behavior, body care and movement, household management, mobility, social interaction, ambulation, alertness behavior, community, work, recreation and pastimes, and eating). The Symptom Distress Scale (McCorkle & Young, 1978) was used to measure nausea, mood, appetite, insomnia, pain, mobility, fatigue, bowel pattern, concentration, and appearance. Ragsdale and Morrow, similar to Lubeck and Fries (1992), reported significant differences across almost all of these subscales when comparing the three groups of subjects and a wide variability among the scale scores at each point. Such findings demonstrate significant variability in health status across the spectrum of HIV infection.

Fawzy et al. (1989) evaluated the QOL and symptoms (measured by Profile of Mood Status [POMS]) in 50 newly diagnosed, relatively healthy AIDS male patients. Psychological distress correlated positively with subjective views of QOL but not with objective measures of health status. QOL was measured with a one-item visual analogue scale from 0 to 10; the mean QOL score was 6.86.

Five of these eight studies examined QOL and HIV infection with AIDS-diagnosed patients in late stages of the illness trajectory. Ragsdale et al. (1992a) and Weitz (1989) used qualitative approaches to explore QOL in late-stage HIV illness. As discussed earlier, Weitz (1989) interviewed 23 males to explore how they managed the uncertainty of HIV infection in their lives. Ragsdale et al. (1992a) interviewed 13 males and 1 female using a grounded theory approach to explore QOL from the viewpoint of the HIV-positive individual. Both studies focused on how the HIV-positive person "controls" his or her illness. O'Brien and Pheifer (1993) also used qualitative methods to follow the physical and psychosocial nursing care needs of patients with HIV infection over a 3-year period as previously described.

Rabkin and associates (1993) evaluated psychological and behavioral QOL in a sample of 53 men living with an AIDS diagnosis for 3 or more years, and judged to be low on mood disorders with little psychiatric distress. The authors reported that physical impairment was unrelated to psychiatric distress or life satisfaction. QOL was measured using the Spitzer (Spitzer et al., 1981) scale, which is completed by the ill person and includes occupational functioning, activities of daily living, perception of own health, support of family and friends as modified by illness status, and outlook. This sample's QOL score suggested that these subjects were essentially healthy but reported widespread dissatisfaction with their sexual lives. Seventy-nine percent reported abstinence in the past month, with a mean of 30 months since the last sexual encounter. "The sexual inhibition of these men contributed to the sense of loneliness and lack of joy that many reported" (p. 167).

Ganz et al. (1993) reported on the QOL in a sample of 318 HIV-positive persons divided into four groups (37% asymptomatic, 20% ARC, 25% AIDS, and 18% AIDS and cancer). QOL as measured by the HOPES scale significantly varied over the severity of HIV infection as predicted. Medical and demographic variables accounted for only 35% of the variance in QOL, suggesting that while measures like clinical status are related to QOL, they are not a substitute for independent assessment of QOL. Although researchers have used a variety of methods and sampled people at different points in the unfolding course of their disease, they share the overriding conclusion that QOL decreases with increasing severity of HIV illness.

HIV-RELATED SIGNS/SYMPTOMS AND QUALITY OF LIFE

Eleven studies were located that examined HIV-related signs/symptoms and QOL. Fix focused on physiological signs and symptoms, and four on psychosocial symptoms. The physiological signs and symptoms included nutrition, diarrhea, pulmonary problems, and sleep disturbances.

Lubeck et al. (1993) have published the most important study on signs/symptoms and QOL. They studied 110 HIV-positive patients with chronic diarrhea with a matched sample of 31 HIV-positive patients over a 12-month period. All subjects had CD4 lymphocytes < 200 mm^3 and thus would qualify as having an AIDS diagnosis based on the current CDC definition. Data were analyzed from the ATHOS database.

QOL was measured by the AIDS Health Assessment Questionnaire, "which covers the following dimensions: use of health services, medications, symptoms and side effects, work loss, disability, global health, energy/fatigue, cognitive functioning, social functioning, and mental health" (p. 479). QOL is defined as the last six dimensions. Chronic diarrhea was defined as "reported diarrhea for greater than or equal to 3 months." Sixty-one percent ($n = 67$) of the patients with chronic diarrhea had no known documented etiological pathogen. The two study groups were similar in functional ability, mental health, cognition, and energy/vitality at the beginning of the study, but the group with chronic diarrhea scored significantly poorer for global health, social contacts, and disease symptoms. During the study, the chronic diarrhea group used more resources, had more expensive inpatient care, and showed significant decreases in ability to work, functional ability, global health, social contacts, and energy levels.

Keithley, Zeller, Szeluga, and Urbanski (1992) reported on the nutritional status, immune function, and QOL for 40 HIV-positive patients attending an outpatient clinic, staged into five categories of disease. They used the Ferrans and Powers (1985) Quality of Life Index and found no changes in QOL over the stages of HIV infection. It is likely that the failure to detect a difference in QOL is due to the small sample size.

Janson-Bjerklie et al. (1992) sorted 201 patients hospitalized with a PCP diagnosis into three categories based on the patients' reports of pulmonary-related problems (pulmonary problems with dyspnea, pulmonary problems without dyspnea, and no pulmonary problems reported). They found no differences among the groups on functional status as measured by the QAM (Holzemer et al., 1993) nor on the one item measures of pain, nausea, and fatigue. Furthermore, patients' self-reports of pulmonary-related problems did not correlate with research-nurse–evaluated QOL measures.

Lovejoy, Paul, Freeman, and Christianson (1991) measured self-care behaviors and symptom distress using validated scales including an 81-item self-care checklist, the Symptom Distress Scale (SDS) and POMS in a sample of 162 HIV-positive men attending an outpatient clinic. The sample self-reported a significant increase in self-care behaviors after learning about their HIV-positive status and relatively low levels of symptom distress. The authors wrote, "despite the relative absence of symptomatology in the sample, there were several identifiable potential correlates of symptom distress such as negative mood states, recent diagnosis of selected HIV-related conditions, functional status, employment status, and an external locus of control" (p. 1183).

Two teams of investigators examined the potential relationship between sleep disturbances and QOL in people with HIV infection. Norman et al. (1992) examined sleep disturbances in HIV-positive asymptomatic males ($n = 14$) with a matched control of 10 HIV-negative males. They reported differences in sleep architecture between the two groups; nonrapid eye movement sleep and rapid eye movement sleep were more evenly dispersed through the night in the HIV-negative controls, probably related to HIV status because no other known explanation could be found. Moeller et al. (1991) examined the reported quality of sleep in 50 HIV-positive (94% males) in all stages of HIV infection. They also reported that sleep disturbances, as measured by the Pittsburg Sleep Quality Index, were correlated with HIV stage of infection.

Four investigators examined psychosocial symptoms, QOL, and HIV infection. Butters et al. (1992) evaluated 140 male AIDS patients receiving palliative care at home in London, England. Using the Support Team Assessment Schedule scale, they measured 17 items of care every 2 weeks until death. Data were collected during initial assessment, 2 weeks later, and near death, focusing on pain control, symptom control, patient anxiety, and practical aid. Symptom control was reported as the most problematic over time. Pain was episodic and resolvable once identified. Practical aid was never a problem for this group of patients.

Brown and Rundell (1993) studied 43 HIV-positive women in the U.S. Air Force to explore potential psychiatric aspects of early HIV infection. Twenty-nine women were interviewed twice. Overall, the group had few identified psychiatric diagnoses or problems. However, many participants (41%) reported that sexual dysfunction increased significantly over time, impairing intimate relationships and detracting from their QOL.

Ostrow et al. (1991) studied potential differences in social support in two samples of African-American ($n = 20$) and white ($n = 20$) males. They found selected racial differences in the role of social support in the mental health of the two groups and in their risk behavior. A positive relationship between perceived adequacy of social support and adoption of safer sexual practices was observed among white but not African-American participants. African-American men also were less likely to be open about their sexual orientation. Although these results may be attributable to racial, ethnic, or cultural differences, the small sample size demands caution in interpretation.

Ragsdale, Kotarba, and Morrow (1992b) reported on work-related activities that improve QOL in a qualitative, grounded-theory study of 19 male, hospitalized AIDS patients. They found that QOL was enhanced when subjects were able to conduct activities important to them. The authors concluded that "quality of life was viewed not as any measurable characteristic of the patients, but as the product of their interactional work" (p. 41). For this study, the concept of work included activities of daily living on the unit, sense of control over the management of their illness, the meaning of "having AIDS," self-identity, comfort and security of environment, and pain management.

Finally, O'Dell et al. (1991) examined the types and degree of disability seen in persons with AIDS at discharge from an acute hospital episode. Caregivers evaluated 37 men using the Functional Independence Measure (FIM). Sixty percent of the patients required human assistance in at least one of the 18 FIM areas, such as stair climbing, ambulation, feeding, and bathing. Disability correlated with length of hospital stay and time since diagnosis. Discharge planning that addresses these disability issues has the potential to enhance the QOL for these patients.

These studies have linked QOL to related symptoms. McMahon and Coyne (1989) provided an excellent overview of the array of potential symptom management areas in patients with HIV. In addition, they discussed the complexity of measuring symptoms and suggest that one should measure frequency, severity, and management strategies for symptoms related both to HIV infection and HIV therapies.

INTERVENTION STUDIES AND QUALITY OF LIFE

Pharmacological Interventions

Twelve pharmacological intervention studies included a measure of QOL as an outcome indicator. Eight examined the QOL in the ZDV clinical trials and four unrelated studies used a QOL outcome measure in clinical trials for anemia, cachexia, Kaposi's sarcoma, and lymphoma.

Fischl et al. (1987) reported the first ZDV double-blind, clinical trial with persons with an AIDS diagnoses. Experimental subjects ($n = 445$) received 250 mg of ZDV every 4 hours, and controls ($n = 137$) took a placebo every 4 hours. QOL was measured at baseline and at 24 weeks with the Karnofsky Performance Scale. These authors suggested that ZDV decreased mortality and morbidity in a selected group of subjects with AIDS. Fischl et al. (1990) also reported on a ZDV clinical trial with subjects who were HIV-positive and asymptomatic. The experimental group ($n = 360$) received ZDV 200 mg orally every 4 hours, and the control group ($n = 357$) took a placebo every 4 hours for 11 months. ZDV was most effective in slowing the onset of an AIDS-defining episode in those subjects with CD4 counts between 200 and 500, and significant differences in adverse reactions were found. QOL was measured by counting symptoms related to ZDV therapy. The ZDV group experienced significantly more malaise or fatigue, nausea and vomiting, bloating, anemia, and dyspepsia.

Wu et al. (1990) measured QOL in 31 AIDS patients in a clinical trial comparing ZDV with a placebo, using the Karnofsky performance measure and the Quality of Well-Being scale. There were no differences between the groups at 1 year, a finding with two possible explanations. First, both groups included subjects with AIDS so they were already scoring relatively low on QOL measures. Also, this study lacks sufficient power to detect differences given the small sample size.

Nordic Medical Research Councils HIV Therapy Group (1992) reported on a randomized trial comparing the efficacy of three daily doses of ZDV (400 mg, $n = 160$; 800 mg, $n = 158$; and 1,200 mg, $n = 156$) in patients with AIDS. Subjects followed for 19 months reported no significant differences among groups on survival or quality of well-being when measured with a one-item visual analogue scale.

Gelber et al. (1992) evaluated the effects of ZDV in mildly symptomatic HIV-positive patients in a randomized clinical trail. The experimental group ($n = 360$) received 1,200 mg of ZDV daily and the control group ($n = 351$) took placebos. After 18 months, the Quality-Adjusted Time Without Symptoms and Toxicity scale (Q-TWIST) showed severe symptoms in 15.1% of the placebo group and 22.8% of the experimental group. The Q-TWIST bases its estimates on Kaplan-Meier curves for time free from adverse events.

De Boer et al. (1993) compared ZDV alone ($n = 16$) with ZDV plus interferon-alpha ($n = 20$) for 1 year, using two multidimensional, nonstandardized QOL measures. Overall, there were few differences between the two groups.

Wu et al. (1993) reported on functional status and well-being in a clinical trial with the experimental group ($n = 36$) taking 200 mg of ZDV 4 times daily and the control group ($n = 34$) taking a placebo. QOL was measured using the 30-item self-report MOS. At baseline, the control group scored significantly higher on selected scales than the control group. At 52 weeks, however, both groups appeared equivalent. In fact, the placebo group scored more positively at 24 weeks. They concluded, "Thus the net effect of high-dose ZDV was to worsen patients' quality of life along a few dimensions at 24 weeks" (p. 455). All eight studies on QOL in ZDV trials showed similar findings: that HIV-positive participants experience significant decrease in QOL when in experimental groups taking high doses of ZDV.

Moyle, Nelson, Hawkins, and Gazzard (1993) reported on the use of didanosine (DDI) in a sample of 151 patients who were intolerant to ZDV. Spitzer's QOL scale was used to measure activity, daily living, health, support, outlook, and total QOL. Overall there were modest improvements in selected QOL measure; however, without a control group, it is impossible to interpret the findings. Significant side effects were noted in the sample, including diarrhea ($n = 19$), peripheral neuropathy ($n = 12$), and pancreatitis ($n = 6$). Thirty-seven patients (25%) were forced to terminate the DDI.

Henry et al. (1992) studied the use of recombinant human erythropoietin in treatment of anemia in subjects in ZDV therapy. The experimental group ($n = 294$) received therapy for up to 12 weeks, and the control group ($n = 307$) did not. The experimental group had a decreased mean number of units of blood transfused per patient compared with the placebo group. The authors report that QOL improved in the experimental group as measured by a one-item VAS on "overall quality of life" with a $p = 0.13$. The study fails to conceptualize or measure QOL adequately. Also, potential side effects or symptoms of the treatment condition were not monitored.

Von Roenn, Murphy, and Wegener (1990) treated cachexia in a sample of 22 AIDS patients with oral megestrol acetate. Twenty-one (95%) of the patients gained weight (average of 7.3 kg) during therapy lasting from 2 to 72 weeks, attributed primarily to the therapy in 18 of these individuals. Interventions that enhance appetite and weight gain would certainly be reasonable related to some aspects of QOL, assuming that the negative side effects are minimal.

Presant et al. (1993) reported on the effects of liposomal daunorubicin treatment of HIV-associated Kaposi's sarcoma. QOL was shown to have improved in the 24 patients in terms of physical performance and emotion when compared with baseline data. QOL was measured with a 21-item, unidentified instrument.

Remick et al. (1993) examined the QOL changes associated with oral combination chemotherapy in the treatment of intermediate-grade and high-grade AIDS-related non-Hodgkin's lymphoma. QOL was assessed in 18 subjects using the Functional Living Index—Cancer and the Brief Symptom Inventory (Derogatis & Melisaratos, 1983). The sample included 7 complete and 4 partial remissions. QOL was measured during times on therapy and off therapy, and no significant differences were found for the 16 subjects with complete data. Unfortunately, this study lacks sufficient power to detect potential differences because of the small sample size.

Surgical Interventions

Diettrich, Cacioppo, Kaplan, and Cohen (1991) studied the outcomes of surgical procedures in a sample of 88 HIV-positive individuals. They reported a mean survival time of 86 weeks for 59 procedures for those subjects who remained alive. They concluded that procedures are indicated to extend patient life or to improve QOL. The authors used no specific QOL scale, however, and failed to show clearly that increased survival is necessarily related to QOL.

Nursing Care Interventions

No nursing intervention studies for HIV infection were located that used QOL as an outcome variable.

SUMMARY AND FUTURE RESEARCH DIRECTIONS

The AIDS epidemic continues to grow. The CDC (Resource Booklet, 1993) reported that 315,390 people have been diagnosed with AIDS and estimated that more than 1 million Americans are infected, a disproportionate number of them people of color and women (Goodkin, Antoni, Helder, & Sevin, 1993). Globally, an estimated 2.2 million persons have been diagnosed with AIDS, and approximately 13 million people are infected. The World Health Organization estimates that by the year 2000 there will be between 30 and 40 million people infected. Primary and secondary prevention, direct nursing care, and enhancement of QOL for these people are our challenges.

Greenfield and Nelson (1992) have documented that in Western societies a paradigm shift from a disease orientation to a focus on healthy functioning and well-being is being experienced. However, problems and issues surrounding the measurement of health status or QOL are complex, and the research findings difficult to interpret. As this chapter makes clear, however, numerous instruments are available to measure different dimensions of QOL in people with HIV/AIDS. Psychometric properties of validity and reliability have been established in these samples. Unfortunately, few women and people of color have been studied. None of the scales has any normative data available for purposes of comparison across treatments, diseases, or settings within the spectrum of HIV infection.

QOL has been monitored across the debilitating spectrum of HIV disease usually by correlating QOL with CD4 counts. Although CD4 counts are understood to be a clinical marker of disease progression, and when less than 200 mm^3 constitute an AIDS-defining diagnosis, they can also be highly variable. Clinical symptomatology does not necessarily correspond to CD4 count. The findings of decreasing QOL over time with HIV infection parallel studies of QOL in other chronic illnesses with few exceptions. Several authors address the importance of sexual functioning when defining QOL in persons with HIV/AIDS. Such a finding suggests the need for more complete assessment and intervention in this area.

Existing QOL scales have been developed by psychologists and physicians from their professional perspectives. Concept-generating work by nurse researchers could yield additional dimensions. Little qualitative, concept-generating work has focused on QOL in HIV/AIDS research. The tendency has been to adopt or revise existing scales, often from the cancer literature, for the AIDS population. Further work is needed to identify, describe, and validate the dimensions of QOL in persons with HIV/AIDS. Few studies have examined QOL in late-stage illness, and many items on scales like the MOS-30 are inappropriate for AIDS patients in hospice care.

Cross-sectional and repeated measures studies of QOL linked to symptoms associated with HIV/AIDS are now appearing in the literature. These studies have included assessments in the areas of chronic diarrhea, nutrition, sleep, and dyspnea. Unfortunately, few studies have moved beyond the descriptive level.

The value of the QOL research in HIV/AIDS pharmacological clinical trials is questionable because the measures of QOL are often limited (e.g., the one-item VAS scale), and the clinical trials have changed the dosage and drug combination too frequently to make trends discernible from the data. However, studies have documented the significant negative effect on QOL from interventions, such as ZDV.

Nursing research on QOL in HIV/AIDS is limited. A few authors have begun important qualitative work on developing a better understanding of the components of QOL for people with HIV/AIDS. One instrument has been specifically developed as an outcome measure for examining the impact of nursing care on QOL in people with AIDS. No intervention studies designed to enhance the QOL for people with AIDS using either nursing care or community-support activities were located.

The need for additional research in the psychometric development of measures of QOL, and their use in clinical trials and clinical practice is clear. Little is known about how QOL differs for men and women, children and adolescents, people of color, immigrants, and so forth. Although there is evidence that QOL diminishes over the course of the illness, it is less clear what concepts are important to monitor in later stages of illness. Further qualitative work to discover and relate relevant conceptualizations of QOL is, therefore, essential.

Zeller, Swanson, and Cohen (1993) have suggested clinical nursing research on symptom management for AIDS patients with respiratory and neurological problems, malnutrition, and opportunistic infections. Their suggestions are closely linked to the research priorities advanced by the National Institute for Nursing Research, National Institutes of Health.

Nurse researchers have initiated clinical trials to demonstrate the effectiveness of nursing care. Although the primary purpose of these studies is to demonstrate resolution of a specific client problem or cost savings, it is crucial that QOL be measured. The inclusion of QOL as an outcome measure for nursing therapeutics is evidence of nursing's commitment to the value of client choices in care and treatment.

ACKNOWLEDGMENTS

The authors acknowledge nursing doctoral students Rose Bianchi and Cheryl Reilly for their library assistance in the preparation of this manuscript.

The preparation of this manuscript was partially supported by NIH-NR02215, Quality of Nursing Care for People with AIDS, 1989–1996, W. L. Holzemer, principal investigator.

REFERENCES

Aaronson, N. K. (1991). Quality of life research in oncology: Past achievements and future priorities. *Cancer, 67*, 839–843.

Bartlett, J. G. (1992). *1992–1993 Recommendations for the medical care of persons with HIV infection. A guide to HIV care from the AIDS care program of the Johns Hopkins Medical Institutions.* New York: Critical Care America.

Beck, A. T., Ward, C. H., Mendelson, M., Mock, J., & Erbaugh, J. (1961). An inventory for assessing depression. *Archives of General Psychiatry, 4*, 53–63.

Bergner, M., Bobbitt, R. A., Carter, W. B., & Gilson, B. S. (1981). The Sickness Impact Profile: Development and final revision of a health status measure. *Medical Care, 19*, 787–805.

Bowling, A. (1991). *Measuring health: A review of quality of life measurement scales.* Philadelphia: Open University Press.

Brown, G. R., & Rundell, J. R. (1993). A prospective study of psychiatric aspects of early HIV disease in women. *General Hospital Psychiatry, 15*, 139–147.

Burgess, A., Dayer, M., Catalan, J., Hawkins, D., & Gazzard, B. (1993). The reliability and validity of two HIV-specific health-related quality of life measures: A preliminary analysis. *AIDS, 7*, 1001–1008.

Butters, E., Higginson, I., George, R., Smits, A., & McCarthy, M. (1992). Assessing the symptoms, anxiety and practical needs of HIV/AIDS patients receiving palliative care. *Quality of Life Research, 1*, 47–51.

Centers for Disease Control. (1993). *HIV/AIDS Surveillance Report* (year-end 1992 ed.). Atlanta, GA: U.S. Department of Health and Human Services.

Cleary, P. D., Fowler, F. J., Weissman, J., Massagli, M. P., Wilson, I., Seage, G. R., Gatsonis, C., & Epstein, A. (1993). Health-related quality of life in persons with acquired immune deficiency syndrome. *Medical Care, 31*, 569–580.

Curtis, A. E., & Fernsler, J. I. (1989). Quality of life of oncology patients: A comparison of patient and primary caregiver reports. *Oncology Nursing Forum, 16*, 49–53.

de Boer, J. B., van Dam, F. S. A. M., Sprangers, M. A. G., Frissen, P. H. J., & Lange, J. M. A. (1993). Longitudinal study of the quality of life of symptomatic HIV-infected patients in a trial of zidovudine versus zidovudine and interferon-alpha. *AIDS, 7*, 947–953.

Derdiarian, A. K., & Schobel, D. (1990). Comprehensive assessments of AIDS patients using the behavioral systems model for nursing practice instrument. *Journal of Advanced Nursing, 15*, 436–446.

Derogatis, L. R., & Melisaratos, N. (1983). The Brief Symptom Inventory: An introductory report. *Psychological Medicine, 13*, 595–605.

Diettrich, N. A., Cacioppo, J. C., Kaplan, G., & Cohen, S. M. (1991). A growing spectrum of surgical disease in patients with human immunodeficiency virus/acquired immunodeficiency syndrome. *Archives of Surgery, 126*, 860–866.

Fava, G. A. (1990). Methodological and conceptual issues in research on quality of life. *Psychotherapy and Psychosomatics, 54*, 70–76.

Fawzy, F. I., Namir, S., Wolcott, D. L., Mitsuyasu, R. T., & Gottlieb, M. S. (1989). The relationship between medical and psychological status in newly diagnosed gay men with AIDS. *Psychiatric Medicine, 7*(2), 23–33.

Ferrans, C. E., & Powers, M. J. (1985). Quality of life index: Development and psychometric properties. *Advances in Nursing Science, 8*(1), 15–24.

Fischl, M. A., Richman, D. D., Grieco, M. H., Gottlieb, M. S., Volberding, P. A., Laskin, O. L., Leedom, J. M., Groopman, J. E., Mildvan, D., Schooley, R. T., Jackson, G. G., Durack, D. T., King, D., & the AZT Collaborative Working Group. (1987). The efficacy of azidothymidine (AZT) in the treatment of patients with AIDS and AIDS-related complex: A double-blind, placebo, controlled trial. *New England Journal of Medicine, 317*, 185–191.

Fischl, M. A., Richman, D. D., Hansen, N., Collier, A. C., Carey, J. T., Para, M. F., Hardy, W. D., Dolin, R., Powderly, W. G., Allan, J. D., Wong, B., Mertgan, T. C., McAuliffe, V. J., Hyslop, N. E., Rhame, F. S., Balfour, H. H., Spector, S. A., Volberding, P., Pettinelli, C., Anderson, A., & the AIDS Clinical Trials Group. (1990). The safety and efficacy of zidovudine (AZT) in the treatment of subjects with mildly symptomatic immunodeficiency virus type 1 (HIV) infection: A double-blind, placebo-controlled trial. *Annals of Internal Medicine, 112*, 727–737.

Foreman, M. D., & Kleinpell, R. (1990). Assessing the quality of life of elderly people. *Seminars in Oncology Nursing, 6*, 292–297.

Fullilove, M. T., Weinstein, M., Fullilove, R. E., Crayton, E. J., Goodjoin, R. B., Bowser, B., & Gross, S. (1990). Race/gender issues in the sexual transmission of AIDS. In P. Volberding & M. A. Jacobson (Eds.), *AIDS clinical review, 1990* (pp. 25–62). New York: Marcel Dekker.

Ganz, P. A., Bernhard, J. & Hurny, C. (1991). Quality-of-life and psychosocial oncology research in Europe: State of the art. *Journal of Psychosocial Oncology, 9*(1), 1–22.

Ganz, P. A., Schag-Coscarelli, C. A., Kahn, B., Peterson, L., & Hirji, K. (1993). Describing the health-related quality of life impact of HIV infection: Findings from a study using the HIV Overview of Problems Evaluation System (HOPES). *Quality of Life Research, 2*, 109–119.

Gelber, R. D., Lenderking, W. R., Cotton, D. J., Cole, B. F., Fischl, M. A., Goldhirsch, A., & Testa, M. A. (1992). Quality-of-life evaluation in a clinical trial of zidovudine therapy in patients with mildly symptomatic HIV infection. *Annals of Internal Medicine, 116*, 961–966.

Glover, J. (1977). *Causing death and saving lives*. New York: Penguin.

Goodinson, S. M., & Singleton, J. (1989). Quality of life: A critical review of current concepts, measures and their clinical implications. *International Journal of Nursing Studies, 26*, 327–341.

Goodkin, K., Antoni, M. H., Helder, L., & Sevin, B. (1993). Psychoneuroimmunological aspects of disease progress among women with human papillomavirus-associated cervical dysplasia and human immunodeficiency virus type 1 co-infection. *International Journal of Psychiatry in Medicine, 23*, 119–148.

Greenfield, S., & Nelson, E. C. (1992). Recent developments and future issues in the use of health status assessment measures in clinical settings. *Medical Care, 30* (Suppl.), MS23–MS41.

Greer, D. S. (1987). Quality of life measurement in the clinical realm. *Journal of Chronic Disorders, 40*, 629–630.

Henry, D. H., Beall, G. N., Benson, C. A., Carey, J., Lone, L. A., Eron, L. J., Fiala, M., Fischl, M. A., Gabin, S. J., Gottlieb, M. S., Kalpin, J. E., Groopman, J. E., Horton, T. M., Jensek, J. G., Levine, R. L., Miles, S. A. Rinehart, J. T., Rios, A., Robbins, W. J., Rickdeschee, J. L., Smith, J. A., Spruano, S. L., Starret, B., Toney, J., Zalusky, R., Abels, R. I., Bryant, E. C., Larholt, K. M., Sampson, A. R., & Rudnick, S. A. (1992). Recombinant human erythropoietin in the treatment of anemia associated with human immunodeficiency virus (HIV) infection and zidovudine therapy. *Annals of Internal Medicine, 117*, 739–748.

Hinds, P. S. (1990). Quality of life in children and adolescents with cancer. *Seminars in Oncology Nursing, 6*, 285–291.

Holzemer, W. L., Henry, S. B., Stewart, A., & Janson-Bjerklie, S. (1993). The Quality Audit Marker: An outcome measure for hospitalized HIV/AIDS patients. *Quality of Life Research, 7*, 99–107.

Holzemer, W. L., Henry, S. B., Reilly, C. A., & Slaughter, R. E. (1994). A comparison of PWA and nurse reports of symptoms. International AIDS Conference, *10*(2), 11 (Abstract No. 338BID).

Jalowiec, A. (1990). Issues in using multiple measures of quality of life. *Seminars in Oncology Nursing,* 6, 271–277.

Janson-Bjerklie, S., Holzemer, W. L., & Henry, S. B. (1992). Patients' perceptions of pulmonary problems and nursing interventions during hospitalization for *Pneumocystis carinii* pneumonia. *American Journal of Critical Care, 1*, 114–121.

Jewett, F. J., & Hecht, F. M. (1993). Preventive health care for adults with HIV infection. *Journal of the American Medical Association, 269*, 1144–1153.

Kaplan, R. M., Anderson, J. P., Wu, A. W., Mathews, W. C., Kozin, F., & Orenstein, D. (1989). The Quality of Well-Being Scale: Applications in AIDS, cystic fibrosis, and arthritis. *Medical Care, 27* (Suppl. 3), S27–S43.

Karnofsky, D. A., & Burchenal, J. H. (1949). The clinical evaluation of chemotherapeutic agents in cancer. In C. M. Macleod (Ed.), *Evaluation of chemotherapeutic agents* (Symposium, Microbiology Section, pp. 191–205). New York: Columbia University Press.

Katz, S. (1987). The science of quality of life. *Journal of Chronic Diseases, 40*, 459–463.

Keithley, J. K., Zeller, J. M., Szeluga, D. J., & Urhanski, P. A. (1992). Nutritional alterations in persons with HIV infection. *Image: Journal of Nursing Scholarship, 24*, 183–189.

Kleinman, A. (1986). Culture, the quality of life and cancer pain. In V. Vjentiafridda, S. Van Dam, R. Yancik, & M. Tamburini (Eds.), *Assessment of quality of life and cancer treatment* (pp. 43–50). Amsterdam: Elsevier Science.

Kleinpell, R. M. (1991). Concept analysis of quality of life. *Dimensions of Critical Care Nursing, 10*, 223–229.

Kober, B., Küchler, T., Broelsch, C., Kremer, B., & Henne-Bruns, D. (1990). A psychological support concept and quality of life research in a liver transplantation program. *Psychotherapy and Psychosomatics, 54*, 117–131.

Koch, U., & Murphy, F. A. (1990). Quality of life in persons with end-stage renal disease in relation to the method of treatment. *Psychotherapy and Psychosomatics, 54*, 161–171.

Künsebeck, H. W., Körber, J., & Freyberger, H. (1990). Quality of life in patients with inflammatory bowel disease. *Psychotherapy and Psychosomatics, 54*, 110–116.

Lemp, G. F., Hirozawa, A. M., Araneta, M. R., Young, K., & Nieri, G. (1991). Improved survival for persons with AIDS in San Francisco. *Proceedings of the VII International Conference on AIDS,* Florence Haley, abstract # TU. C. 41 7(1), 66.

Lovejoy, M. C., Paul, S., Freeman, E., & Christianson, B. (1991). Potential correlates of self-care and symptom distress in homosexual/bisexual men who are HIV seropositive. *Oncology Nursing Forum, 18*, 1175–1185.

Lubeck, D. P., Bennett, C. L., Mazonson, P. D., Fifer, S. K., & Fries, J. F. (1993). Quality of life and health service utilization among HIV-infected patients with chronic diarrhea. *Journal of Acquired Immune Deficiency Syndromes, 6*, 478–484.

Lubeck, D. P., & Fries, J. F. (1992). Changes in quality of life among persons with HIV infection. *Quality of Life Research, 1*, 359–366.

Lubeck, D. P., & Fries, J. F. (1993). Health status among persons infected with human immunodeficiency virus. *Medical Care, 31*, 269–276.

Marshall, P. A. (1990). Cultural influences on perceived quality of life. *Seminars in Oncology Nursing, 6*, 278–284.

McCorkle, R., & Young, K. (1978). Development of a symptom distress scale. *Cancer Nursing, 1*, 373–378.

McMahon, K. M., & Coyne, N. (1989). Symptom management in patients with AIDS. *Seminars in Oncology Nursing, 5*, 289–301.

McNair, D. M., Lorr, M., & Droppelman, L. F. (1971). *EDITS manual for the profile of moods states*. San Diego: Educational and Industrial Testing Service.

McSweeney, A. J., Grant, I., Heaton, R. K., Adams, K. M., & Timms, R. M. (1982). Life quality of patients with chronic obstructive pulmonary disease. *Archives of Internal Medicine, 142*(3), 473–478.

Moeller, A. A., Oechsner, M., Backmund, H. C., Popescu, M., Emminger, C., & Holsboer, F. (1991). Self-reported sleep quality in HIV infection: Correlation to the stage of infection and zidovudine therapy. *Journal of Acquired Immune Deficiency Syndromes, 4*, 1000–1003.
Moore, P. A. (1991). Treating HIV infections as a chronic disease. *AIDS Patient Care, 5*, 133–139.
Moore, R. D., Hidalgo, J., Sugland, B. W., & Chaisson, R. E. (1991). Zidovudine and the natural history of the acquired immunodeficiency syndrome. *New England Journal of Medicine, 324*, 1412–1416.
Mor, V., & Guadadnoli, E. (1988). Quality of life measurement: A psychometric tower of Babel. *Journal of Clinical Epidemiology, 41*, 1055–1058.
Morris, J. N., Suissa, S., Sherwood, S., Wright, S. M., & Greer, D. (1986). Last days: A study of the quality of life of terminally ill cancer patients. *Journal of Chronic Diseases, 39*, 47–61.
Moyle, G. J., Nelson, M. E., Hawkins, D., & Gazzard, B. G. (1993). The use and toxicity of didanosine (ddI) in HIV antibody-positive individuals intolerant to zidovudine (AZT). *Quarterly Journal of Medicine , 86*, 155–163.
Muthny, F. A., Koch, U., & Stump, S. (1990). Quality of life in oncology patients. *Psychotherapy and Psychosomatics, 54*, 145–160.
Nordic Medical Research Councils HIV Therapy Group. (1992). Double blind dose-response study of zidovudine in AIDS and advanced HIV infection. *British Medical Journal, 504*, 13–17.
Norman, S. E., Chediak, A. D., Freeman, C., Kiel, M., Mendez, A., Duncan, R., Simoneau, J., & Nolan, B. (1992). Sleep disturbances in men with asymptomatic human immunodeficiency (HIV) infection. *Sleep, 15*, 150–155.
O'Brien, M. E., & Pheifer, W. G. (1993). Physical and psychosocial nursing care for patients with HIV infection. *Nursing Clinics of North America, 28*, 303–316.
O'Dell, M. W., Crawford, A., Bohi, E. S., & Bonner, F. J., Jr. (1991). Disability in persons hospitalized with AIDS. *American Journal of Physical Medicine Rehabilitation, 70*, 91–95.
Olesen, M. (1990). Subjectively perceived quality of life. *IMAGE: Journal of Nursing Scholarship, 3*, 187–190.
Ostrow, D. G., Whitaker, R. E. D., Frasier, K., Cohen, C., Wan, J., Frank, C., & Fisher, E. (1991). Racial differences in social support and mental health in men with HIV infection: A pilot study. *AIDS Care, 3*, 55–62.
Ott, C. R., Sivarajan, E. S., Newton, K. M., Almes, M. J., Bruce, R. A., Bergner, M., & Gilson, B. S. (1983). A controlled randomized study of early cardiac rehabilitation: The Sickness Impact Profile as an assessment tool. *Heart & Lung, 12*, 162–170.
Padilla, G. V., Presant, C., Grant, M. M., Metter, G., Lipsett, J., & Heide, F. (1983). Quality of Life Index for patients with cancer. *Research in Nursing & Health, 6*, 117–126.
Presant, C. A., Scolaro, M., Kennedy, P., Blayney, D. W., Flanagan, B., Lisak, J., & Presant, J. (1993). Liposomal daunorubicin treatment of HIV-associated Kaposi's sarcoma. *The Lancet, 341*, 1242–1243.
Rabkin, J. G., Remien, R., Katoff, L., & Williams, J. B. W. (1993). Resilience in adversity among long-term survivors of AIDS. *Hospital and Community Psychiatry, 44*, 162–167.

Ragsdale, D., Kotarba, J. A., & Morrow, J. R., Jr. (1992a). Quality of life of hospitalized persons with AIDS. *IMAGE: Journal of Nursing Scholarship, 24*, 259–265.

Ragsdale, D., Kotarba, J. A., & Morrow, J. R., Jr. (1992b). Work-related activities to improve quality of life in HIV disease. *Journal of the Association of Nurses in AIDS Care, 3*(1), 39–44.

Ragsdale, D., & Morrow, J. (1990). Quality of life as a function of HIV classification. *Nursing Research, 39*, 355–359.

Remick, S. C., McSharry, J. J., Wolf, B. C., Blanchard, C. G., Eastman, A. Y., Wagner, H., Portuese, E., Wighton, T., Powell, D., Pearce, T., Horton, J., & Ruckdeschel, J. C. (1993). Novel oral combination chemotherapy in the treatment of intermediate-grade and high-grade AIDS-related non-Hodgkin's lymphoma. *Journal of Clinical Oncology, 11*, 1691–1702.

Resource Booklet (1993). *Time to Act! World AIDS Day, 1 December 1993*. Washington, DC: American Association for World Health.

Rockey, P. H., & Griep, R. J. (1980). Behavioral dysfunction in hyperthyroidism: Improvement with treatment. *Archives of Internal Medicine, 140*, 1194–1197.

Schag-Coscarelli, C. A., Ganz, P. A., Kahn, B., & Peterson, L. (1992). Assessing the needs and quality of life of patients with HIV infection: Development of the HIV Overview of Problems-Evaluation System (HOPES). *Quality of Life Research, 1*, 397–413.

Siegrist, J., & Junge, A. (1989). Background material for the workshop on QALYs. *Social Science and Medicine, 29*, 463–468.

Slevin, M. L., Plant, H., Lynch, D., Drinkwater, J., & Gregory, W. M. (1988). Who should measure quality of life, the doctor or the patient? *British Journal of Cancer, 57*, 109–112.

Spitzer, W. O. (1987). State of science, 1986: Quality of life and functional status as target variables for research. *Journal of Chronic Diseases, 40*, 465–471.

Spitzer, W. O., Dobson, A. J., Hall, J., Chesterman, E., & Levi, J. (1981). Measuring the quality of life of cancer patients. *Journal of Chronic Diseases, 34*, 585–597.

Stewart, A. L., & Ware, J. E., Jr. (Eds.). (1992). *Measuring functioning and well-being: The medical outcomes study approach*. Durham, NC: Duke University Press.

Stewart, A. L., Hays, R. D., & Ware, J. E., Jr. (1988). The MOS short-form general health survey: Reliability and validity in a patient population. *Medical Care, 26*, 724–735.

Troidl, H., Kusche, J., Vestweber, K., Eypasch, E., Koeppen, L., & Bouillon, B. (1987). Quality of life: An important endpoint both in surgical practice and research. *Journal of Chronic Diseases, 40*, 523–528.

Varricchio, C. G. (1990). Relevance of quality of life to clinical nursing practice. *Seminars in Oncology Nursing, 6*, 255–259.

Vermund, S. H. (1991). Changing estimates of HIV-1 seroprevalence in the United States. *Journal of NIH Research, 3*(7), 77–81.

Von Roenn, J. H., Murphy, R. L., & Wegener, N. (1990). Megestrol acetate for treatment of anorexia and cachexia associated with human immunodeficiency virus infection. *Seminars in Oncology, 17*, 13–16.

Wachtel, T., Piette, J., Mor, V., Stein, M., Fleishman, J., & Carpenter, J. (1992). Quality of life in persons with human immunodeficiency virus infection:

Measurement by the medical outcomes study instrument. *Annals of Internal Medicine, 116*, 129–137.

Wallston, K. A., Burger, C., Smith, R. A., & Baugher, R. J. (1988). Comparing the quality of death for hospice and non-hospice cancer patients. *Medical Care, 26*, 177–182.

Weitz, R. (1989). Uncertainty and the lives of persons with AIDS. *Journal of Health and Social Behavior, 30*, 270–281.

Williams, J. B. W., & Rabkin, J. G. (1991). The concurrent validity of items in the Quality of Life Index in a cohort of HIV-positive and HIV-negative gay men. *Controlled Clinical Trials, 12*, 129S–141S.

Wu, A. W., Matthews, W. C., Brysk, L. T., Atkinson, J. H., Grant, I., Abramson, I., Kennedy, C. J., McCutchan, J. A., Spector, S. A., & Richman, D. D. (1990). Quality of life in a placebo-controlled trial of zidovudine in patients with AIDS and AIDS-related complex. *Journal of Acquired Immune Deficiency Syndromes, 3*, 683–690.

Wu, A. W., Rubin, H. R., Matthews, W. C., Ware, J. E. Jr., Brysk, L. T., Hardy, W. D., Bozzette, S. A., Spector, S. A., & Richman, D. D. (1991). A health status questionnaire using 30 items from the medical outcomes study: Preliminary validation in persons with early HIV infection. *Medical Care, 29*, 786–798.

Wu, A. W., Rubin, H. R., Mathews, W. C., Brysk, L. M., Bozette, S. A., Hardy, W. D., Atkinson, J. H., Grant, I., Spector, S. A., McCutchan, J. A., & Richman, D. D. (1993). Functional status and well-being in a placebo-controlled trial of zidovudine in early symptomatic HIV infection. *Journal of Acquired Immune Deficiency Syndromes, 5*, 452–458.

Yancik, R., & Yates, J. W. (1986). Quality-of-life assessment of cancer patients: Conceptual and methodologic challenges and constraints. *The Cancer Bulletin, 38*, 217–222.

Zeller, J. M., Swanson, B., & Cohen, F. L. (1993). Suggestions for clinical nursing research: Symptom management in AIDS patients. *Journal of the Association of Nurses in AIDS Care, 4*, 13–17.

Chapter 2

Physical Health of Homeless Adults

ADA M. LINDSEY
SCHOOL OF NURSING
UNIVERSITY OF CALIFORNIA, LOS ANGELES

CONTENTS

Although the existence and plight of homeless people have been chronicled throughout history, only within the last decade, has some attention in the United States been focused on the health status and health care issues of this growing, disenfranchised, vulnerable population. Researchers and other authors, in the past 10 or 12 years, have been adding to the knowledge base about homeless populations and their health care needs (Brickner, Scharer, Conanan, Elvy, & Savarese, 1985; Institute of Medicine, 1988; Lindsey, 1992a, 1992b). Most studies are reported after 1985.

This research review is centered on the physical health of homeless adults. There also is a body of research on the physical health of homeless children and adolescent youth and a growing body of research focused on the mental health of homeless people, but review of these areas of study is beyond the scope of this chapter. Mental health was examined in some of the research in this review, and the reason for including the work was that the research also was focused on some aspect of physical health.

The search strategies used to access the research for this review included computerized on-line searches of MEDLINE (for January 1980 to September 1993), and the Cumulative Index to Nursing and Allied Health Literature (CINAHL) (for January 1983 to September 1993) using the key words homeless and health. A manual search of the CINAHL was done for 1980 through 1982. The MEDLINE search resulted in 670 citations with most ($n = 433$) occurring for 1990 to 1993. This list was reduced by excluding citations for foreign studies, nonresearch articles, and those dealing with homeless and mental health and homeless children and adolescent youth. The MEDLINE search was cross-referenced against a chapter entitled "Health Issues Among the Homeless" in the book *Homelessness: An Annotated Bibliography* (Henslin, 1993a, 1993b). The studies included for this review were from holdings available in the UCLA libraries or those available in on-line abstract form. Some additional published studies available in the author's own reference collection were included. Not included in this review of research articles are the research findings on various aspects of health of homeless adults that are summarized in book chapters and in special journal issues devoted to perspectives of homelessness (Brickner et al., 1985; Brickner, Scharer, Conan, Savarese, & Scanlan, 1990; Homelessness, 1991; Hunter, 1993; Jahiel, 1992; Robertson & Greenblatt, 1992; Vladeck, 1990; Wood, 1992; Wright & Weber, 1987). Articles in which homeless health-related research is reviewed also are not described here (Berne, Dato, Mason, & Rafferty, 1990; Fischer & Breakey, 1991; Garrett, 1989; Lindsey, 1992b; Stephens, Dennis, Toomer, & Holloway, 1991). A more extensive manual search including reviews of references cited by the investigators and use of citations in review articles may have resulted in uncovering additional research. All literature searches and retrieval were completed by a graduate research assistant.

Physical health of homeless adults, although a somewhat delimited focus, represents a broad spectrum of topical areas. In an attempt to develop a sense of coherence about the state of knowledge evolving from this body of research, the studies chosen for this review on physical health were classified into six categories: general health problems, specific health problems, factors affecting physical health, health risks, health care needs and health status, and special health problems (tuberculosis, substance abuse, and HIV infection). A second major categorization is physical health care services. This category includes studies in which use, barriers to access, and models of delivery of care to homeless adults were examined. A total of 78 studies were reviewed.

GENERAL HEALTH PROBLEMS

Research included in this categorization were studies focused on determining, in a global way, the most frequent physical health problems experienced by homeless adults. Most of the 15 studies reviewed in this category were descriptive, and a comparison group was used in only 4 of the studies.

Nurse researchers have reported findings about the physical health problems of homeless individuals seeking care in clinics where nurses provide care or in nurse-managed clinics that serve this population (Abdellah, Chamberlain, & Levine, 1986; Bowdler, 1989; Brecht, Lindsey, & Stuart, 1991; Gottesman, Lewis, Lindsey, & Brecht, 1993; Lindsey, 1989; Reuler, Bax, & Sampson, 1986; Stanhope, 1989; Stanhope & Blomquist, 1989; Wright et al., 1987). From 1,184 evaluations of a Portland, Oregon, sample, the most common physical health problems were dermatological conditions, need for general evaluation, musculoskeletal pain, and respiratory and gastrointestinal problems (Reuler et al., 1986). Using charts of 6,235 individuals in a New York City study, the most frequently cited problems were drinking or drug abuse (32.6%), trauma (30.7%), upper respiratory conditions (27.8%), chronic lung disease (20.6%), and limb disorders (19.8%) (Wright et al., 1987). During a 34-month period (1985–1987), 7,369 homeless individuals had more than 21,000 encounters recorded in a downtown Los Angeles nurse-managed clinic (Lindsey, 1989). The three most frequent conditions were acute nasopharyngitis (14.8%), need for tuberculosis (TB) screening (11.3%), and open wounds/lacerations (10.4%). For a small sample ($N = 90$) from Richmond, the five most frequent diagnoses were mental illness (53%), respiratory system diseases (50%), infections and parasitic disorders (33%), diseases of the nervous system (23%), and injuries and poisonings (21%)(Bowdler, 1989). In these four studies, researchers used existing clinical records; the samples were taken from those homeless persons who sought health care. Thus, the findings may not be representative of the general homeless population. Information about the onset of the problems in relation to time of becoming homeless was not reported in these studies.

Using a Los Angeles–area beach community-based sample of 529 homeless people, Gelberg and Linn (1989) conducted an interview and a screening physical examination with limited blood testing to determine the physical health of this population. This community-based sampling strategy has the potential to uncover health care problems of homeless persons who may not be included in sampling from clinical or shelter populations. In a second report of findings from this study of 529 homeless adults, variability in 12 physical health measures was assessed according to demographic characteristics of age, gender, ethnicity, total length of time homeless, and work status (Gelberg & Linn, 1992). Age and gender contributed most to the explanation of differences in physical health of this sample. As expected, older individuals were more likely than younger persons to have a chronic disease and functional disability, and men were more likely than women to be substance abusers. This sample had a wide variety of physical health problems. Using the same sample, they reported on the differences in health between the older (50–78 years) and younger (18–49 years) age homeless adults (Gelberg, Lind, & Mayer-Oakes, 1990). The older group, in addition to functional disabilities and chronic disease, were more likely to have elevated blood pressure, creatinine and cholesterol, and less likely to be drug users than the younger age group. The older group had a higher proportion of whites and veterans, and reported having no social contact for a month.

In four research reports, the health problems of homeless adults were compared with those of nonhomeless adults (Ferenchick, 1991, 1992; Gelberg, Linn, Usatine, & Smith, 1990; Morris & Crystal, 1989). The homeless adults ($N = 464$) in one study had more functional limitations, dermatological problems, seizures, chronic obstructive pulmonary disease, serious visual and dental problems, and more social isolation than did the poor nonhomeless sample who sought care in the same clinic (Gelberg, Linn, Usatine, & Smith, 1990). Although the same sample was used for multiple reports, this study was strengthened by the community-based sampling and incorporation of comparative methodology (homeless vs. nonhomeless adults). In a retrospective study using medical records, the medical problems of homeless and nonhomeless adults who sought care in an outpatient clinic serving the medically indigent were examined (Ferenchick, 1991). Homeless adults ($N = 150$) more often sought care for cuts and gynecological problems than the nonhomeless sample ($N = 154$) and were more likely to be diagnosed as alcoholic. In contrast to the findings reported for the Gelberg, Linn, Usatine, and Smith (1990) study, this investigator found no other significant differences in the occurrence of other health problems in the two groups. The medical problems of homeless and nonhomeless adults ($N = 475$) who sought care during a 1-year period in an ambulatory clinic serving the medically indigent were compared in a third study (Ferenchick, 1992). Using interviews and medical records, no significant differences between the groups in age, gender, and ethnicity were found. Similar to the previous report, the homeless adults had a higher prevalence of injuries and gynecological problems than did the nonhomeless group. The homeless adults also had more dental problems and were more likely to be alcohol abusers. Unlike the reports by Gelberg, Linn, Usatine, and Smith (1990), this investigator concluded there are more similarities than differences in the medical problems experienced between the homeless and nonhomeless adults. However, the homeless adults were reported to have a higher prevalence of illness. Sampling homeless and nonhomeless adults who use the same clinics provides additional information about possible differences in health care problems. However, because homeless populations are not homogeneous, it is possible that the differences in findings from populations sampled from different clinics in different geographical regions reflect this heterogeneity.

A retrospective review of inpatient medical records of medically indigent adults who were hospitalized in San Diego County during a 2-year period (1985, 1986) revealed that 5.3% ($N = 226$) were homeless adults (Morris & Crystal, 1989). The most common discharge diagnosis for the homeless group was diseases and disorders of the skin: 21.2% compared with 8.7% for the nonhomeless indigent. Cellulitis was the most prevalent dermatological condition of the homeless adults. The status of homelessness compared with housed also was more frequently associated with the discharge diagnostic category of substance use and substance-induced organic mental disorders. From these few comparative studies, differences in health problems were identified for homeless adults, and these problems were different by setting of the study.

In Baltimore, Breakey and colleagues studied 298 men and 230 women randomly selected from shelters, jails, and missions and subsequently randomly selected 203 subjects from the larger group to undergo psychiatric and physical examinations (Breakey et al., 1989). Baseline data were obtained by interviews of the initial sample. From this baseline interview, the investigators found this sample had considerable evidence of disaffiliation and substance abuse. The physical and psychiatric examinations of the subsample confirmed the high prevalence of alcohol abuse disorders, mental illnesses and other psychiatric disorders, and a range of physical health problems. This study is notable because of the use of random selection of this difficult-to-sample population.

One recent study conducted by nurse researchers was conceptualized from a community health framework using the classification scheme of the Omaha Visiting Nurse Association (Reilly, Grier, & Blomquist, 1992). Health problems were categorized into four domains of community health practice. The data were collected in a nurse-managed clinic (Lexington, Kentucky) during an 18-month period during 6,668 visits by 1,064 patients. A mean of 1.93 health problems per visit was encountered from the total of 12,900 health problems identified. Regardless of age or gender, the four most frequent primary health problems identified involved circulation, integument, respiration, and pain. They also had problems with nutrition, vision, and the neuromusculoskeletal system. Similar to findings of other studies, the older patients had more health problems that were chronic; they also had a higher average number of clinic visits than did the younger adults. Substance misuse was identified frequently as a secondary problem for clinic visits by younger men. In contrast to findings of some other studies, only 13% of the health problems assessed in this sample were classified in the psychosocial domain suggesting less focus on mental health problems. Strengths of this descriptive study included the use of a community health framework, the examination of the health problems by age and gender, the length of time of data collection, and the large sample size.

Using a 58-item questionnaire with a large sample ($N = 1{,}008$) of homeless adult men from three shelters in Santa Clara County California, investigators asked whether physical illnesses and injuries were present when they first became homeless or whether the problems contributed significantly to their loss of shelter (Winkleby & Fleshin, 1993). Of the sample, 42% were combat- ($N = 173$) and noncombat- ($N = 250$) exposed veterans. The veterans were more likely to report alcohol abuse before loss of shelter than were the nonveterans ($N = 585$). Those veterans who were combat-exposed were more likely to have a higher prevalence of physical injuries and more psychiatric hospitalizations before becoming homeless than the other veterans and the nonveterans. Although this study included a large sample, the results were based on self-reports of the homeless adults in response to questions on alcohol intake, injuries, and psychiatric hospitalization, and were based on recall and comparison of information before and after they became homeless. This sample was obtained from a shelter population. However, this represents a single study determining onset of health problems in relation to onset of becoming homeless.

Another way to determine health problems of homeless adults was used for a San Francisco population (Centers for Disease Control, 1991b). Between 1985 and 1990, the causes of their deaths were characterized.

In general, the state of knowledge about the most frequent physical health problems of homeless adults has been derived predominantly from convenience samples of people in shelters or who have sought care in a clinic or who have been hospitalized. There was only one community-based sample. Most of the studies had a large sample size, and some studies were longitudinal. Follow-up of this addressless population is difficult to achieve. There was a limited number of studies where comparisons of physical health problems between homeless and poor nonhomeless adults have been done. Whether poor nonhomeless adults is the best comparative group to use remains controversial. Although some findings across studies about the most frequent physical health problems were similar, there also were notable differences that possibly reflect the nonhomogenity of this population in and across geographical regions. The dissimilarities in findings may also reflect differences in the clinic populations, the shelter populations, the community-based populations, and the hospitalized populations sampled. There were no intervention studies. Once the most common health problems are identified for a representative sample, interventions need to be designed and examined for their effectiveness in preventing or decreasing the incidence of the health problem, or in ameliorating recurrence or adverse consequences in this difficult-to-care-for population.

SPECIFIC HEALTH PROBLEMS

Nine research reports are reviewed under this category in four groups: reproductive health problems, other specific health problems, nutritional status, and dental problems. They are studies of diverse specific health problems, and there is an absence of coherent development of knowledge in this body of work. With one exception, nutritional status, they were discrete single studies.

Reproductive Health Problems. Killion (1988) conducted a qualitative study to examine the coexistence of pregnancy and homelessness in black women. She used participant observations, focused observations, interviews, life histories, diaries, and documents to describe how a sample of black women in Los Angeles coped with the consequences of coexisting pregnancy and homelessness. Based on a nurse-practitioner practice model, Shuler (1991) studied the family planning needs of 50 homeless women who sought care in a downtown Los Angeles family planning clinic. Contraception use was reported by slightly more than one third (34%), thus the majority was at risk for unintended pregnancy and sexually transmitted diseases. Most (84%) desired birth control; those least likely to use contraception were black cocaine users. More than one half used alcohol (56%) or street drugs (52%), and 30% reported engaging in prostitution. To determine the incidence of sexually transmitted disease and Papanicolaou (Pap) smear results, Johnstone and colleagues reviewed clinical records of 104 female homeless clients who received care from a mobile women's health unit in Chicago (Johnstone, Tornabene, & Marcinak, 1993). They found that 30% of the Pap smears had abnormal findings; atypia and inflammation were the most common, with trichomoniasis representing 26%. Chlamydia (3%) and gonorrhea (6%) also were reported. Although these are single, descriptive studies with convenience sampling, and other methodological limitations, it is apparent from the findings, homeless women need regular access to gynecological care.

Other Specific Health Problems. Medical directors of health clinics serving homeless adults in large U.S. cities were surveyed to determine the management of hypertension for the homeless being seen in these clinics (Kinchen & Wright, 1991). The investigators compared the responses of the 65 responding medical directors with data from surveys of clinicians in "normal" clinical practice. They concluded that although the therapeutic goals were similar for the homeless and nonhomeless adults, medical practice was adapted to the unique circumstances of the homeless hypertensives.

Communicable disease problems as represented by diarrheal illness and control measures were assessed by survey in 73 government-funded shelters for battered women and their children across five regions in 15 states (Gross & Rosenberg, 1987). Although this represents a study in which the specific health problem was more child focused than adult, it is reflective of need for attention to health problems that arise in a shelter environment. Fewer than one half of the shelter directors acknowledged screening potential residents for communicable diseases before admission to the shelter. Twelve percent of the directors reported outbreaks of diarrheal illness that affected more than 10 residents. Few shelters had a place designed for diapering. Although most of the shelter staff had first-aid training, only 5% of the 73 shelters had health care workers. The need for attention to basic hygiene and health care practices in this group of shelters was identified. This is one study where the findings have immediate application to practice, particularly in community health nursing. Further study of other types of shelters is needed to assess the magnitude of other potentially problematic communicable diseases and the existence of appropriate control measures. Although not specified as research, Smith described an educational project designed as an intervention to teach parents in a shelter for the homeless about the treatment of diarrhea and dehydration in infants and children (Smith, 1988). The project was evaluated to be successful, and the intervention has been implemented in other shelters.

Nutritional Status. The nutritional adequacy of the diets of homeless individuals has been examined (Drake, 1992; Luder, Boey, Buchalter, & Martinez-Weber, 1989; Luder, Ceysens-Okada, Koren-Roth, & Martinez-Weber, 1990). Additional nutritional adequacy studies are reviewed elsewhere (Wiecha, Dwyer, & Dunn-Strohecker, 1991). Luder and colleagues studied nutritional status indicators in 55 homeless adults (Luder et al., 1989). In addition to determining that the quality of the nutritional intake was inadequate, the anthropometric measures of these subjects were significantly different from the U.S. general population distributions. The findings reflected decreased levels of lean body mass and increased levels of body fat, including elevated serum cholesterol levels. They cautioned that the nutritional status of these homeless adults may place them at increased risk of developing nutrition-associated conditions. In another study of 96 homeless persons, 90% reported they got enough to eat, but the investigators reported a low score on dietary adequacy (Luder et al., 1990). The diet records showed a high level of cholesterol and saturated fat intake, and the serum cholesterol levels of 82% of the subjects were above the desired level of 200 mg/dL. More than one third (39%) of the subjects showed evidence of hypertension and obesity. The investigators concluded that although the homeless subjects obtained a sufficient quantity of food, the shelter meals required modification to meet recommended nutritional adequacy criteria. Drake studied the nutritional status and the nutritional adequacy of the diets of 96 single homeless mothers and their 192 dependent children (Drake, 1992). These subjects, similar to those in the previously cited studies, felt they were getting enough food to eat. However, this whole group was found to be consuming less than 50% of the Recommended Dietary Allowances (RDA) of several substances, such as iron, folic acid, magnesium, and zinc; the women also were eating less than 50% of the RDA for calcium. Similar to the previously cited studies, this group also was eating more than the desirable amounts of fats. The need to modify shelter meals was identified. The inadequate nutrient intake of children may put them at risk for growth and development delays.

Dental Problems. Using the 529 community-based homeless sample, Gelberg and colleagues reported findings on the dental health of their subjects (Gelberg, Linn, & Rosenberg, 1988). Their homeless sample was only one half as likely to have had a dental visit in the previous year compared with the general population, although 27% reported experiencing a toothache within the past month. The homeless sample had more grossly decayed teeth than the general population. The best predictor of missing teeth was age. Older homeless adults had more dental problems than the younger homeless. The investigators concluded that although their homeless sample had lower use of dental services than the general population, they had more dental pathosis.

Research Gaps. From this review of disparate studies categorized as specific health problems, the lack of collection of studies on any one physical health problem is apparent (except for the few studies on nutritional adequacy). The studies are descriptive; only one project reported on an educational intervention (for diarrhea and dehydration). No standardized instruments were used. Convenience samples were used, and only a few included comparison data or groups. There obviously are tremendous gaps in the state of knowledge in how specific health problems are experienced and managed in homeless adults.

FACTORS AFFECTING HEALTH

Four studies were reviewed that addressed factors that may affect the physical health of homeless adults. In one study, the onset of morbidity was examined (Winkleby & White, 1992). Data were collected from a sample of 1,399 homeless adults in three shelters in Santa Clara County, California. The investigators compared characteristics of the individuals with and without physical and other health problems when they initially became homeless. According to the self-report data, 45.6% of the sample had no impairments at the time they became homeless. This group with no impairments when they became homeless was younger or was more likely to be of minority status than those individuals who reported having impairments at the time of becoming homeless. Those with no impairments at the time of becoming homeless were over time likely to develop psychiatric and addictive problems. These investigators suggested that homelessness is a factor that influences the health of some adults, that is, homelessness contributes to development of physical health problems.

In New Jersey, some sheltered care facilities are regulated and licensed by the state, whereas homeless shelters serving as temporary residences are not licensed (Knight, Mason, Christopher, Beck, & Toughill, 1991). Knight and colleagues conducted a study to determine if the state policies regulating licensure of sheltered care facilities reflected differences in the physical, psychological, and social health status of the populations served. They found those in homeless shelters had higher incidence of respiratory, gastrointestinal, integumentary, and substance-abuse problems than the residents in other types of facilities. However, these temporary residences for homeless people were not licensed in New Jersey. They suggest that health assessment and monitoring also should be required for temporary residences similar to that required in other residential facilities. This state policy is a factor that has the potential of influencing the health of homeless adults.

In a third study, the readability of patient instruction sheets used by a clinic serving a homeless population was determined and compared with the average reading level of a sample of 70 homeless individuals (Roskamp, 1987). Only 14.3% of the sample read at a level that allowed them to comprehend all of the patient instruction sheets. The mean readability of the instruction sheets was 10.5, and although the mean educational level of the sample was 11.3, their average reading level was 7.9. Thus, the level of reading difficulty of printed patient instruction materials (comprehension of and adherence to instruction) also has the potential of influencing the health status of this population.

Another factor that affects the health status of the homeless population is their degree of compliance in taking prescribed medications. Two nurse investigators studied the perceived factors that enhance or diminish the compliance of 61 urban homeless adults in taking medications (Nyamathi & Shuler, 1989). For one third of the sample, the compliance rate ranged from about one half to not at all. Structural variables, such as lack of a place to store the medications and difficulty obtaining the prescribed medications, were cited as deterrents. Being close to a health clinic, understanding need for the medication, and being able to carry the medication enhanced compliance.

These investigations of factors that affect health also represent discrete studies (e.g., the fact of being homeless, reading level of health-related instruction materials, result of being in a shelter without health regulation, and barriers in adherence to taking prescribed medications). This body of work is at the descriptive level and represents only a beginning. However, two of the studies have immediate potential for application: the examination of the reading level of patient instruction sheets and the state policy involved in health-related regulation of temporary shelters for homeless individuals. Given the paucity of studies in this category, considerably more work is required to develop the knowledge base about factors affecting the health status of homeless people.

HEALTH RISKS

Although health risks represent a category of research, for the six studies included here, health risks have been conceptualized from a different perspective in each study. For example, in one study gender differences in health risks and reported physical symptoms were compared between a survey sample of 100 homeless adults and the general population (Ritchey, La Gory, & Mullis, 1991). In another study, the risk factors for ill health were conceptualized more from an environmental perspective (place of "residence," access to heat, running water, bathing facility, and poverty level) (Winkleby, 1990). This was a survey study comparing the risk factors for ill health of a sample of 71 homeless poor with data of nonhomeless poor from the 1980 California census and a 1982 California Behavioral Risk Factor Survey. Most (about 90%) homeless people reported having no access to basic necessities, such as heated rooms and hot running water, and they were less likely to get preventive health care than the nonhomeless poor individuals. Vredevoe, Brecht, Shuler, and Woo (1992) conceptualized risk factors for disease as smoking, drug and alcohol use, obesity, and sedentary lifestyle. These investigators analyzed the International Classification of Diseases diagnosis categories from the clinical records of 1,252 homeless clients seeking care in a downtown Los Angeles nurse-managed clinic for relationships with the identified risk factors. The risk factors were predictive of health problems.

A 44-item high-risk smoking practices questionnaire was developed and used in interviews of 58 predominately male, multiethnic homeless individuals (Aloot & Vredevoe, 1993). Significant high-risk smoking practices were identified, such as sharing the same cigarette among smokers (85%); remaking cigarettes from discarded butts, filters, street drugs, and fresh loose tobacco (71%); smoking collected butts (61%); and adding street drugs to rerolled cigarettes (17%). These unconventional behaviors place these homeless individuals at greater risk for exposure to toxins trapped in tobacco remains and filters, and increase risk of transmitting infectious diseases.

Health risks of homeless black men seeking services during one month from a Dade County Florida Community Homeless Assistance Plan were assessed by survey (Centers for Disease Control, 1991a). Health behaviors and health risks were identified from self-report data from interviews of a convenience sample of 100 homeless men in a shelter in Utah (Mason, Jensen, & Boland, 1992). In this study health risks were conceptualized as incidence of disease, particularly related to hypertension, diabetes, and mental illness. The health behaviors included assessment of exercise, diet, substance use, behaviors related to AIDS, and use of the health care system. In this sample, 31 reported a diagnosis of hypertension, 8 were diabetics, and 20 had been treated for mental illness during the past year; thus, almost 60% of the sample were assessed as having a health risk, but few reported compliance with the prescribed therapeutic regimen, which clearly puts them at additional risk for related health problems.

Similar to the research reviewed in the previous categories, the studies in this category also remain at the descriptive level and lack conceptual congruence across studies. There was also lack of use of standardized instruments across studies, presumably because of the paucity of such measures for the variables being addressed in this nonhomogeneous vulnerable population. Although risk factors were the focus of these studies, synthesis of results across studies was not possible because of the disparate nature of the variables conceptualized as risk factors.

HEALTH CARE NEEDS AND HEALTH STATUS

Although the major focus of the 14 studies included in this category centers on determining health care needs and the health status of homeless adults, they also represent rather diverse perspectives. However, three of the studies were undertaken to obtain data to support the development of nurse-managed clinics to serve homeless populations (Bowdler & Barrell, 1987; Malloy, Christ, & Hohlock, 1990; Skelly, Getty, Kemsley, Hunter, & Shipman, 1990).

Using an ethnographic approach, Kinzel (1991) interviewed 14 residents of single-room occupancy (SRO) hotels and 16 transients in downtown Spokane, Washington, for the purpose of comparing their self-perceived health concerns. Both groups reported not feeling healthy, with the transient group more often reporting health problems associated with living on the street, and they more frequently used emergency departments for acute problems than did the SRO group. The investigator suggested from the findings that if health care needs are to be met, location of services needs to be variable according to the homeless population to be served. In a study of 40 homeless people conducted in Baltimore, investigators suggested that to meet the needs of homeless people, health care services need to be appropriate to the different types of homelessness (marginal, recent, and chronic) (Belcher, Scholler-Jaquish, & Drummond, 1991). In another study, unmet health care needs of women were identified by a survey of 43 shelters in Chicago (Barge &

Norr, 1991). Self-care requisites were identified in a study of elderly homeless men (Harris & Williams, 1991). This is one of a few studies that referenced any theoretical model.

The three studies assessing the health needs of homeless people as a basis for developing a nurse-managed clinic were conducted in three locations: Richmond, Virginia, Buffalo, New York, and Charleston, South Carolina (Bowlder & Barrell, 1987; Malloy et al., 1990; Skelly et al., 1990). In the Richmond study, data were collected from a survey approach (interviews of 70 homeless people in one shelter), from a key informant approach (telephone survey of 16 key service providers), and from an indicator approach (audit of 45 charts from a free clinic) (Bowdler & Barrell, 1987). In the Buffalo study, data on perceived health care needs were collected from interviews of 124 homeless individuals in one shelter (Skelly et al., 1990). For the Charleston study, 51 homeless adults seeking shelter were interviewed using the Basic Shelter Inventory instrument (Malloy et al., 1990). This is one of the few studies identifying a theoretical model; they referred to social disaffiliation as being a potential basis for intervention for underserved populations. These three studies, like others, revealed that homeless people perceive they have health care problems and need health care services. Most did not have a regular service for health care and tended to use emergency departments.

In the remaining seven studies in this category, researchers examined the perceived health status of homeless adults. Four of the studies sampled populations in Los Angeles (Gelberg & Linn, 1988; Linn & Gelberg, 1989; Robertson & Cousineau, 1986; Ropers & Boyer, 1987). One third of a sample of 238 homeless reported their health as poor or fair, and more than half had no regular source of care (Robertson & Cousineau, 1986). Using a perceived health status index for in-depth interviews of 269 homeless, the best predictors of poor health were length of unemployment, level of education, gender, and number of nights spent in a shelter (Ropers & Boyer, 1987). Data from a community-based sample of 529 homeless were used to determine the relationship between previous use of mental health services and their physical health status, perceived needs, and other factors (Gelberg & Linn, 1988). These investigators also asked this sample to prioritize their five basic needs (Linn & Gelberg, 1989). The top priority was good health; the sample also identified the needs of steady income, permanent job, permanent home, and regular meals.

In two of the studies, aging or elderly homeless people were used as the sample to examine physical well-being or health (Cohen, Teresi, & Holmes, 1988; Reilly, 1991). Comparing male street dwellers in the Bowery section of New York City with nonstreet dwellers, the street dwellers scored worse on all the physical health scales used (Cohen et al., 1988). Some variables associated with poor health were stress, unfulfilled needs, and being a young-older age. In the other study, the investigator examined the relationship between health and space and time use in 74 homeless individuals (Reilly, 1991). General health status, functional health status, and symptom status were included in the health status measures. Both functional health status and general health status were correlated positively with distance traveled in a 24-hour period. The investigator concluded that the relationships between health and space and time use provided some support that health is a capability constraint in this elderly homeless sample. This is one of the few studies reviewed that was conceptualized from a theoretical perspective.

The last study in this category does not actually reflect a homeless sample per se; however, 26% of the sample were homeless individuals (Barter, 1990). It is included because it is one of the few studies in which standardized instruments were used. Perceived health status was measured using two instruments (General Health Rating Index [Barter, 1990] and the Sickness Impact Profile [Bergner, Bobbitt, Carter, & Gilson, 1981]). These instruments were completed by 76 medically indigent adults using a primary care clinic in Marin County, California. The investigator found that unemployment more than any other demographic variable affected the perceived health status. Less education also was associated with lower scores on their perceived health status.

Although this category of studies reflects a collection of research focused on a topical area, health care needs, and health status, there is inadequate depth in the knowledge base because the questions addressed in these studies are not comparable, the same or similar measures have not been used, nor do they build on previous work, and the samples, although all were homeless adults, are dissimilar. None of these samples were selected randomly. A few studies employed comparative methods, and all were descriptive. One incorporated standardized instruments allowing more confidence in the findings. Unlike most studies in this review, there were several studies in this category that were based on a theoretical model. Generally the use of a theoretical base or construction of a framework helps the investigator in determining and maintaining conceptual congruence throughout the study and facilitates a more systematic development of a knowledge base. However, in the studies that were based on a theoretical model, the models used were all different, so again any synthesis or building of knowledge are precluded. Thus, the studies in this category, similar to those in the other categories, represent beginning work in developing an understanding about the physical health of homeless adults.

SPECIAL PROBLEMS

Tuberculosis

Four studies were focused on various aspects of tuberculosis in homeless individuals. One study examined the compliance and adverse reactions to an isoniazid preventive regimen offered to 64 men who had been exposed to an outbreak of tuberculosis in a shelter (Nazar-Stewart & Nolan, 1992). Of the 47 who began the preventive regimen, only 23 completed it; only one of those beginning the regimen experienced a hepatotoxic reaction. The investigators concluded from this longitudinal study that directly supervised isoniazid therapy can be used in a preventive regimen. One report summarized 17 case studies of Ohio homeless shelter residents who had clinically active tuberculosis (Centers for Disease Control, 1990). In a third report, the incidence of drug-resistant tuberculosis in homeless individuals admitted to a Texas Health Department facility was examined (Morris & McAllister, 1992). Of the 26 homeless with culture-verified tuberculosis, 7 patients had tuberculosis resistant to one or more antituberculosis drugs. Drug-resistant tuberculosis was identified in another study using a sample of homeless individuals in Boston (Barry et al., 1986). After finding 26 cases of tuberculosis in a homeless population, the investigators developed a tuberculosis screening program for homeless people housed in three of the largest Boston shelters during a four-night period. Each person was asked to have a chest radiograph and a tuberculin skin test. Symptomatic persons ($N = 217$) were requested to provide a sputum specimen. From almost 750 sheltered people, a total of 586 participated in the TB screening program. Following administration of the skin test to 362 homeless people, only 187 skin test recipients were located in 2 days. A total of 465 had a chest radiograph; although 24 films were suspicious, 4 cases of tuberculosis were confirmed. The investigators comment on the cost of case finding.

These cumulative findings suggest that tuberculosis is a special problem among homeless populations and represents a potential public health problem if cases are undetected and if there is increased incidence of drug-resistant tuberculosis. Again, these studies, although focusing on tuberculosis in homeless individuals, also are all different. However, they illustrate some general problems in studying this population. For example, in the first study in which a preventive intervention was incorporated, the difficulty in adherence to the prevention regimen was demonstrated. In the last study, the cost-effectiveness of a screening/case-finding intervention for this population was raised as an issue. Only slightly more than one half of the skin test recipients returned for skin test reading; from the 586 who were screened, 4 cases were confirmed. In these studies, interventions were incorporated, and outcomes were examined.

HIV Infection

Some aspect of HIV infection was examined in seven studies incorporating homeless adults in the samples. Christiano and Susser (1989) conducted a study of 23 pregnant women residing in a hotel for homeless in New York City to determine their knowledge and perceptions of HIV infection. They talked with each woman at least seven times during an 8-week period in an informal unstructured way. They found a high level of ignorance about how to avoid HIV infection. There was a lack of condom use, and only three knew that AIDS could be transmitted to the fetus by an HIV-positive mother. The investigators concluded that the sample had incomplete or inaccurate information about HIV infection, engaged in unprotected sexual contact, and were at risk for HIV infection.

HIV risk factors in homeless minority women were determined in three studies (Nyamathi, 1991, 1992; Nyamathi, Bennett, Leake, Lewis, & Flaskerud, 1993). Nyamathi categorized 460 black women as being at high, moderate, or low risk for HIV infection to determine what psychosocial factors were associated with risk level (Nyamathi, 1992). Those in high-risk groups reported having greater use of intravenous drugs, having a partner who uses IV drugs, having been diagnosed with a sexually transmitted disease, having multiple sex partners without condom use, and providing sexual intercourse for money or drugs. Those at high risk (65%) were differentiated from the other two risk levels by use of emotion-focused coping, lower self-esteem, greater depression, and greater severity of concerns. The women were tested for HIV antibodies, and 6 were HIV-positive; 4 of these were in the high-risk group. These findings have implications for identifying those women at greater risk for HIV infection and developing an intervention program. In a sample of 581 homeless (68.5%) or drug rehabilitation program (31.5%) minority women, Nyamathi investigated the relationship of self-esteem, sense of coherence, and support availability with high-risk behavior for HIV infection and other factors (Nyamathi, 1991). These variables accounted for only 10% of the variance in high-risk activities. In the third study,

Nyamathi and colleagues administered survey instruments to 1,173 impoverished women of color who were in homeless shelters or in drug recovery programs to determine their AIDS-related knowledge, perceptions, and risk behaviors (Nyamathi et al., 1993). The investigators found differences in those variables based on ethnicity and level of acculturation of the women. They concluded there is a need for culturally sensitive AIDS prevention programs and that sessions need to be separate for women of different ethnicity and acculturation level.

Of the remaining three studies in this category, one reported the HIV seropositive prevalence from the records of 90 men discharged from a New York City shelter program for homeless psychiatric male patients (Susser, Valencia, & Conover, 1993). From the 90 records, 62 had an HIV serostatus recorded; 12 of those were HIV positive (19.4%). A study was conducted to profile the AIDS patients appearing in West Virginia (Patton, 1989). The profile compiled suggested the typical AIDS patient in West Virginia is a native son but was infected out of state, is in an advanced stage of the disease, is under the age of 30, and is homeless. The last study in this category tested the effectiveness of two interventions, a specialized and a traditional AIDS counseling program for impoverished women of color (Nyamathi, Leake, Flaskerud, Lewis, & Bennett, 1993). The sample of 858 women (African-American and Latina) were residing in 1 of 10 homeless shelters or in 1 of 11 drug recovery programs. Of the 858 women, 448 participated in the specialized program, and 410 participated in the traditional program. The intervention interval was a 2-week period; significant improvements occurred in women exposed to either intervention. Although there were some differences between the two groups, the specialized program was not more effective than the traditional program. Thus, the nursing interventions, regardless of content, influenced positively the outcome variables (cognitive, behavioral, and psychological). The investigators concluded that the findings supported the framework used to guide this study, the Comprehensive Health Seeking and Coping Paradigm (developed previously by Nyamathi). This study represents an important development in the body of work related to homeless individuals and physical health, testing the effectiveness of two interventions on specified outcomes.

This group of studies, like most others in this review, represents beginning work. The work of Nyamathi and colleagues is an exception; by using the same at-risk population for several studies, by using some standardized instruments, by examining related questions across studies, by exploring relationships among variables, and by testing the effectiveness of an intervention in one study, there is evidence of a sense of coherent effort to develop the knowledge base. More critical analysis may suggest opportunities to strengthen and build on this base, but at least there is base for extension.

Substance Abuse

Two of the eight studies reviewed in this category focused on drug use and risk for HIV infection (el-Bassel & Schilling, 1991; Siegal et al., 1991). Those in the first study sample were not exclusively homeless people; the investigators studied the behavioral factors that put IV drug users at risk for acquiring and transmitting HIV (Siegal et al., 1991). Homeless shelter residence was one of the three factors significantly related to HIV infection in a sample of 855 Ohio adults not in drug treatment. The second study obtained data from a sample of 108 African-American males participating in a free lunch program; this sample had a history of drug use, and almost 70% were homeless (el-Bassel & Schilling, 1991). The purpose was to determine relationships among drug use, sexual activity, use of AIDS prevention practices, and perceived risk of AIDS. A large majority (75%) perceived themselves to be at risk for AIDS.

Using data collected from homeless health care projects in 16 of the 19 cities that participated in the Robert Wood Johnson/The Pew Charitable Trusts–funded Health Care for the Homeless Program, Wright and colleagues compared the health problems of the adult homeless identified as possible alcohol abusers with the health problems of the adult homeless (Wright, Knight, Weber-Burdin, & Lam, 1987). In their analysis they used data from clients seen at least twice ($N = 11{,}886$). Alcohol abuse was reported for approximately 23% of the population. Mental illness was significantly more common among alcohol abusers than nonabusers; alcohol abusers also had higher rates of drug abuse. Peripheral vascular disease, hypertension, gastrointestinal disorders, and trauma were the most frequent major physical health problems. The rates for these disorders were higher in the alcohol abusers than in the homeless nonabusers. Indicators of substance abuse and mental health status were compared for 214 homeless adults and 250 nonhomeless poor individuals from a population who sought care at a community clinic (Linn, Gelberg, & Leake, 1990). The homeless group was more likely to have been arrested for drinking, to have been hospitalized for alcohol or mental health problems, and to have experienced delirium tremens than the nonhomeless poor clinic users. Another group of investigators using a 57-page interview protocol collected data from 1,260 men and women residing in New York City public shelters (Struening, Padgett, Pittman, Cordova, & Jones, 1991). The purpose was to develop a typology based on measures of substance use and mental disorders.

A comparison of the prevalence and severity of alcoholism was done for a Los Angeles inner-city sample of homeless adults and a housed sample matched by demographic characteristics with the homeless group (Koegel & Burnam, 1988). The prevalence of alcoholism (measured by the National Institute of Mental Health [NIMH] Diagnostic Interview Schedule [Robins, Helzer, Croughan, & Ratcliff, 1981]), the prevalence of psychiatric disorders, and the severity of drinking patterns were greater in the homeless sample than in the housed group. Other important differences in the two groups were described. This study is one of the few reviewed that used a known instrument and compared variables across a homeless and nonhomeless sample. Prevalence of alcohol and drug abuse and psychiatric hospitalization were studied in a cross-sectional survey of more than 1,400 adults using three shelters in northern California county (Winkleby, Rockhill, Jatulis, & Fortmann, 1992). These investigators used selected items from the NIMH Diagnostic Interview Schedule to assess substance abuse. They compared their data with three different nonhomeless populations, and they examined the reliability of responses from a small subset of the sample by reinterview methodology. Substance abuse was 15% to 33% lower before individuals became homeless.

The last study in this group did not focus on a homeless sample but reported that homeless persons did as well as nonhomeless people who participated in an outpatient clinical trial of drug therapy for alcoholism (O'Connor, Gottlieb, Kraus, Segal, & Horowitz, 1991). They reported a 45% rate of treatment failure for a sample of 179 patients; withdrawal symptom severity and higher craving were associated with higher rates of treatment failure. This study represents one of the few in which investigators attempted to determine the effectiveness of an intervention on outcome.

Although few studies of substance abuse have been included here, it is likely more research has been done and could be accessed through a search for studies of mental health and substance abuse in homeless populations. Although important, inclusion of that body of research is beyond the scope of this review. Strengths of the studies included in this category are the use of a standardized instrument, use of comparison groups, use of data from multiple sites, and examination of an outcome. Similar to other categories of studies, synthesis of findings is not possible because the purposes of the studies were individually unique.

PHYSICAL HEALTH CARE SERVICES

Eleven studies were classified as focusing on physical health care services for homeless adults. These are reviewed in three groups: utilization of physical health care services, barriers to access to these services, and models of delivery of health care services to this vulnerable population.

Utilization

Three examples of utilization studies included a retrospective chart review to determine cost and rate of hospitalization for an urban Honolulu homeless population; a description of use of medical, alcohol, drug, and other services by residents of New York City homeless shelters; and record of use of public health care facilities before the deaths of 18 homeless people in Atlanta (Hanzlick & Lazarchick, 1989; Martell et al., 1992; Padgett, Struening, & Andrews, 1990). In one other study of system utilization, the referral appointment keeping of 118 homeless Seattle women was examined (Schlossstein, St. Clair, & Connell, 1991). They were being screened for health care needs. Symptom severity was associated with referral keeping. In a fifth study, investigators examined the relationship of emergency department use, and substance abuse and mental health problems (Padgett & Struening, 1991). They used survey data from 1,152 homeless adults in New York shelters. The most frequent reason given for the last emergency department use was traumatic injury. More than 27% reported using the emergency department in the past 6 months. The investigators suggested that substance abuse and presence of mental disorders influenced use.

Barriers to Access

In a study of barriers to access, human service providers were queried about their perceptions of barriers to health care services for homeless individuals (Hunter, Getty, Kemsley, & Skelly, 1991). A comparison of barriers to medical care was evaluated for 194 homeless families from 10 Los Angeles shelters and 196 nonhomeless poor families from the same geographical regions of the city (Wood & Valdez, 1991). More homeless families were uninsured, less likely to report having a regular provider for preventive care or sick care, and more likely to use emergency services for health care than the housed poor families. The investigators concluded that homeless families have more problems than do nonhomeless poor families in accessing health care. Although not a research paper, Cousineau & Lozier (1993) describe problems of access to health care for homeless people that may continue even with health care reform.

Models of Delivery of Care

In four studies, aspects of or models of delivery of physical health care services to homeless adults were assessed. The engagement techniques used in a program for homeless and marginally housed elderly were described (Cohen, Onserud, & Monaco, 1992). In a follow-up evaluation of 132 individuals, the number of service encounters, type of presenting problem, and perceived level of social support were the strongest predictors of outcome.

Patient care and staffing patterns of the 157 clinics that receive federal funding for the purpose of providing care to homeless individuals were studied (Doblin, Gelberg, & Freeman, 1992). From telephone interviews with the medical directors of these clinics, they reported that 75% of the clinics provided care only to homeless patients and that they saw an average of 96 homeless people per week. Ten percent of the clinics had no physician staff; an additional third had physician staff for 5 hours per week or fewer. Nurse practitioners were employed in 80% of these federally funded clinics serving homeless clients. The investigators concluded with a strong caution that these clinics were in danger of losing their ability to provide high quality care due to severe budget constraints. A second concern related to their continued viability in the federal budget since assessment of quality was not being done and they were therefore vulnerable to further budget cuts.

Hunter and colleagues conducted a national survey to identify evaluation criteria used in programs of health care for homeless clients (Hunter, Crosby, Ventura, & Warkentin, 1991). They described the difficulty of developing a comprehensive list of those agencies that provide health care services to the homeless. Data were collected from one group ($N = 96$) by telephone and from a second group ($N = 156$) by a mail survey. Of these 252 providers, 163 completed the survey. The survey revealed key areas recommended by providers as being useful as evaluation criteria—for example, structural elements, processes of health care services delivery, and cost. Because many of the projects are grant funded, they participated in the preparation of annual reports documenting the user profile; the care provided; and, to some extent, the costs but not necessarily the cost-effectiveness. The investigators recognize the need to have outcome indicators of effectiveness in evaluating health care programs serving homeless clients.

In another evaluation study, telephone interviews were conducted with informants from 19 agencies across the U.S. providing health care to homeless clients to determine what types of HIV infection prevention and education programs had been developed for the homeless and the assessment of effectiveness of these programs in reducing HIV infection in homeless clients (Fetter & Larson, 1990). In reality, the questions could not be answered for the cities or projects as a whole because of the variability in the homeless populations and the projects, and because the number of homeless who are HIV-infected remains unknown. The report, however, provided insight into the magnitude of the problem. The projects provided testing, counseling, and referral for those at high risk for HIV infection.

This group of studies included using a different method; telephone interviews were used for data collection. There is some controversy about the credibility of data obtained from this technique. Descriptions of how and what information is to be obtained is critical. Retrospective chart reviews were used for data collection in several of the studies in this classification. Thus, credibility of the results is predicated on the quality and completeness of patient records (which remains unknown) and whether the desired information was recorded. In one study, a conclusion was stated but was not based on the variables studied; it reflected an interpretative opinion. Similar to the studies included under other categories, the research reviewed under physical health care services represents beginning work. Because homeless adults are a sizable, significant population who may have problems accessing health care and frequently resorts to use of emergency services for care, this represents a critical area requiring additional research. There is particular need for studies testing the effectiveness of diverse models of care on the issues of access, adherence to a therapeutic regimen, and health care outcomes for this population.

CONCLUSIONS AND DIRECTIONS FOR FUTURE RESEARCH

The body of work reported in the past 10 or more years, with few exceptions, has not had an accumulation of effort by single or multiple investigators. The more typical pattern is the single research report. Perhaps this is a reflection of the fairly recent focus on homeless health care, but it is problematic in terms of building and extending the body of knowledge. What also is notable in this collection of work is the many disciplines represented by the investigators contributing to this field. There is a definite presence of nurse investigators adding to the state of knowledge about the health of homeless individuals (Lindsey, 1992b).

Almost all of the studies were descriptive, and few cited were based on an underlying theoretical framework. There was a considerably diverse conceptualization of variables studied. Most of the studies did not use any standardized instruments for data collection. Many used a survey approach, and many included use of clinical records for data collection. Only a few studies used a longitudinal design for data collection. Given the nature of this population, it is difficult to do longitudinal or follow-up studies. Challenges for research with homeless people and sampling issues also have been identified by others (Brickner et al., 1991; Fischer & Breakey, 1991; Institute of Medicine, 1988; Lindsey, 1992a, 1992b; Maurin, 1986; Maurin, Russell, & Hitchcox, 1989; Sergi, Murray, & Cotanch, 1989; Vredevoe, Shuler, & Woo, 1992).

Many of the studies used a sample from one setting (e.g., either a shelter or a clinic serving homeless people), and thus the samples may not reflect the total homeless population. A few studies compared the variables studied in their homeless sample with the general U.S. population or with a housed low-income sample. However, a housed sample may not provide the best comparison group. More comparative studies need to be done to determine how and if homeless people differ from others in terms of health and health care issues. This information is needed to provide direction for the design of effective health care services for this vulnerable population.

Some differences in health status were found to be related to age, gender, and length of time homeless. There also may be differences by ethnic group. These areas require further exploration as they have potential to impact the health status and provision of health care to the nonhomogeneous homeless populations.

Because of the beginning state of research development for this population, it was difficult to provide an integrative synthesis of findings. As yet, there is not a "coherent whole." It is possible that some of the studies could have been categorized differently or have been included in more than one category. However, because of the emerging nature of this work, it is unlikely such cross-categorization would influence dramatically the lack of a coherent synthesis. Some of the findings can provide direction for rather immediate clinical application. For example, findings from several studies showed evidence that primary health care can be provided to this population by nurses in nurse-managed clinics.

Because of the long-term consequences, additional research must focus on the health of homeless adults: (a) those who are at greater risk for infectious, communicable diseases, such as HIV infection, tuberculosis, and sexually transmitted disease; (b) those who are drug or alcohol abusers; and (c) those who have chronic illnesses. Additional research on the access to and provision of health care services to this vulnerable population is needed, particularly testing effectiveness of interventions, different models of delivery of health care, and the resulting health care outcomes. There is need to find ways to engage the homeless in seeking and following prescribed health care regimens. These research issues and directions are the challenges for the next decade of work.

ACKNOWLEDGMENTS

I want to acknowledge the able assistance of Jenny Cashman in the literature search and retrieval process, and Sharadha Viswanathan and Marla Crow in the preparation of the manuscript.

REFERENCES

Abdellah, F. G., Chamberlain, J. G., & Levine, I. S. (1986). Role of nurses in meeting needs of the homeless: Summary of a workshop for providers, researchers, and educators. *Public Health Reports, 101*, 494–498.

Aloot, C., Vredevoe, D. L., & Brecht, M. (1993). Evaluation of high risk smoking practices used by the homeless. *Cancer Nursing, 16*, 123–130.

APA Council of Representatives. (1991). Resolution on homelessness. *American Psychologist, 46*, 1108.

Barge, F. C., & Norr, K. F. (1991). Homeless shelter policies for women in an urban environment. *Image—The Journal of Nursing Scholarship, 23*, 145–149.

Barry, M. A., Wall, C., Shirley, L., Bernardo, J., Schwingl, P., Brigandi, E., & Lamb, G. (1986). Tuberculosis screening in Boston's homeless shelters. *Public Health Reports, 101*, 487–494.

Barter, M. A. (1990). *Analysis of the perceived health status of the adult medically indigent population in Marin County*. Unpublished doctoral dissertation, University of San Francisco, San Francisco, CA.

Belcher, J. R., Scholler-Jacquish, A., & Drummond, M. (1991). Three stages of homelessness: A conceptual model for social workers in health care. *Health and Social Work, 16*, 87–93.

Bergner, M., Bobbit, R. A., Carter, W. B., & Gilson, B. S. (1981). The Sickness Impact Profile: Development and final revision of a health status measure. *Medical Care, 19*, 787–805.

Berne, A. S., Dato, C., Mason, D. J., & Rafferty, M. (1990). A nursing model for addressing the health needs of homeless families. *Image—The Journal of Nursing Scholarship, 22*, 8–13.

Bowdler, J. E. (1989). Health problems of the homeless in America. *Nurse Practitioner, 14*(7), 44–51.

Bowdler, J. E., & Barrell, L. M. (1987). Health needs of homeless persons. *Public Health Nursing, 4*, 135–140.

Breakey, W. R., Fischer, P. J., Kramer, M., Nestadt, G., Romanoski, A. J., Ross, A., Royall, R. M., & Stine, O. C. (1989). Health and mental health problems of homeless men and women in Baltimore. *Journal of American Medical Association, 262*, 1352–1357.

Brecht, M.-L., Lindsey, A. M., & Stuart, I. (1991). *Health care needs of the homeless in Los Angeles* (California Policy Seminar Report). Berkeley: University of California.

Brickner, P. W., Scharer, L. K., Conanan, B., Elvy, A., & Savarese, M. (Eds.). (1985). *Health care of homeless people*. New York: Springer Publishing.

Brickner, P. W., Scharer, L. K., Conanan, B. A., Savarese, M. & Scanlan, B. C. (Eds.). (1990). *Under the safety net: The health and social welfare of the homeless in the United States*. New York: W. W. Norton.

Centers for Disease Control. (1990). Tuberculosis among residents of shelters for the homeless—Ohio. *Morbidity and Mortality Weekly Report, 40*, 869–871.

Centers for Disease Control. (1991a). Characteristics and risk behaviors of homeless black men seeking services from the Community Homeless Assistance Plan—Dade County, FL. *Morbidity and Mortality Weekly Report, 40*, 865–868.

Centers for Disease Control. (1991b). Deaths among homeless persons—San Francisco. *Morbidity and Mortality Weekly Report, 40*, 877–880.

Christiano, A., & Sussser, I. (1989). Knowledge and perceptions of HIV infection among homeless pregnant women. *Journal of Nurse-Midwifery, 34*, 318–322.

Cohen, C. I., Onserud, H., & Monaco, C. (1992). Project rescue: Serving the homeless and marginally housed elderly. *Gerontologist, 32*, 466–471.

Cohen, C. I., Teresi, J. A., & Holmes, D. (1988). The physical well-being of old homeless men. *Journal of Gerontology, 43*(Suppl.), S121–S128.

Cousineau, M., & Lozier, J. N. (1993). Assuring access to health care for homeless people under national health care. *American Behavioral Scientist, 36*, 857–870.

Doblin, B. J., Gelberg, L., & Freeman, H. E. (1992). Patient care and professional staffing patterns in McKinney Act clinics providing primary care to the homeless. *Journal of American Medical Association, 267*, 698–701.

Drake, M. A. (1992). The nutritional status and dietary adequacy of single homeless women and their children in shelters. *Public Health Reports, 107*, 312–319.

el-Bassel, N., & Schilling, R. F. (1991). Drug use and sexual behavior of indigent African American men. *Public Health Reports, 106*, 586–590.

Ferenchick, G. S. (1991). Medical problems of homeless and nonhomeless persons attending an inner-city clinic: A comparative study. *American Journal of the Medical Sciences, 301*, 379–382.

Ferenchick, G. S. (1992). The medical problems of homeless clinic patients: A comparative study. *Journal of General Internal Medicine, 7*, 294–297.

Fetter, M. S., & Larson, E. (1990). Preventing and treating human immunodeficiency virus infection in the homeless. *Archives of Psychiatric Nursing, 4*, 379–383.

Fischer, P. J., & Breakey, W. R. (1991). The epidemiology of alcohol, drug, and mental disorders among homeless persons. *American Psychologist, 46*, 1115–1128.

Garrett, G. R. (1989). Alcohol problems and homelessness: History and research. *Contemporary Drug Problems, 16*, 301–332.

Gelberg, L., & Linn, L. S. (1988). Social and physical health of homeless adults previously treated for mental health problems. *Hospital and Community Psychiatry, 39*, 510–516.

Gelberg, L., & Linn, L. S. (1989). Assessing the physical health of homeless adults. *Journal of American Medical Association, 262*, 1973–1979.

Gelberg, L., & Linn, L. S. (1992). Demographic differences in health status of homeless adults. *Journal of General Internal Medicine, 7*, 601–608.

Gelberg, L., Linn, L. S., & Mayer-Oakes, S. A. (1990). Differences in health status between older and younger homeless adults. *Journal of the American Geriatrics Society, 38*, 1220–1229.

Gelberg, L., Linn, L. S., & Rosenberg, D. J. (1988). Dental health of homeless adults. *Special Care in Dentistry, 8*, 167–172.

Gelberg, L., Linn, L. S., Usatine, R. P., & Smith, M. H. (1990). Health, homelessness, and poverty: A study of clinic users. *Archives of Internal Medicine, 150*, 2325–2330.

Gottesman, M. M., Lewis, M. A., Lindsey, A. M., & Brecht, M.-L. (1993). Evolution and population characteristics of a nurse-managed health center for the homeless and high-risk low income families. In J. K. Hunter (Ed.), *Nursing and health care for the homeless* (pp. 33–49), Albany, NY: State University of New York Press.

Gross, T. P., & Rosenberg, M. L. (1987). Shelters for battered women and their children: An under-recognized source of communicable disease transmission. *American Journal of Public Health, 77*, 1198–1201.

Hanzlick, R., & Lazarchick, J. (1989). Health care history and utilization for Atlantans who died homeless. *Journal of the Medical Association of Georgia, 78*, 205–208.

Harris, J. L., & Williams, L. K. (1991). Universal self-care requisites as identified by homeless elderly men. *Journal of Gerontological Nursing, 17*(6), 39–43.

Henslin, J. M. (1993a). *Homelessness: An annotated bibliography* (Vol. 1, New York: Garland. pp. 1–597.

Henslin, J. M. (1993b). *Homelessness: An annotated bibliography* (Vol. 2, New York: Garland. pp. 1–1054).

Hunter, J. K. (Ed.). (1993). *Nursing and health care for the homeless*. Albany: State University of New York Press.

Hunter, J. K., Crosby, F. E., Ventura, M. R., & Warkentin, L. (1991). A national survey to identify evaluation criteria for programs of health care for homeless. *Nursing & Health Care, 12*, 536–542.

Hunter, J. K., Getty, C., Kemsley, M., & Skelly, A. H. (1991). Barriers to providing health care to homeless persons: A survey of providers' perceptions. *Health Values, 15*(5), 3–11.

Institute of Medicine. (1988). *Homelessness, health and human needs*. Washington, DC: National Academy Press.

Jahiel, R. I. (1992). *Homelessness: A prevention-oriented approach*. Baltimore: The Johns Hopkins University Press.

Johnstone, H., Tornabene, M., & Marcinak, J. (1993). Incidence of sexually transmitted diseases and Pap smear results in female homeless clients from the Chicago Health Outreach Project. *Health Care for Women International, 14*, 293–299.

Killion, C. M. (1988). Black, homeless and pregnant. *Proceedings of the West Virginia Nurses' Association Research Symposium* (pp. 259–264). Morgantown, WV: West Virginia Nurses Association.

Kinchen, K., & Wright, J. D. (1991). Hypertension management in health care for the homeless clinics: Results from a survey. *American Journal of Public Health, 81*, 1163–1165.

Kinzel, D. (1991). Self-identified health concerns of two homeless groups. *Western Journal of Nursing Research, 13*, 181–194.

Knight, K., Mason, D. J., Christopher, M. A., Beck, T. L., & Toughill, E. (1991). A comparison of the health status of residents of sheltered care facilities in Monmouth County, New Jersey. *Public Health Nursing, 8*, 182–189.

Koegel, P., & Burman, M. A. (1988). Alcoholism among homeless adults in the inner city of Los Angeles. *Archives of General Psychiatry, 45*, 1011–1018.

Lepkowski, J. M. (1991). Sampling the difficult-to-sample. *Journal of Nutrition, 121*, 416–423.

Lindsey, A. M. (1989). Health care for the homeless. *Nursing Outlook, 37*, 78–81.

Lindsey, A. M. (1992a). Health care for the homeless. In L. Aiken, & C. Fagin (Eds.), *Charting nursing's future: Agenda for the 1990's*, pp. 381–401. Philadelphia: Lippincott.

Lindsey, A. M. (1992b). Nursing research serving the underserved: Homeless health care. *Communicating Nursing Research, 25*, 55–72.

Linn, L. S., & Gelberg, L. (1989). Priority of basic needs among homeless adults. *Social Psychiatry and Psychiatric Epidemiology, 24*, 23–29.

Linn, L. S., Gelberg, L., & Leake, B. (1990). Substance abuse and mental health status of homeless and domiciled low-income users of a medical clinic. *Hospital and Community Psychiatry, 41*, 306–310.

Luder, E., Boey, E., Buchalter, B., & Martinez-Weber, C. (1989). Assessment of the nutritional status of urban homeless adults. *Public Health Reports, 104*, 451–457.

Luder, E., Ceysens-Okada, E., Koren-Roth, A., & Martinez-Weber, C. (1990). Health and nutrition survey in a group of urban homeless adults. *Journal of the American Dietetic Association, 90*, 1387–1392.

Malloy, C., Christ, M. A., & Hohloch, F. J. (1990). The homeless: Social isolates. *Journal of Community Health Nursing, 7*, 25–36.

Martell, J. V., Seitz, R. S., Harada, J. K., Kobayashi, J., Sasaki, V. K., & Wong, C. (1992). Hospitalization in an urban homeless population: The Honolulu Urban Homeless Project. *Annals of Internal Medicine, 116*, 299–303.

Mason, D. J., Jensen, M., & Boland, D. L. (1992). Health behaviors and health risks among homeless males in Utah. *Western Journal of Nursing Research, 14*, 775–790.

Maurin, J. T. (1986). Knowledge gaps which can be addressed through nursing research. In *Role of nurses in meeting the health/mental health needs of the homeless* (pp. 67–76). Washington, DC: American Public Health Association.

Maurin, J. T., Russell, L., & Hitchcox, M. (1989). Obstacles to research analysis. *Journal of Psychosocial Nursing, 27*(6), 19–23.

Morris, J. T., & McAllister, C. K. (1992). Homeless individuals and drug-resistant tuberculosis in south Texas. *Chest, 102*, 802–804.

Morris, W., & Crystal, S. (1989). Diagnostic patterns in hospital use by an urban homeless population. *Western Journal of Medicine, 151*, 472–476.

Nazar-Stewart, V., & Nolan, C. M. (1992). Results of a directly observed intermittent isoniazid preventive therapy program in a shelter for homeless men. *American Review of Respiratory Disease, 146*(1), 57–60.

Nyamathi, A. M. (1991). Relationship of resources to emotional distress, somatic complaints, and high-risk behaviors in drug recovery and homeless minority women. *Research in Nursing & Health, 14*, 269–277.

Nyamathi, A. M. (1992). Comparative study of factors relating to HIV risk level of black homeless women. *Journal of Acquired Immune Deficiency Syndromes, 5*, 222–228.

Nyamathi, A., Bennett, C., Leake, B., Lewis, C., & Flaskerud, J. (1993). AIDS related knowledge, perceptions, and behaviors among impoverished minority women. *American Journal of Public Health, 83*, 65–71.

Nyamathi, A. M., Leake, B., Flaskerud, J., Lewis, C., & Bennett, C. (1993). Outcomes of specialized and traditional AIDS counseling programs for impoverished women of color. *Research in Nursing & Health, 16*, 11–21.

Nyamathi, A., & Shuler, P. (1989). Factors affecting prescribed medication compliance of the urban homeless adult. *Nurse Practitioner, 14*(8), 47–54.

O'Connor, P. G., Gottlieb, L. D., Kraus, M. L., Segal, S. R., & Horowitz, R. I. (1991). Social and clinical features as predictors of outcome in outpatient alcohol withdrawal. *Journal of General Internal Medicine, 6*, 312–316.

Padgett, D. K., & Struening, E. L. (1991). Influence of substance abuse and mental disorders on emergency room use by homeless adults. *Hospital and Community Psychiatry, 42*, 834–838.

Padgett, D., Struening, E. L., & Andrews, H. (1990). Factors affecting the use of medical, mental health, alcohol, and drug treatment services by homeless adults. *Medical Care, 28*, 805–821.

Patton, M. (1989). The virus in our midst. *West Virginia Medical Journal, 85*(3), 92–97.

Reilly, F. E. (1991). *Health, space use, and time use by homeless elderly people.*. Unpublished doctoral dissertation, University of Kentucky, Lexington.

Reilly, F. E., Grier, M. R., & Blomquist, K. (1992). Living arrangements, visit patterns, and health problems in a nurse-managed clinic for the homeless. *Journal of Community Health Nursing, 9*, 111–121.

Reilly, E., & McInnis, B. N. (1985). Boston Massachusetts: The Pine Street Inn Nurses' Clinic and Tuberculosis Program. In P. W. Brickner, L. K. Scharer, B. Conanan, A. Elvy, & M. Savarese (Eds.), *Health Care of Homeless People* (pp. 291–299). New York: Springer Publishing.

Reuler, J. B., Bax, M. J., & Sampson, J. H. (1986). Physician house call services for medically needy, inner-city residents. *American Journal of Public Health, 76*, 1131–1134.

Ritchey, F. J., La Gory, M., & Mullis, J. (1991). Gender differences in health risks and physical symptoms among the homeless. *Journal of Health and Social Behavior, 32*, 33–48.

Robertson, M. J., & Cousineau, M. R. (1986). Health status and access to health services among the urban homeless. *American Journal of Public Health, 76*, 561–563.

Robertson, M. J., & Greenblatt, M. (1992). *Homelessness: A national perspective*. New York: Plenum.

Robins, L. N., Helzer, J. E., Croughan, J., & Ratcliff, K. S. (1981). National Institute of Mental Health Diagnostic Interview Schedule. *Archives of General Psychiatry, 38*, 381–389.

Ropers, R. H., & Boyer, R. (1987). Perceived health status among the new urban homeless. *Social Science and Medicine, 24*, 669–678.

Roskamp, D. A. (1987). *Comparison of the reading levels of a homeless population and readability levels of printed self-care instruction sheets.* Unpublished doctoral dissertation, University of California, Los Angeles.

Schlossstein, E., St. Clair, P., & Connell, F. (1991). Referral keeping in homeless women. *Journal of Community Health, 16*, 279–285.

Sergi, J. S., Murray, M., & Cotanch, P. H. (1989). An understudied population: The homeless. *Oncology Nursing Forum, 16*(1), 113–114.

Shuler, P. (1991). *Homeless women's holistic and family planning needs (Parts 1 and 2).* Unpublished doctoral dissertation, University of Michigan, Ann Arbor.

Siegal, H. A., Carlson, R. G., Falck, R., Li, L., Forney, M. A., Rapp, R. C., Baumgartner, K., Myers, W., & Nelson, M. (1991). HIV infection and risk behaviors among intravenous drug users in low seroprevalence areas in the Midwest. *American Journal of Public Health, 81*, 1642–1644.

Skelly, A. H., Getty, C., Kemsley, M., Hunter, J., & Shipman, J. (1990). Health perceptions of the homeless: A survey of Buffalo's City Mission. *Journal of the New York State Nurses Association, 21*(2), 20–24.

Smith, L. G. (1988). Home treatment of mild, acute diarrhea and secondary dehydration of infants and small children: An educational program for parents in a shelter for the homeless. *Journal of Professional Nursing, 4*, 60–63.

Stanhope, M. K. (1989). An innovative approach to nursing care of the homeless (p. 307). *Sigma Theta Tau International 30th Biennial Convention scientific sessions book of abstracts.*

Stanhope, M., & Blomquist, K. B. (1989). An innovative approach to nursing care of the homeless. In *Nursing care for vulnerable populations* (Ninth Annual Research Conference Southern Council in Collegiate Education for Nursing) [Abstract]. Lexington, KY: Southern Regional Education Board.

Stephens, D., Dennis, E., Toomer, M., & Holloway, J. (1991). The diversity of case management needs for the care of homeless persons. *Public Health Reports, 106*, 15–19.

Struening, E., Padget, D. K., Pittman, J., Cordova, P., & Jones, M. (1991). A typology based on measures of substance abuse and mental disorder. *Journal of Addictive Diseases, 11*(1), 99–117.

Susser, E., Valencia, E., & Conover, S. (1993). Prevalence of HIV infection among psychiatric patients in a New York City men's shelter. *American Journal of Public Health, 83*, 568–570.

Vladeck, B. C. (1990). Health care and the homeless: A political parable for our time. *Journal of Health Politics, Policy and Law, 15*, 305–317.

Vredevoe, D. L., Brecht, M., Shuler, P., & Woo, M. (1992). Risk factors for disease in a homeless population. *Public Health Nursing, 9*, 263–269.

Vredevoe, D. L., Shuler, P., & Woo, M. (1992). The homeless population. *Western Journal of Nursing Research, 14*, 731–740.

Wiecha, J., Dwyer, R. J. T., & Dunn-Strohecker, M. (1991). Nutrition and health services needs among the homeless. *Public Health Reports, 106*, 364–374.

Winkleby, M. A. (1990). Comparison of risk factors for ill health in a sample of homeless and nonhomeless poor. *Public Health Reports, 105*, 404–410.

Winkleby, M. A,. & Fleshin, D. (1993). Physical, addictive and psychiatric disorders among homeless veterans and nonveterans. *Public Health Reports, 108*, 30–36.

Winkleby, M. A., Rockhill, B., Jatulis, D., & Fortmann, S. P. (1992). The medical origins of homelessness. *American Journal of Public Health, 82*, 1394–1398.

Winkleby, M. A., & White, R. (1992). Homeless adults without apparent medical and psychiatric impairment: Onset of morbidity over time. *Hospital and Community Psychiatry, 43*, 1017–1023.

Wood, D. (1992). *Delivering health care to homeless persons*. New York: Springer Publishing.

Wood, D., & Valdez, R. B. (1991). Barriers to medical care for homeless families compared with housed poor families. *American Journal of Diseases of Children, 145*, 1109–1115.

Wright, J. D., Knight, J. W., Weber-Burdin, E., & Lam, J. (1987). Ailments and alcohol: Health status among drinking homeless. *Alcohol Health and Research World, 11*(3), 23–27.

Wright, J. D., Rossi, P. H., Knight, J. W., Weber-Burdin, E., Tessler, R. C., Stewart, C. E., Geronimo, M., & Lam, J. (1987). Homelessness and health: The effects of life style on physical well-being among homeless people in New York City. *Research in Social Problems and Public Policy, 4*, 41–72.

Wright, J. D., & Weber, E. (1987). *Homelessness and health*. New York: McGraw-Hill.

Chapter 3

Child Sexual Abuse: Initial Effects

SUSAN J. KELLEY
SCHOOL OF NURSING
GEORGIA STATE UNIVERSITY

CONTENTS

Sexual abuse of children is a significant social and health issue. Research on the prevalence of sexual abuse during childhood speaks to the urgency of the problem. In a large, nationally representative survey of 2,626 American adults, a childhood history of sexual abuse was disclosed by 27% of women and 16% of men (Finkelhor, Hotaling, Lewis, & Smith, 1990). It was not until the late 1970s that child sexual abuse (CSA) was recognized as a serious societal problem. Systematic knowledge development on the problem did not begin to appear in the literature until the mid-1980s, however.

Research on the effects of CSA generally is divided into the proximate or initial effects during childhood and the long-term effects experienced in adulthood. This chapter focuses on the immediate effects of CSA and provides a critical analysis of the research literature that has evolved in this area.

This review is limited to databased inquiries that employed standardized measures to assess impact of CSA; included subjects 18 years of age and younger; and included groups of nonabused children or normative data to make comparisons. Case studies and nonquantitative reports were excluded. Sample sizes in the studies reviewed varied from 10 to 369, with most including 50 or more sexually abused subjects.

Studies published in nursing, medical, psychology, and interdisciplinary journals were included. Computer searches from 1970 through 1993 were conducted on MEDLINE, PsychLit, and CINAHL. A hand search was conducted of the six abuse-related interdisciplinary journals for their entire years of publication through 1993 (*Child Abuse and Neglect: The International Journal; Journal of Interpersonal Violence; Victimology; Journal of Family Violence; Violence and Victims;* and *Journal of Child Sexual Abuse*). The "ancestry" and "invisible college" approach also were used to retrieve information. The ancestry approach involves tracking citations from one article to another; the invisible college approach involves communicating with known experts in the topic area to obtain obscure publications and materials in press (Cooper, 1982).

This chapter begins with an introduction to the state of the science in childhood sexual abuse research, including a discussion of the methodological limitations of the work to date. The specific review is divided into the following categories: effects of sexual abuse in childhood; variables associated with increased impact; and promising areas for future research. A summary and recommendations for future research directions then are presented.

OVERVIEW OF RESEARCH ON EFFECTS OF CHILD SEXUAL ABUSE

Research on the effects of CSA has included small and large samples, descriptive studies of questionable validity, and ones that were rigorous and empirically sound. The earliest work on CSA largely was retrospective and focused primarily on the long-term effects of CSA as experienced in adulthood. Since the 1980s there has been a dramatic increase in the number of studies concentrating on the effects of CSA during childhood. It was not until the mid-1980s that rigorous studies of the impact of CSA appeared in the literature. In the last 5 years, this area of research has increased tremendously.

Early research on CSA was plagued with small sample sizes, lack of comparison groups, and failure to use standardized measures. More recently, sample sizes have increased, and researchers have used nonabused, normal children, as well as nonabused clinical (psychiatrically disturbed) children in comparison groups. Another improvement has been the use of standardized measures to examine the impact of CSA. However, most studies employing standardized measures have, until recently, relied almost exclusively on parent report instruments typically completed by mothers. This single-informant approach is potentially problematic in that findings from several studies suggested that reports of their sexually abused children's behaviors may be biased by the mothers' own reactions to the abuse (Cohen & Mannarino, 1988; Everson, Hunter, Runyan, Edelsohn, and Coulter, 1989; Mannarino & Cohen, 1986; Mannarino, Cohen, & Gregor, 1989; Mannarino, Cohen, & Berman, 1994b; Newberger, Gremy, Waternaux, & Newberger, 1993).

A methodological improvement employed by some researchers of late is the use of multiple informants to measure subjects' response to CSA. This approach uses child self-report, projective and observational measures, therapist reports, and parental reports. An example of this approach is found in the study conducted by Waterman, Kelly, Oliveri, and McCord (1993) in which the researchers used a combination of parent, child, and therapist report measures to assess victim impact in a sample of 97 children sexually abused in day care centers.

In the first wave of methodologically sound research on the immediate effects of CSA conducted in the 1980s, researchers used standardized measures and comparison groups to validate the negative effects of CSA empirically. Studies demonstrated increased global problems, such as increased behavioral and emotional problems in sexually abused children when compared with normal, nonabused children. A limitation to this approach was the difficulty in differentiating the abuse-specific effects of CSA abuse from intervening variables, such as family functioning, maternal support, and negative life events. Only a small proportion of studies in this first wave of research examined the relationship between the level of psychological disturbance and abuse-related variables (i.e., relationship of child to offender, severity of abuse, and the child's age and gender). Thus, a second wave of child sexual abuse research sought to determine factors that mediate the impact of CSA as well as to identify abuse-specific effects of CSA. Recently, researchers have developed instruments to measure abuse-specific sequelae (Friedrich, Grambsch, Broughton, Kuipers, & Beilke, 1991; Lanktree & Briere, 1992; Mannarino, Cohen, & Berman, 1994a).

A third wave of research, still in an early stage of development, comprises prospective longitudinal studies that examine how the sequelae of CSA are manifested over time, and what facilitates or hinders recovery.

A problem extant in studies of the impact of CSA is that samples generally comprised children reported to child protective services for CSA and children receiving therapy for the effects of CSA. Thus, only children formally identified as abused were included in studies, posing problems with generalizability of findings to sexually abused children who remain hidden. Likewise, those most severely affected by CSA are referred for treatment, thereby overestimating the symptomatology associated with CSA in the general population. Consequently, findings of studies on the impact of CSA reviewed herein cannot be generalized to unreported victims. Another methodological limitation in research on the effects of CSA is the failure of most researchers to measure preabuse factors, such as psychological disturbances that may have antedated the abuse.

In addition to the methodological issues discussed earlier, research on the effects of CSA has been hindered by statistical issues. Many of the studies conducted to date had small sample sizes that limited statistical power and decreased the likelihood of detecting differences among groups of abused and nonabused subjects. Small samples also restricted many researchers from using multivariate statistics. Use of multivariate analyses is critical in research on the effects of CSA because investigators use multiple measures of psychological functioning, and CSA effects are multiple and interrelated.

The following review of the research on the effects of CSA must be viewed within the context of the preceding constraints.

EFFECTS OF SEXUAL ABUSE IN CHILDHOOD

Behavior Problems

Investigators have found that sexually abused children display a variety of disturbed behaviors immediately following disclosure of abuse. The most frequently reported initial effect of CSA was increased behavior problems (Adams-Tucker, 1982; Cohen and Mannarino, 1988; Einbender & Friedrich, 1989; Friedrich, Beilke, & Urquiza, 1988; Friedrich, Urquiza, and Beilke, 1986; Gomes-Schwartz, Horowitz, and Sauzier, 1985; Kelley, 1989, 1992; Lipovsky, Saunders, & Murphy, 1989; Mannarino, Cohen, & Gregor, 1989; Mannarino, Cohen, & Berman, 1994b; Tong, Oates, & McDowell, 1987; Waterman et al., 1993). These investigators used the parent version of the Child Behavior Checklist (CBCL) (Achenbach & Edelbrock, 1983) to measure behavior problems, with the exception of studies conducted by Gomes-Schwartz et al. (1985) and Adams-Tucker (1982) in which the Louisville Behavior Checklist (Miller, 1981) was used to measure child behavior problems. Although not all of these studies reported the proportion of children scoring in the clinical range in behavior problems on the CBCL, those that did indicated that a significant proportion of sexually abused children have behavior problem scores that fall in the clinical range (Einbender & Friedrich, 1989; Friedrich et al., 1986; Kelley, 1989; Waterman et al., 1993). Scores in the clinical range indicate severe disturbance; less than 2% of children in the general population would be expected to fall in the clinical range. Behavior problems on the CBCL are divided into two domains: internalizing and externalizing problems. Internalizing problems include withdrawal, depression, and anxiety, whereas externalizing problems include behaviors, such as aggression, hyperactivity, and distractability.

Self-Esteem

Comparisons of self-esteem levels between groups of sexually abused children and nonabused children using standardized self-report measures of self-esteem have yielded equivocal results. Cohen and Mannarino (1988) studied self-esteem in 24 sexually abused females, aged 6 to 12 years, using the Piers-Harris Children's Self-Concept Scale (Piers & Harris, 1969) and found no differences between subjects' scores and normative data. When Lipovsky et al. (1989) compared self-esteem scores of 37 victims of father-daughter incest and 41 nonabused siblings aged 11 years and older, no significant differences were found; both groups reported significant problems related to self-esteem. However, when Tong et al. (1987) examined self-esteem levels of 45 sexually abused children aged 8 to 18 years, they found that sexually abused girls had significantly lower self-esteem scores than the comparison group of nonabused girls. Interestingly, no differences were found on levels of self-esteem between the sexually abused boys and the comparison group of nonsexually abused boys in this sample.

Three studies of sexually abused adolescents (Cavaiola & Schiff,

1989; German, Habenicht, & Futcher, 1990; Orr & Downs, 1985) found lower self-esteem scores in sexually abused adolescents than in comparison or normative groups on standardized measures of self-esteem. In their study of adolescent incest victims, German et al. (1990) found that sexually abused subjects ($n = 40$) scored significantly lower in overall self-concept than the female adolescents from the normative group on the Piers-Harris Children's Self-Concept Scale. Cavaiola and Schiff (1989) compared four groups on self-esteem: physically abused chemically dependent adolescents; sexually abused chemically dependent adolescents; nonabused chemically dependent adolescents; and nonabused, nonchemically dependent adolescents. The four groups comprised males and females aged 13 to 18 years old. Using the Tennessee Self-Concept Scale (Fitts, 1965), Cavaiola and Schiff (1989) found that sexually and physically abused, chemically dependent adolescents demonstrated significantly lower self-esteem than both comparison groups of nonabused adolescents. It is important to note that no differences were found on self-esteem scores between the sexually abused children and physically abused children; both groups scored low in self-esteem. Orr and Downes (1985) found poorer self-esteem scores in a group of sexually abused adolescent females ($n = 20$) when compared with a group of acutely medically ill, nonabused adolescent females ($n = 20$) using the Offer Self-Image Questionnaire for Adolescents (Offer, Ostrov, & Howard, 1977).

The results of these studies suggest that age and gender influence the relationship between CSA and self-esteem with school-aged females and adolescent males, and females appearing more vulnerable to lowered self-esteem. Inasmuch as low self-esteem has been found more frequently in older children, it is likely that low self-esteem is associated with an increase in awareness of the stigmatizing nature of CSA. There are several alternative explanations for the conflicting results from studies on the impact of CSA on self-esteem. First is the possibility that the conflicting results are related to measurement problems because several different self-esteem measures were used in the various studies. Another possible reason for discrepant findings among studies is that this area of social-emotional functioning is not always negatively impacted by CSA.

Depression and Anxiety

Numerous researchers have examined depression and anxiety among sexually abused children. In their sample of 24 sexually abused females, Cohen and Mannarino (1988) found no differences on self-report measures of depression and anxiety when comparing sexually abused subjects' scores to normative data. Lipovsky and colleagues (1989) compared child-reported depression and anxiety scores between victims of father-daughter sexual abuse ($n = 40$) and nonabused siblings ($n = 40$). Sexually abused subjects scored higher in depression than the comparison group of nonabused siblings; however, no significant differences were found on anxiety scores. Sansonnet-Hayden, Haley, Marriage, and Fine (1987) compared depression scores of 17 sexually abused psychiatrically hospitalized adolescents to 37 nonsexually abused psychiatric inpatient adolescents and found that the sexually abused adolescents scored higher on depressive symptomatology. Wozencraft, Wagner, and Pelegrin (1991) studied depression in a sample of 65 sexually abused children using the Children's Depressive Inventory (CDI) (Finch, Saylor, & Edwards, 1985) and found that the sexually abused children described themselves as experiencing significantly higher levels of depression than was reported by members of a normative sample. In addition, older victims and those whose mothers were less compliant with treatment were more likely to have CDI scores that were above the 90th percentile.

Thus, most studies examining depression as an outcome variable of CSA reported increased levels of depressive symptomatology in children who were victims of CSA. These findings were consistent across studies despite differences in the ages of children in the samples and in instruments used to measure depression. The nonsignificant findings between CSA children and normative values in Cohen and Mannarino's (1988) study may be related to the small sample size ($n = 24$) and lack of a matched comparison group. The large normative data set may contain wide standard deviations that obscures differences with the small CSA sample.

Posttraumatic Stress Disorder

Some clinicians and researchers have placed the sequelae of CSA within the context of posttraumatic stress disorder (PTSD). PTSD is characterized by repetitive or reexperiencing phenomena, autonomical hyperarousal, and phobic or avoidance behaviors. Reported rates of PTSD among sexually abused children vary considerably across studies. Deblinger, McLeer, Atkins, Ralphe, and Foa (1989) examined the prevalence of PTSD symptoms in a retrospective chart review of 29 child psychiatric inpatients with a history of sexual abuse. Of these children, 20.7% met the *Diagnostic and Statistic Manual* (3rd ed., rev.) (DSM III-R) (American Psychiatric Association, 1987) criteria for PTSD compared with 6.9% of a matched group of physically abused children and 10.3% of a matched group of nonabused children. It is important to note that these differences were not statistically significant. To minimize potential investigator bias, a research assistant blind to the purpose of the study examined the medical records for documentation of the presence or absence of symptoms of PTSD. In addition, interrater reliability was established for symptom occurrence (Deblinger et al., 1989).

McLeer, Deblinger, Atkins, Foa, and Ralphe (1988) studied the effects of CSA in 31 children being treated on an outpatient basis. The researchers found that 48.4% of subjects met the DSM III-R criteria for PTSD based on data obtained from structured interviews with subjects. Kiser et al. (1988) reported that 9 out of 10 children in their sample of children sexually abused in a day care setting met the DSM III-R criteria of PTSD based on therapists' ratings. It is important to note that because of the young age of the children, the therapists' ratings were based on parent reports and clinical impressions in addition to child self-reports. In Waterman et al.'s study (1993) of children abused in day care centers, 83% of children in the ritualistic sexual abuse group and 36% in the sexual abuse group met the DSM III-R diagnostic criteria for PTSD based on therapists' ratings of PTSD symptoms.

Interpretation of these findings must be made with caution because of differences among studies in how symptoms of PTSD were measured and because reliability procedures were not reported by most of the researchers. Because assessment for PTSD requires the subjects' verbalization of thoughts and feelings related to a specific trauma (i.e., sexual abuse in these studies), it is not feasible for evaluators to be blind to group assignment when interviews are used to determine if the subject meets the diagnostic criteria for PTSD. In addition, interpretation of symptoms and statements by evaluators is necessary. Thus, the possibility for investigator bias exists when studying PTSD. Further studies, using larger samples and reliable and valid measures of PTSD symptoms, are warranted to determine the prevalence of PTSD in sexually abused children. Videotapes rated independently by trained observers and with calculations of interrelated reliabilities would be a major step forward for this line of research.

Sexualized Behaviors

The studies cited previously do not necessarily determine the abuse-specific effects of CSA because behavior problems, low self-esteem, depression, and PTSD also have been reported in studies of physically abused and psychiatrically disturbed children. Therefore, it is important for researchers to attempt to determine abuse specific effects of CSA.

Researchers have repeatedly found that sexually abused children display more sexualized behaviors than comparison groups of nonabused children, physically abused children, and psychiatrically disturbed, nonabused children. To date, increased sexualized behavior is the only symptom that has consistently differentiated sexually abused children from physically abused children and nonabused clinical comparison groups. White, Halpin, Strom, and Santilli (1988) compared a group of 2- to 6-year-old sexually abused children ($n = 17$) to a group of nonreferred children ($n = 23$) and a group of neglected children ($n = 18$) on a modified version of the Minnesota Child Development Inventory (Ireton & Thwing, 1972). They found that sexually abused children demonstrated higher levels of sexualized behaviors; in particular, these children more often masturbated in social and stressful situations.

Several investigators used the six-item Sex Problem scale of the Child Behavior Checklist (CBC) (Achenbach & Edelbrock, 1983) to examine sexualized behaviors. They found significantly higher scores on the Sex Problem scale with groups of sexually abused children when compared with groups of nonsexually abused children (Cohen & Mannarino, 1988; Einbender & Friedrich, 1989; Mannarino et al., 1989). As Friedrich (1993) noted, problems exist with the empirically derived Sex Problems scale of the CBC because: (a) it does not include all of the six items directly related to sexual behavior contained in the CBC; and (b) it includes several other items related to peer relations and verbal expression. In addition, the Sex Problems scale is not applicable for each gender and age profile of the CBC. In an attempt to remedy this problem, several investigators have used the six items of the CBC related to sexual behavior as a separately derived scale and found increased sexual behaviors in sexually abused children when compared with nonsexually abused children (Friedrich, Beilke, & Urquiza, 1987; Friedrich et al., 1988; Friedrich & Luecke, 1988; Kelley, 1989).

In a study conducted by Gomes-Schwartz, Horowitz, and Cardarelli (1990), sexualized behaviors differentiated between sexually abused children and nonsexually abused psychiatric controls using the Louisville Behavior Checklist (LBC) (Miller, 1981), whereas other scales of the LBC failed to differentiate between the groups.

Sexual behavior problems have proved to be a useful discriminating variable to distinguish groups of sexually abused children from groups of nonsexually abused children. A major methodological advancement in the study of the effects of CSA was the development of the 35-item Child Sexual Behavior Inventory (CSBI) to assess sexualized behaviors in sexually abused children (Friedrich et al., 1991). Friedrich and colleagues (1991) conducted a large-scale, community-based survey using the CSBI to assess the frequency of sexual behaviors in normal preadolescent children and to measure the relationship of these behaviors to age, gender, socioeconomic, and family variables. The sample consisted of 880, 2- through 12-year-old children, with no known history of CSA. Examples of sexualized behaviors included child puts mouth on genitals, masturbates with objects, and imitates intercourse. The frequency of sexual behaviors varied widely, with more aggressive sexual behaviors and sexual behaviors imitative of adults being rare. Older children were found to be less sexual in their behaviors than younger children. Increased sexual behaviors were found to be related to increased general behavior problems as measured by the CBD and to family nudity; they were not found to be related to socioeconomic variables.

Friedrich et al. (1992) later used the CSBI to compare a sample of 276 sexually abused children to the normative sample ($n = 880$) described earlier. The CSBI total score differed significantly between the two groups, with sexually abused children demonstrating a greater frequency of total sexual behaviors than did the normative sample. In addition, the CSBI differentiated the sexual abuse group from the nonsexual abuse group on 27 of the 35 individual items. One limitation of the CSBI is that it is a parent report measure, and as previously discussed, parents may be biased in their ratings of their abused children's behaviors. Also, it is likely that as children grow older, they are less likely to display inappropriate sexualized behaviors in the presence of parents.

Research using direct observation of children's sexualized behaviors has been limited to the use of anatomical dolls. Findings from multiple studies indicated that sexually abused children display more sexualized behaviors than nonsexually abused children when playing with anatomical dolls (Jampole & Weber, 1987; Sivan, Schor, Koeppl, & Noble, 1988; White, Strom, Santilli, & Halpin, 1986).

VARIABLES ASSOCIATED WITH SEVERITY OF EFFECTS

Researchers have examined preabuse, abuse-related, and postabuse variables to determine which types of experiences place victims of CSA at increased risk for greater psychological disturbance. Such information is important for clinicians treating sexually abused children.

Abuse-related variables have been studied more extensively than preabuse or postabuse variables. Abuse-related variables typically examined in relation to differential impact include age, gender, severity of abuse, use of physical force, relationship of offender to child, victim, and time elapsed between assessment and end of abuse. A problem inherent with this approach is that these factors are often interrelated. For instance, early age at time of onset is often related to abuse by a family member. Penetration (severity of abuse) occurs more often with older victims. Likewise, increased victim age is correlated with longer duration of abuse. Unfortunately, most studies conducted to date have not employed sample sizes large enough to control statistically for these intercorrelated variables. Only a few researchers have attempted to control statistically for the interaction of abuse-related variables (Conte & Schuerman, 1987; Mennen, 1993; Morrow & Sorell, 1989).

Preabuse Factors

Only one investigator to date has examined the relationship between preabuse factors and psychological symptomatology in sexually abused children. Mannarino, Cohen, and Berman (1994) studied preabuse factors in a sample of 94 sexually abused children. Comparison groups of clinical controls ($n = 89$) and normal controls ($n = 75$) were also included in the study. Results indicated that the sexually abused and clinical control groups had significantly more developmental and psychiatric problems and more past stressors than the normal group. Presence of prior developmental and psychiatric problems in sexually abused children was associated with increased behavioral and emotional problems, self-reported depressive symptoms, and lower self-esteem after disclosure. The researchers theorized that sexual abuse may exacerbate the negative psychological impact of preexisting problems and that past stressors may make children more vulnerable to sexual abuse.

Abuse-Related Factors

Age. Although the age of the victim was the variable examined most often in CSA studies, findings on the relationship between children's age and impact of CSA remain inconclusive. One set of investigators reported that school-aged children were more negatively affected by sexual abuse than preschool-aged children or adolescents (Gomes-Schwartz et al., 1990), whereas another investigator reported that older children and adolescents were more negatively affected (Adams-Tucker, 1982). Wolfe, Gentile, and Wolfe (1989) reported that younger children were more symptomatic. Age may, however, explain qualitative differences in symptomatology. Friedrich and colleagues (1986) found that victim age was related to type of behavior problems with younger children displaying more internalizing behaviors and older children displaying more externalizing behaviors (Friedrich et al., 1986). Wozencraft et al. (1991) found suicide ideation to be more common in older victims. Yet another study failed to find a relationship between age at time of assessment and degree of symptomatology (Einbender & Friedrich, 1989). The inconsistencies in these findings may be related to idiosyncratic reactions or to different manifestations of the effects of CSA at various stages of social, emotional, and cognitive development.

Gender. The small numbers of males included in most studies of CSA conducted to date has made comparisons between the genders difficult. In a study of sexual abuse of children in day care centers Kelley (1989) found no difference in severity of impact between sexually abused male ($n = 30$) and female ($n = 37$) subjects as measured by the parent version of the CBCL. In addition there were no significant differences on the internalizing or externalizing dimensions of the CBCL when males and females were compared. In contrast, Friedrich and colleagues (1986) found sexually abused girls to be more internalizing in their behaviors, whereas sexually abused males were found to be more externalizing in their behaviors. As previously described, Tong et al. (1987) found self-esteem to be more negatively impacted in sexually abused girls than in boys. In addition, sexually abused girls in their sample also scored higher in behavior problems on the parent and teacher reports of the CBCL, but not on self-reports of the CBCL. The authors of the study theorize that the increased impact observed in the female subjects may be related to the relationship of the subject to the perpetrator, with girls more likely to have been abused by a relative or acquaintance, and males more likely to have been abused by a stranger. This illustrates the difficulty previously mentioned in sorting out the effects of intercorrelated variables. Thus, research conducted to date has inadequately addressed potential differences in male and female reactions to CSA.

Severity of Abuse. More intrusive forms of sexual abuse, especially those involving penetration, have been found in numerous studies to be associated with increased severity of impact (Friedrich et al., 1986, 1987). Conte and Schuerman (1987) found that an increase in the number of types of abuse, including penetration, was related to increased psychological disturbance. In a study conducted by Mennen (1993) penetration predicted higher levels of distress on depression and self-worth measures in a sample of 75 sexually abused girls aged 6 to 18 years.

Morrow (1991) studied attributions of 84 female adolescent incest victims and found internal or self-blaming attributions to be more common in those who experienced intercourse. Morrow and Sorrell (1989) examined self-esteem as measured by the Rosenberg Self-Esteem Scale (Rosenberg, 1979), depression as measured by the Beck Depression Inventory (Beck, 1961), and antisocial and self-injurious behaviors as measured by the Negative Behaviors Checklist (Morrell & Sorrell, 1989) in a sample of 101 sexually abused adolescents. Results of multiple regression analysis revealed that severity of abuse was the single most powerful predictor of distress levels, with intercourse being associated with lower self-esteem, higher levels of depression, and greater numbers of antisocial and self-injurious behaviors (Morrow & Sorell, 1989).

Mannarino, Cohen, Smith, and Moore-Motily (1991) found on a 1-year follow-up that sexually abused girls ($n = 73$) who had been subjected to intercourse had significantly more symptomatology than those who had experienced less intrusive forms of sexual abuse. Those who were subjected to intercourse had increased depressive symptoms as measured by the Children's Depression Inventory (Kovacs, 1985); anxiety symptoms, as measured by the State-Trait Anxiety Inventory for Children (Spielberger, 1973); self-esteem problems, as measured by the Piers-Harris Children's Self-Concept Scale (Piers & Harris, 1969), and behavioral difficulties, as measured by the Child Behavior Checklist (Achenbach & Edelbrock, 1983). Teams of investigators found no relationship between level of psychological trauma and severity of abuse (Einbender & Friedrich, 1989; Wozencraft et al., 1991).

Physical Force. Most researchers reported that use of physical force is related to increased psychological disturbance. Conte and Shuerman (1987) reported that physical restraint of the victim during abuse was associated with increased severity of impact. Morrow and Sorell (1989) also reported increased impact in a sample of sexually abused adolescents when physical force was used. In Mennen's study (1993) physical force predicted higher levels of depression and lower self-worth scores when the perpetrator was not a father figure and lower levels of distress when the abuser was a father figure. This differential effect may be related to attribution of blame in that it may be easier to blame a father-figure perpetrator, as opposed to oneself, when physical force is used.

Relationship to Offender. Increased closeness in the relationship between the victim and offender has been found to be associated with increased sequelae in numerous studies, with abuse by a father or father figure frequently reported as having the most serious impact (Adams-Tucker, 1982; Conte & Schuerman, 1987; Friedrich et al., 1986). For instance, Wozencraft et al. (1991) found suicide ideation, as measured by the CDI, to be more common in subjects sexually abused by relatives. McLeer et al. (1988) reported that children sexually abused by biological fathers were more likely to meet the criteria for PTSD (75%) than those sexually abused by a trusted adult who was not the father figure (25%). In contrast, Mennen (1993), failed to find increased impact when the perpetrator was a father or father figure.

Limitations in the research conducted to date examining the relationship of the perpetrator to the child victim include inconsistencies among studies in definitions of "father figure." Another limitation is the assumption that a particular category of relationship is necessarily equated with the child's emotional closeness to the perpetrator. Two studies indicated that extrafamilial sexual abuse has serious negative consequences for children. In Kelley's (1989) study of 67 children sexually abused in day care centers the subjects had behavior problem scores comparable with those reported in samples of children sexually abused by relatives. The implication is that the relative-nonrelative distinction is not always an adequate predictor of sexual abuse sequelae. Burgess, Hartman, McCausland, and Powers (1984) examined stress responses in children and adolescents abused by nonfamily members in sex rings (a group of adults who provide children for hire as prostitutes) and found that 75% demonstrated negative psychological and social adjustment. Use of a standardized measure to determine subjects' emotional closeness to the perpetrators would help clarify the link between relationship of the offender and level of impact.

Time Elapsed Since Abuse. Although most studies have reported decreased symptomatology with increased lapse in time between abuse and time of data collection (Friedrich et al., 1986, 1987; Waterman et al., 1993) other studies found no decrease in symptomatology over time (McLeer et al., 1988; Wolfe et al., 1989).

Postabuse Factors

The preabuse and abuse-related variables discussed earlier provide insight into how reactions to CSA may vary; yet because these variables are unalterable after the fact, they provide minimal direction for intervention. Therefore, it is crucial to identify factors that attenuate the impact of CSA so that interventions can be directed accordingly. Mediators of impact of CSA identified in research findings include family conflict, maternal support, and attribution style.

Family Conflict. Waterman et al. (1993) found that the least negatively impacted children in their sample of children abused in day care centers were those whose families had lower numbers of family stressors, coping styles that involved actively mobilizing resources, families who were close but not enmeshed, and families that resolved problems without a great deal of overt anger and conflict. Thus, interventions directed toward decreasing stress or increasing positive coping strategies in families may facilitate children's recovery from CSA.

Maternal Support. Investigators who examined maternal support following disclosure of sexual abuse consistently found that maternal support played a critical role in mitigating the negative impact of CSA (Conte & Schuerman, 1987; Everson et al., 1989; Friedrich et al., 1987; Gomes-Schwartz et al., 1990; Kelley, 1990; Morrow & Sorell, 1989; Waterman et al., 1993). Maternal support involves believing the child's disclosure of sexual abuse, providing emotional support, and protecting the child from subsequent abuse.

In Everson et al.'s (1989) study less than one half of mothers of incest victims ($n = 84$) were supportive of their children. Maternal support predicted psychological functioning in children, with children who are believed and supported faring much better. Mothers were more supportive of their children if the offenders were ex-spouses than if they were men with whom the women had current relationships. Children who were removed from the home and placed in foster or institutional care after discovery of the sexual abuse were more likely to have mothers who were nonsupportive. In addition, when level of maternal support was examined in mothers of children removed from the home, levels of maternal support continued to be related to children's psychological functioning. In Morrow and Sorell's (1989) study, lower self-esteem and higher depression levels were associated with negative responses of mothers to the CSA disclosure.

The findings from these studies clearly indicated that intervention aimed at supporting mothers and helping them to believe, support, and protect their children facilitates the child's recovery following disclosure of sexual abuse.

Attribution Style. Morrow (1991) studied attributions of female adolescent incest victims ($n = 84$) and found that attribution style was related to self-esteem and depression, with subjects being significantly more depressed and reporting lower self-esteem when they attributed the abuse to something about themselves (internal attribution) rather than an external reason (external attribution). Wolfe et al. (1989) also found sexually abused children's attribution style to be correlated with depressive symptoms. These findings supported the clinical goal of alleviating self-blame and negative self-perceptions in victims of CSA.

Summary of Factors Associated With Increased Severity of Effects

In summary, many variables, including preabuse, abuse-related, and postabuse variables, influence the severity of impact of sexual abuse. Psychological and developmental problems before the sexual abuse negatively influence psychological adjustment to CSA. Findings from most studies reviewed indicated that closeness of the relationship between victim and offender, severity of abuse, and use of physical force are associated with increased negative impact. The influences of age, gender, and time elapsed since abuse are still unclear and warrant further study. Several investigators found that lack of maternal support, family conflict, and self-blaming attributions following sexual abuse exacerbated the negative sequelae of CSA.

TRAUMAGENIC DYNAMICS MODEL

Investigators have found that reactions to CSA are multifaceted and influenced by a variety of intervening variables. Thus, no single symptom profile or syndrome related to the impact of CSA has been supported. The most comprehensive, empirically validated conceptual model accounting for the multifaceted effects of CSA is the Traumagenic Dynamics Model proposed by Finkelhor and Browne (1985, 1986). This model has been empirically supported by investigators studying the effects of CSA.

According to the Traumagenic Dynamics Model, CSA has a variety of effects, depending on the characteristics of the abuse, on four main areas of children's development: sexuality, ability to trust in personal relationships, self-esteem, and sense of their ability to affect the world. Four distinct types of mechanisms account for the variety of effects. The mechanisms are traumatic sexualization, betrayal, stigmatization, and powerlessness. The presence and forms of these mechanisms vary in different abuse situations.

Traumatic sexualization refers to conditions in sexual abuse under which a child's sexuality is shaped in developmentally inappropriate and interpersonally dysfunctional ways (Finkelhor, 1987). As previously described, numerous studies have found increased sexualized behaviors in sexually abused children, thus empirically validating the mechanism of traumatic sexualization. In betrayal, the second dynamic, children discover that someone in whom they trust has caused them harm. The dynamic of betrayal encompasses not only the child's experience with the offender but also with nonoffending family members. For instance, many sexually abused children experience a sense of betrayal when they find their mothers will not believe or protect them. Symptoms traced to betrayal include depression and anxiety, both of which have been documented by researchers. Stigmatization, the third dynamic, refers to the negative messages about the self, such as guilt, shamefulness, and worthlessness that are communicated to the child around the abusive experience. Lowered self-esteem, reported by many investigators, is related to the stigmatization of CSA. Powerlessness, the fourth dynamic, results from the child's sense of control and efficacy being repeatedly overruled, from intrusion of body space, and from coercion and threats. Symptoms of PTSD, especially fear and anxiety, observed in many victims of CSA, seem to be connected to the powerlessness experienced by child victims.

Although findings from several of the studies on CSA reviewed in this chapter collectively support the Traumagenic Dynamics Model, only one in-depth study was designed with a goal of testing this model. Findings from one of the most extensive studies of the impact of CSA strongly supported the Traumagenic Dynamics Model (Waterman et al., 1993). Because the model is multifactorial, only researchers who design comprehensive studies, such as the one of Waterman et al., will be capable of testing the validity of the Traumagenic Dynamics Model. Further testing of this model will improve our understanding of the impact of CSA.

PROMISING AREAS OF RESEARCH

Development of Abuse-Specific Measures

An encouraging development in the study of the effects of CSA is the development of several abuse-related assessment measures. Conte and Schuerman (1987) developed a behavior checklist comprising behaviors frequently observed in sexually abused children. Wolfe et al. (1989) developed the Sexual Abuse Fear Evaluation subscale (SAFE) and the Children's Impact of Traumatic Events Scale-Revised (CITES) to assess posttraumatic stress symptoms. The CSBI, developed by Friedrich and colleagues (1991) and previously discussed in the section on sexualized behaviors, has excellent psychometric properties.

Lanktree and Briere (1992) devised the Trauma Symptom Checklist for Children (TSC-C), a 54-item self-report measure for children 8 years of age and older, to assess dimensions of trauma. It consists of six subscales (Anxiety, Depression, Post-Traumatic Stress, Sexual Concerns, Dissociation, and Anger). Although developed to assess acute childhood trauma of various types, the items in the TSC-C were written to be sensitive to sexual abuse in particular.

Mannarino et al. (1994a) have recently developed the Children's Attributions and Perceptions Scale (CAPS) to assess perceptions and attributions believed to be particularly relevant to sexually abused children, and that are not measured by existing instruments. The CAPS consists of 18 items and four subscales: feeling different from peers; personal attributions for negative events, perceived credibility, and interpersonal trust.

These measures have been successful in differentiating groups of sexually abused children from groups of nonsexually abused children. In addition the TSC-C was found to be sensitive to decreases in symptomatology over time in a group of sexually abused children receiving abuse-focused psychotherapy (Lanktree, Briere, & de Jonge, 1993). Because the TSC-C, CAPS, CITES, and SAFE are child self-report measures they avoid the potential bias associated with reliance on parent report measures.

Longitudinal Designs

One of the more promising advancements in CSA research has been the implementation of longitudinal studies. To date, there are several longitudinal studies on the effects of CSA (Everson et al., 1989; Goodman et al,. 1992; Gomes-Schwartz et al., 1990; Mannarino et al., 1991; Runyan, Everson, Edelsohn, Hunter, & Coulter, 1988). The longest period, however, that children were followed was 5 years (Waterman et al., 1993), with most researchers studying the effects of CSA for only 12 to 18 months. Symptoms of emotional distress were noted to decrease over time in most studies (Gomes-Schwartz et al. 1990; Goodman et al., 1992; Mannarino et al., 1991; Runyan et al., 1988; Waterman et al., 1993).

CONCLUSIONS AND FUTURE RESEARCH DIRECTIONS

In conclusion, research on the effects of CSA has become increasingly more sophisticated during the past decade. Investigators found that sexually abused children develop significant psychological problems including behavior problems; lowered self-esteem; depression; inappropriate sexual behaviors; and, in some instances, PTSD. The research findings reviewed here indicate that there are a multitude of factors that influence the psychological adjustment of children to sexual abuse. These include preabuse conditions, abuse-related factors, and postabuse factors.

Despite advances in empirically validating psychological disturbances in sexually abused children, we are still unclear whether the symptoms that sexually abused children display can be attributed to the sexual abuse per se, or to psychological impairment that may have antedated the abuse, abuse-related factors, and postabuse factors.

To date, most research conducted on the effects of CSA has been cross-sectional, examining symptomatology at a single point. Prospective, longitudinal studies would help to determine the effects of CSA at different stages of development and to discover what factors contribute to recovery. The most methodologically sound approach to studying the effects of CSA would be to design a prospective, longitudinal study in which a large cohort of normal, nonabused children are followed from birth. Because of the high prevalence rates of CSA in our society (Finkelhor et al., 1990), a substantial number of these children would subsequently become sexually abused. Data would be collected before abuse for baseline purposes, at time of disclosure, and periodically after the abuse. The sexually abused and nonabused children within this cohort could be compared on multiple dimensions of development, including social, emotional, and cognitive development. Such a design, however, would be expensive and time-consuming. Conversely, lifelong trauma from and treatment for CSA is expensive and time-consuming.

Inclusion of multiple comparisons groups, such as physically abused children, nonabused siblings, and psychiatrically disturbed children, may help investigators sort out some of the abuse-specific effects of CSA. The inclusion of comparison groups of children who have experienced traumatic events other than abuse, such as injury in a motor vehicle accident, may help determine how sexual abuse differs in impact from other traumatic events in childhood (Kelley, 1991). Employment of multiple informants and multiple measures, especially the newly developed measures of abuse-specific effects of CSA would strengthen future studies. Equally important is the inclusion of larger sample sizes to allow for adequate statistical power and application of multivariate statistical analyses.

REFERENCES

Achenbach, T. M., & Edelbrock, C. S. (1983). *The child behavior checklist manual*. Burlington, VT: University of Vermont.

Adams-Tucker, C. (1982). Proximate effects of sexual abuse in childhood: A report on 28 children. *American Journal of Psychiatry, 139*, 1252–1256.

American Psychiatric Association. (1987). *Diagnostic and statistical manual of mental disorders* (3rd ed., rev.). Washington, DC: American Psychiatric Association.

Beck, A. T., Ward, C., Mendelson, M., Mock, J., & Erbaugh, J. (1961). An inventory for measuring depression. *Archives of General Psychiatry, 4*, 561–571.

Burgess, A. W., Hartman, C. R., McCausland, M. P., & Powers, P. (1984). Response patterns in children and adolescents exploited through sex rings and pornography. *American Journal of Psychiatry, 141*, 656–662.

Cavaiola, A. A., & Schiff, M. (1989). Self-esteem in abused chemically dependent adolescents. *Child Abuse and Neglect: The International Journal, 13*, 327–334.

Cohen, J. A., & Mannarino, A. P. (1988). Psychologic symptoms in sexually abused girls. *Child Abuse and Neglect: The International Journal, 12*, 571–577.

Conte, J. R., & Shuerman, J. R. (1987). Factors associated with an increased impact of child sexual abuse. *Child Abuse and Neglect: The International Journal, 11*, 201–211.

Cooper, H. M. (1982). Scientific guidelines for conducting integrative research reviews. *Review of Educational Research, 52*, 291–302.

Deblinger, E., McLeer, S. V., Atkins, M. S., Ralphe, D., & Foa, E. (1989). Posttraumatic stress in sexually abused, physically abused, and nonabused children. *Child Abuse and Neglect: The International Journal, 13*, 403–408.

Einbender, A. J., & Friedrich, W. N. (1989). Psychological functioning and behavior of sexually abused girls. *Journal of Consulting and Clinical Psychology, 57*, 155–157.

Everson, M. D., Hunter, W. M., Runyan, D. K., Edelsohn, G. A., & Coulter, M. L. (1989). *American Journal of Orthopsychiatry, 59*, 197–207.

Finch, A. J., Saylor, C. F., & Edwards, G. L. (1985). Children's depression inventory: Sex and grade norms for normal children. *Journal of Consulting and Clinical Psychology, 53*, 424–425.

Finkelhor, D. (1987). The trauma of child sexual abuse: Two models. *Journal of Interpersonal Violence, 2*, 348–366.

Finkelhor, D., & Browne, A. (1985). The traumatic impact of child sexual abuse: A conceptualization. *American Journal of Orthopsychiatry, 55*, 530–541.

Finkelhor, D., & Browne, A. (1986). Initial and long-term effects: A conceptual framework. In D. Finkelhor (Ed.), *A sourcebook on child sexual abuse* (pp. 180–198). Newbury Park, CA: Sage.

Finkelhor, D., Hotaling, G., Lewis, I. A., & Smith, S. (1990). Sexual abuse in a national survey of adult men and women: Prevalence, characteristics and risk factors. *Child Abuse and Neglect: The International Journal, 14*, 19–28.

Fitts, W. R. (1965). *Manual for the Tennessee self-concept scale*. Nashville, TN: Counselor Records and Tests.

Friedrich, W. N. (1993). Sexual victimization and sexual behavior in children: A review of recent literature. *Child Abuse and Neglect: The International Journal, 17*, 59–66.

Friedrich, W. N., Beilke, R. L., & Urquiza, A. J. (1987). Children from sexually abusive families: A behavioral comparison. *Journal of Interpersonal Violence, 3*, 21–28.

Friedrich, W. N., Beilke, R. L., & Urquiza, A. J. (1988). Behavior problems in young sexually abused boys: A comparison study. *Journal of Interpersonal Violence, 3*, 21–28.

Friedrich, W. N., Grambsch, P., Broughton, D., Kuipers, J., & Beilke, R. L. (1991). Normative sexual behavior in children. *Pediatrics, 88*, 456–464.

Friedrich, W. N., Grambsch, P., Damon, L., Hewitt, S., Koverola, C., Lang, R., Wolfe, V., & Broughton, D. (1992). The child sexual behavior inventory: Normative and clinical findings. *Psychological Assessment, 4*, 303–311.

Friedrich, W. N., & Luecke, W. J. (1988). Young school-age sexually aggressive children. *Professional Psychology: Research and Practice, 19*, 155–164.

Friedrich, W. N., Urquiza, A. J., & Beilke, R. L. (1986). Behavioral problems in sexually abused young children. *Journal of Pediatric Psychology, 11*, 47–57.

German, D. E., Habenicht, D. J., & Futcher, W. G. (1990). Psychological profile of the female adolescent incest victim. *Child Abuse and Neglect: The International Journal, 14*, 429–438.

Gomes-Schwartz, B., Horowitz, J., & Sauzier, M. (1985). Severity of emotional distress among sexually abused preschool, school-age, and adolescent children. *Hospital and Community Psychiatry, 36*, 503–508.

Gomes-Schwartz, B., Horowitz, J., & Cardarelli, A. P. (1990). *Child sexual abuse: The initial effects*. Newbury Park, CA: Sage.

Goodman, G. S., Taub, E. P., Jones, D. P. H., England, P., Port, L. K., Rudy, L., & Prado, L. (1992). Testifying in court: Emotional effects on child sexual assault victims. *Monographs of the Society for Research in Child Development, 57* (5, Serial No. 229).

Ireton, H., & Thwing, E. (1972). *Minnesota Child Development Inventory*. Minneapolis: Behavioral Systems.

Jampole, L., & Weber, M. K. (1987). An assessment of the behavior of sexually abused and nonabused children with anatomically correct dolls. *Child Abuse and Neglect: The International Journal, 11*, 187–192.

Kelley, S. J. (1989). Stress responses of children to sexual abuse and ritualistic abuse in day care centers. *Journal of Interpersonal Violence, 4*, 502–513.

Kelley, S. J. (1990). Parental stress response to sexual abuse and ritualistic abuse in day care centers. *Nursing Research, 39*, 25–29.

Kelley, S. J. (1991). Methodological issues in child sexual abuse research. *Journal of Pediatric Nursing, 6*, 21–29.

Kelley, S. J. (1992). Child maltreatment, stressful life events, and behavior problems in school-aged children in residential treatment. *Journal of Child and Adolescent Psychiatric Nursing, 5*, 5–13.

Kiser, L. J., Ackerman, B. J., Brown, E., Edwards, N. B., McColgan, E., Pugh, R., & Pruitt, D. B. (1988). Post-traumatic stress disorder in young children: A reaction to purported sexual abuse. *Journal of the American Academy of Child and Adolescent Psychiatry, 27*, 645–649.

Kovacs, M. (1985). Children's depression inventory: CDI. *Cycle Pharmacology Bulletin, 21*, 995–998.

Lanktree, C., & Briere, J. (1992, January). *Further data on the Trauma Symptom Checklist for Children (TSC-C): Reliability, validity, and sensitivity to treatment*. Paper presented at the San Diego Conference on Responding to Child Maltreatment, San Diego.

Lanktree, C., Briere, J., & de Jonge, J. (1993, August). *Effectiveness of therapy for sexually abused children: Changes in Trauma Symptom Checklist for Children (TSC-C) Scores*. Paper presented at the annual meeting of the American Psychological Association, Toronto, Ontario, Canada.

Lipovsky, J. A., Saunders, B. E., & Murphy, S. M. (1989). Depression, anxiety, and behavior problems among victims of father-child sexual assault and nonabused siblings. *Journal of Interpersonal Violence, 4*, 452–468.

Mannarino, A. P., & Cohen, J. A. (1986). A clinical-demographic study of sexually abused children. *Child Abuse and Neglect: The International Journal, 10*, 17–23.

Mannarino, A. P., Cohen, J. A., & Berman, S. R. (1994a). The children's attributions and perceptions scale: A new measure of sexual abuse related factors. *Journal of Clinical Child Psychology, 23*, 204–211.

Mannarino, A. P., Cohen, J. A., & Berman, S. R. (1994b). The relationship between preabuse factors and psychological symptomatology in sexually abused girls. *Child Abuse and Neglect: The International Journal, 18*, 63–71.

Mannarino, A. P., Cohen, J. A., & Gregor, M. (1989). Emotional and behavioral difficulties in sexually abused girls. *Journal of Interpersonal Violence, 4*, 437–541.

Mannarino, A. P., Cohen, J. A., Smith, J. A., & Moore-Motily, S. (1991). Six- and twelve-month follow-up of sexually abused girls. *Journal of Interpersonal Violence, 6*, 494–511.

McLeer, S. V., Deblinger, E., Atkins, M. S., Foa, E. B., & Ralphe, D. L. (1988). *Journal of the American Academy of Child and Adolescent Psychiatry, 27*, 650–654.

Mennen, F. E. (1993). Evaluation of risk factors in childhood sexual abuse. *Journal of the American Academy of Child and Adolescent Psychiatry, 32*, 934–939.

Miller, L. C. (1981). *Louisville behavior checklist*. Los Angeles: Western Psychological Services.

Morrow, K. B. (1991). Attributions of female adolescent incest victims regarding their molestation. *Child Abuse and Neglect: The International Journal, 15*, 477–483.

Morrow, K. B., & Sorell, G. T. (1989). Factors affecting self-esteem, depression and negative behaviors in sexually abused female adolescents. *Journal of Marriage and Family, 51*, 677–786.

Newberger, C. M., Gremy, I. M., Waternaux, C. M., & Newberger, E. H. (1993). Mothers of sexually abused children: Trauma and repair in longitudinal perspective. *American Journal of Orthopsychiatry, 63*, 92–102.

Offer, D., Ostrov, E., & Howard, K. (1977). *The Offer Self-image Questionnaire for Adolescents: A manual*. Chicago: Michael Reese Hospital and Medical Center.

Orr, D. P., & Downes, M. C. (1985). Self-concept of adolescent sexual abuse victims. *Journal of Youth and Adolescence, 14*, 401–410.

Piers, E. V., & Harris, D. B. (1969). *The Piers-Harris children's self-concept scale*. Nashville, TN: Counselor Recordings and Tests.

Rosenberg, M. (1979). *Conceiving the self*. New York: Basic Books.

Runyan, D. K., Everson, M. D., Edelsohn, G. A., Hunter, W. M., & Coulter, M. L. (1988). Impact of legal intervention on sexually abused children. *Journal of Pediatrics, 113*, 647–653.

Sansonnet-Hayden, H., Haley, G., Marriage, K., & Fine, S. (1987). *Journal of the American Academy of Child and Adolescent Psychiatry, 26*, 753–757.

Sivan, A. B., Schor, D. P., Koeppl, G. K., & Noble, L. D. (1988). Interaction of normal children with anatomical dolls. *Child Abuse and Neglect: The International Journal, 12*, 295–304.

Spielberger, C. D. (1973). *Manual for the State-Trait Anxiety Inventory for Children*. Palo Alto, CA: Consulting Psychologist Press.

Tong, L., Oates, K., & McDowell, M. (1987). Personality development following sexual abuse. *Child Abuse and Neglect: The International Journal, 11*, 371–383.

Waterman, J., Kelly, R. J., Oliveri, M. K., & McCord, J. (1993). *Behind the playground walls: Sexual abuse of children in preschools*. New York: Guilford.

White, S., Halpin, B. M., Strom, G. A., & Santilli, G. (1988). Behavioral comparisons of young sexually abused, neglected, and nonreferred children. *Journal of Clinical Child Psychology, 17*, 53–61.

White, S., Strom, G. A., Santilli, G., & Halpin, B. M. (1986). Interviewing young sexual abuse victims with anatomically correct dolls. *Child Abuse and Neglect: The International Journal, 10*, 519–529.

Wolfe, V. V., Gentile, C., & Wolfe, D. A. (1989). The impact of sexual abuse on children: A PTSD formulation. *Behavior Therapy, 20*, 215–228.

Wozencraft, T., Wagner, W., & Pellegrin, A. (1991). Depression and suicidal ideation in sexually abused children. *Child Abuse and Neglect: The International Journal, 15*, 505–511.

Chapter 4

Neuro-behavioral Effects of Childhood Lead Exposure

HEIDI VONKOSS KROWCHUK
SCHOOL OF NURSING
THE UNIVERSITY OF NORTH CAROLINA AT GREENSBORO

CONTENTS

Childhood lead poisoning is recognized as the most important preventable pediatric environmental health problem in the United States (Centers for Disease Control [CDC], 1991). Despite recognition of this problem and the publication of prevention strategies, childhood exposure to lead continues to be widespread. There is little disagreement that high levels of lead exposure in children result in symptomatic lead poisoning, the effects of which are deleterious to every body system (e.g., mental retardation, altered hemoglobin synthesis, nephropathy, encephalopathy), and may result in death (Chisolm, 1971; Perlstein & Attala, 1966). Since the mid-1970s, researchers have reported not only metabolic changes that occur in children exposed to low and moderate levels of lead, but some also have demonstrated serious and irreversible neurobehavioral sequelae associated with this exposure. However, there remains debate over the neurobehavioral consequences of low to moderate exposure levels (at which clinical signs of lead poisoning are not evident) in children (Ernhart, Morrow-Tlucak, Wolf, Super, & Drotar, 1989; Needleman & Gatsonis, 1990; Ruff & Bijur, 1989).

Virtually all children in the United States are exposed to lead from a number of environmental sources (American Academy of Pediatrics [AAP], 1987). In 1990, the Environmental Protection Agency (EPA) estimated that approximately 3 million children in the United States had blood lead levels high enough potentially to affect their neurological and behavioral development (EPA, 1992). Although some children develop symptomatic lead poisoning, the majority remain asymptomatic. However, the damaging effects of exposure to environmental lead, such as learning disabilities, hyperactivity, and poor motor coordination, are said to be continuing to take their toll (Lin-Fu, 1992; Rabin, 1989).

Investigation into all aspects of childhood lead poisoning (e.g., the epidemiology of the disease, the pathophysiology of the disease, the preventive aspects of the disease) has occurred. Because it would be impossible to review critically all of the volumes of literature published about low-level lead poisoning for this chapter, the choice was made to review only those studies pertaining to the neurobehavioral consequences of low-level lead exposure. Using computerized MEDLINE and Cumulative Index of Nursing and Allied Health Literature (CINAHL) subject searches (1983–1994), as well as manual searches of *Index Medicus* (1979–1994), CINAHL (1979–1994), and *Dissertation Abstracts* (1979–1994), studies related to lead exposure and children's neurological and behavioral development were identified. Only those studies published from 1979 to the present were reviewed, because studies conducted before 1979, for the most part, examined samples with high blood lead levels (> 50 μg/dL), and they drew inferences about lead effects on neurobehavioral development from data on subjects with symptomatic toxicity. Studies conducted since 1979 have focused primarily on the effects of low to moderate lead exposure on physical and neurobehavioral development.

Studies reviewed originated in the disciplines of medicine, toxicology, physiology, and biochemistry. Not one nursing study was identified using the retrieval procedures listed earlier. However, despite an extensive search, it is possible that some studies were missed. Also, manuscripts from conference proceedings were not included in the search.

The review begins with an overview of the problem of lead poisoning, followed by a review of the studies that have included investigation of the neurobehavioral effects of low-level lead exposure in infants and children. The chapter concludes with recommendations for research.

OVERVIEW OF LEAD POISONING

Historical Perspective

Childhood lead poisoning was first described over a century ago by Gibson, a physician who encountered a case of peripheral paralysis in a young child and compared the case to chronic lead poisoning in adults (Gibson, Love, Hardie, Bancroft, & Turner, 1892). Twelve years later Gibson (1904) discovered that the source of the lead poisoning was household paint. Unfortunately, Gibson's important observations were ignored, and until the mid-1940s, the prevailing view was that once a child survived the acute phase of lead poisoning, there were no lasting central nervous system effects (McKhann, 1933). This opinion finally was challenged by Byers and Lord (1943) who studied 20 lead-poisoned children and found that 10 had encephalopathy, a common sequela of lead toxicity, and 19 had learning or behavior disorders, such as short attention span and impulsiveness. Byers and Lord postulated that lead poisoning produces long-term neurological deficits in children, even when central nervous system symptoms are absent. A few epidemiological studies (McLaughlin, 1956; Thurston, Middlekamp, & Mason, 1955) followed from their work; however, it was not until the early 1970s that epidemiological and cross-sectional studies of low-level lead exposure were conducted.

These early studies of lead exposure involved simple comparisons of a lead-exposed group and a control group on intelligence test measures; significant differences usually were found. As experience accumulated and research strategies became more sophisticated, researchers began to assess the influence of covariates, such as socioeconomic status, parental education, and parental intelligence using multiple regression techniques (Gatsonis & Needleman, 1992). Though conflicting results were common, lead exposure and neurobehavioral deficit remained significantly associated (Gatsonis & Needleman, 1992).

Defining Lead Poisoning

Since 1970, the accumulated information on the sources of lead, its effects on humans (especially infants and children), and the determination of safe lead thresholds has increased substantially. Before 1960, a blood lead level about 60 μg/dL of whole blood was considered toxic (Chisolm & Harrison, 1956). By the late 1970s, the toxic level was determined to be 30 μg/dL of whole blood (PbB); in 1985, the CDC further shifted the toxicity level to 25 μg/dL PbB, and in 1991, faced with strong scientific evidence that the adverse health effects of lead exposure occur at even lower blood lead levels, the CDC set the toxic level at 10 μg/dL PbB (CDC, 1991).

The CDC (1991) has developed a categorical approach to defining lead poisoning according to PbB concentration. Within each classification identified, specific interventions are recommended. The six classes and interventions they identify are

1. *Class I.* PbB ≤ 9 μgdL—not lead poisoned
2. *Class IIA.* PbB 10 to 14 μg/dL—rescreen and initiate prevention activities
3. *Class IIB.* PbB 15 to 19 μg/dL—initiate nutritional and educational interventions, rescreen, and, if elevation continues, investigate environment and initiate environmental intervention
4. *Class III.* PbB 20 to 44 μg/dL—initiate environmental evaluation and remediation and initiate medical evaluation; consider pharmacological intervention to chelate lead
5. *Class IV.* PbB 45 to 69 μg/dL—requires medical, pharmacological, and environmental intervention
6. *Class V.* PbB ≥ 70 μg/dL—medical emergency requires immediate intervention (CDC, 1991)

The potential effects of low-level exposure (PbB 10 to 44 μg/dL) are the focus of this chapter. Lead is a poison that affects almost every body system; however, it is most damaging to the developing nervous systems and brains of fetuses, infants, and young children (AAP, 1987, 1993; CDC, 1991; Moore, 1980). The Agency for Toxic Substances and Disease Registry (1988) reports that the adverse health effects of lead begin at blood levels of about 4 to 10 μg/dL and include reduced gestational age, reduced birthweight, and neurobehavioral and developmental deficits. As the blood lead level rises, nerve conduction is reduced (25–30 μg/dL), hemoglobin synthesis is impaired (40 μg/dL), peripheral neuropathies develop (50–70 μg/dL), and encephalopathy results when the level reaches 80 to 100 μg/dL. Death is the consequence of a blood lead level that reaches 150 μg/dL.

Sources of Lead Exposure

Lead-Based Paint. The most common source of childhood lead exposure is lead-based paint (CDC, 1991). Children at higher risk of exposure are those living in substandard (dilapidated or deteriorated) housing constructed before 1960, when interior lead-based paint was commonly used (AAP, 1987). Exterior lead-based paint was available until the mid-1970s; although currently not available for residential use, it still is used in maritime, farm, and outdoor equipment.

Soil/Dust. Other sources of lead exposure include soil and dust in children's play areas. Lead is a component of soil and dust; in industrialized and urban areas, lead found in soil is in the form of particulate matter (i.e., powdered paint and atmospheric fallout of lead particles), a form that is easily ingested (Agency for Toxic Substances and Disease Registry, 1988). The fine particles blown off soil constitute dust; the concentration of lead in dust usually exceeds that in soil (Lin-Fu, 1992). Elevated lead concentrations in outdoor dust can result from sandblasting painted exterior surfaces (Landrigan, Baker, & Himmelstein, 1982). Elevated lead concentrations in indoor dust may result from improper removal of interior lead-based paint (Needleman & Bellinger, 1991).

Airborne Lead. Before reducing the amount of lead in gasoline, one of the major sources of exposure was from airborne lead in automobile emissions (EPA, 1986). However, studies have documented a decrease in blood lead levels associated with the removal of lead in gasoline (Annest, Pirkle, & Makuc, 1983; Hayes et al., 1994; Rabinowitz & Needleman, 1982); and airborne lead is now considered a minor source of exposure for children.

Food. Food is another source of lead exposure to children. Airborne lead particles deposited in soil contaminate crops; lead pesticides compound the problem (Mahaffey, 1990). However, most lead contamination of food occurs in processing (Lin-Fu, 1992). Until the early 1980s, lead solder in food cans was a major source of exposure (Lamm & Rosen, 1974; Mitchell & Aldous, 1979; Jelinek, 1982).

Water. Drinking water is another source of lead exposure; the major source of the lead is household plumbing made from lead pipes or containing lead solder joints. Lead pipes and solder present problems for all drinking water, but especially for water which is acidic (soft or plumbosolvent water). Large amounts of lead can leach from plumbing exposed to plumbosolvent water, resulting in significant increases in blood lead levels in those who consume the water (EPA, 1987).

Placental Transfer. Placental transfer is an important and not commonly explored source of infant lead exposure. Lead is rapidly transferred across the placenta to the developing fetus, and umbilical cord PbB levels are highly correlated with maternal PbB levels (Scanlon, 1971; Silbergeld, 1991). Furthermore, cord PbB levels not only reflect the transfer of maternal lead from exposure during pregnancy but also reflect the transfer of maternal lead stores mobilized from bone as a result of pregnancy (Silbergeld, 1991; Thompson, Robertson, &

Fitzgerald, 1985). Researchers have demonstrated that for infants whose birthweight is less than 2,500 g, placental lead levels almost triple the levels found in infants whose birthweight is greater than 4000 g (Ward, Watson, & Bryce-Smith, 1987).

Miscellaneous Sources. Other sources of lead exposure for children include colored ink in bread wrappers, children's books, and newsprint; batteries, cosmetics (children touch their mother's faces and subsequently ingest the lead when they put their fingers in their mouths), fishing weights, and antique toys painted with leaded paint (AAP, 1987; Lin-Fu, 1992; Needleman & Bellinger, 1991). Folk remedies used by many immigrants also are a continuing source of lead poisoning in children (CDC, 1992).

Exposure Determination

When lead is inhaled or ingested, it is deposited in both the hard tissues (long-term sites) and soft tissues (short-term sites) of the body. The half-life of lead deposited in soft tissue is about 30 days, and the half-life of lead deposited in hard tissue (such as bone) is 5.1 years (Mushak, 1992b). Therefore, when measuring lead exposure, the concentration of lead can be determined from whole blood, which demonstrates acute exposure; or from bone, which demonstrates chronic or long-term exposure. Researchers have used shed deciduous teeth as a measure of lead content in bone (Bellinger & Needleman, 1992; Mushak, 1992a). However, the reliability and validity of using this bone has been questioned, because the accumulation of dentine lead varies with tooth location in the jaw and dentition type (Paterson et al., 1988). New techniques for measuring bone lead currently are being developed. However, lead levels obtained from whole blood (venous samples) are still the most commonly used and interpretable biological index of lead exposure available (Bellinger & Needleman, 1992; Piomelli, Rosen, Chisolm, & Graef, 1984).

NEURODEVELOPMENTAL EFFECTS OF CHILDHOOD LEAD EXPOSURE

Cross-Sectional Studies

The neurobehavioral effects of lead exposure in children are particularly notable because of the sensitivity of the developing central and peripheral nervous system and the irreversibility of lead-associated injury to the system. In early lead-poisoning studies, researchers described neurological impairment resulting from high levels of PbB in children. It is now well documented that severe exposure in children (PbB > 80 μg/dL) can cause encephalopathy characterized by ataxia, impairment of consciousness, coma, and seizures (Perlstein & Attala, 1966). Consequently, recent research has focused on the neurobehavioral effects of low-level lead exposure (PbB ≤ 44 μg/dL), and many researchers have conducted cross-sectional investigations to study these effects.

In 1979, in a study considered the first to control adequately for confounding variables (e.g., socioeconomic status, maternal age at subjects' birth, maternal educational level, parental intelligence quotient [IQ]) associated with lead exposure, Needleman and his colleagues studied the deciduous teeth of 2,335 clinically asymptomatic for lead toxicity school-aged children with no known elevated lead exposure. A dose-response relationship was found in the study subjects between level of exposure and the outcome measures of IQ scores, speech and language ability, attention span, and classroom behavior. When confounding variables were controlled, significant differences were found in all outcome measures between those children classified as having high dentine lead levels (≥ 24 parts per million; mean PbB = 35.5 ± 10.1 μg/dL) and those with low dentine lead levels (≤ 6 parts per million; mean PbB = 23.8 ± 6.0 μg/dL).

These researchers used reliable, valid, and sensitive measures of neurobehavioral performance. They controlled for confounding variables that are known to affect development and used reliable and valid procedures to determine lead exposure in the subjects. Although these researchers attempted to control for sample selection bias (the population consisted of 3,329 first and second graders in two Massachusetts cities of which 70% [$n = 2{,}335$] comprised the initial lead exposure sample), complex exclusion criteria and classification procedures resulted in a total of 270 subjects tested and 158 subjects included in the final data analysis. This suggests that the sample was not representative of the population.

In a follow-up of these children, the researchers reported that children in the high-lead (mean PbB = 35.5 ± 10.1 μg/dL) group were significantly more likely to have had academic difficulty (i.e., held back a grade in school) (Bellinger, Needleman, Bromfield, & Mintz, 1984), and at 18 years of age, they had lower class rank, poorer vocabulary and grammatical reasoning scores, poorer hand-eye coordination, and more absenteeism in the final year of school than did those 18-year-olds with low dentine lead levels in early childhood. Furthermore, when confounding variables were controlled, high dentine lead levels in early childhood were associated with reading disability and failure to graduate from high school (Needleman, Schell, Bellinger, Leviton, & Allred, 1990).

The sample used in the follow-up study at 18 years of age consisted of 132 of the 270 subjects tested at 6 to 7 years of age. Significant differences in confounding variables (paternal education, maternal IQ, maternal education) were noted between those tested and those not tested at 18 years of age, suggesting that selection bias existed and therefore, findings could be attributed to this bias.

In another group of studies that used designs similar to those of Needleman et al. (1979), Yule, Landsdown, Millar, and Urbanowicz (1981) investigated cognitive outcomes (IQ, reading, and spelling scores) in 166 British school children classified as high (PbB range 13–32 μg/dL) or low (PbB range 4–12 μg/dL) lead exposure based on PbB levels. When age, socioeconomic status, and gender were controlled, the researchers found significant differences between the groups; elevated blood lead levels were negatively associated with IQ levels. However, in better designed replication studies where representative samples were used, lead level had no statistically significant effect on IQ, though it did have a significant effect on reaction time (Lansdown, Yule, Urbanowicz, & Hunter, 1986; Yule & Lansdown, 1983). Consistent with the Needleman et al. (1979) findings, teacher ratings of children's nonadaptive classroom behavior were positively related to level of lead exposure.

In 1990, Needleman and Gatsonis conducted a metaanalysis of cross-sectional studies that used multiple regression analysis with lead level (either PbB or dentine lead level) as the main effect and IQ, measured by the Stanford-Binet IQ Scale (Terman & Merrill, 1973), the Wechsler Intelligence Scale–Revised (Wechsler, 1974), the McCarthy Scale (McCarthy, 1972), or the British Ability Scale as the dependent variable, and controlled for covariates (e.g., socioeconomic and familial factors). Although the researchers selected 24 cross-sectional studies (published from 1972–1987) as the sample for their metaanalysis, 12 studies had to be excluded from the analysis for methodological reasons. Excluded studies were characterized by (a) a lack of consistency in the protocol for determining lead exposure; for instance, some studies included samples in which lead exposure had been measured by analyzing either PbB (a measure of short-term exposure) or teeth (a measure of chronic exposure); (b) use of unreliable or nonvalid instruments to measure the outcome variable (e.g., use of screening tests to measure neuropsychological deficits); (c) failure to control for confounding variables; (d) small sample sizes; (e) biases in sample selection; and (f) failure to consider the potential effects of measurement error (Gatsonis & Needleman, 1992; Needleman & Gatsonis, 1990). The 12 studies included in the meta-analysis (Ernhart, Landa, & Wolf, 1985; Fergusson, Fergusson, Horwood, & Kinzett, 1988; Fulton et al., 1987; Hansen, Trillingsgaard,

Beese, Lyngbye, & Grandjean, 1989; Hatzakis, Kokevi, & Katsouyanni, 1987; Lansdown et al., 1986; Needleman, Geiger, & Frank, 1985; Pocock, Ashby, & Smith, 1987; Schroeder, Hawk, Otto, Mushak, & Hicks, 1985; Winneke et al., 1983; Yule et al., 1981) were not without methodological problems; however, the shortcomings of these 12 were minor compared to those excluded.

In their meta-analysis, Needleman and Gatsonis (1990) separated the analyses into type of tissue measured (i.e., dentine lead or PbB). Joint *p* values were derived using both the Fisher and the Mosteller and Bush methods (Hedges & Okin, 1985; Rosenthal, 1984) for combining probabilities. The combined *p* value for the PbB group was $< .0001$; for the dentine lead group, the combined *p* value was $< .004$ (Needleman & Gatsonis, 1990). The meta-analysis indicted that low-level lead exposure and intellectual deficit were negatively associated, despite some methodological problems in the studies reviewed. Considered singly, none of the 12 studies could provide definitive confirmation that low-level lead exposure in children is associated with a lower IQ level. However, as the researchers point out, the findings from the meta-analysis are consistent with findings from both experimental studies conducted on animals and current prospective studies conducted with cohorts of children (Needleman & Gatsonis, 1990).

In other cross-sectional studies, researchers have investigated the relationship between PbB or dentine lead level and neuropsychological deficit. Using a convenience sample of 201 African-American mother-child pairs from the Baltimore Soil Lead Abatement Demonstration Project clinic, Sciarillo, Alexander, and Farrell (1992) examined the relationship between child behavior and PbB level. Child behavior was operationalized as the total behavior problem scores on the Achenbach (1986) Child Behavior Checklist. The researchers controlled for socioeconomic and familial variables (e.g., maternal age, maternal education level) known to confound the relationship between lead exposure and neurobehavioral deficit, and also included maternal depression as a possible confounder. Lead concentrations were determined from clinic data (all children had routine venipunctures done to assess PbB), and the children were divided into two groups (a low-exposed and a high-exposed group) for analysis. Using multiple logistic regression, the researchers determined that children in the high-exposed group (PbB > 15 μg/dL) were 2.7 times more likely to have behavior problems, such as aggression, hyperactivity, and delinquency, than were those in the low-exposed (PbB ≤ 15 μg/dL) group. Maternal depression was the most influential confounding variable contributing to the child's total behavior problem score in both the multiple linear and logistic regression procedures employed; however, the lead effect remained statistically significant when the maternal depression was controlled.

The findings of this study are consistent with the finding that children with known lead toxicity (PbB > 40 μg/dL) have increased motor activity (David, Clark, & Voeller, 1972; David, Hoffman, Sverd, Clark, & Voeller, 1976). However, the children enrolled in this study and defined as "high exposed" had low to moderate PbB levels (mean PbB = 27.8 μg/dL, *SD* = 10.4). Caution must be used in generalizing the results of this study to other samples or populations. The sample used was a nonprobability sample; furthermore, the outcome variable, child behavior, was a maternal report measure. Although not statistically significant, mothers whose children were in the high-exposed group had more symptoms of depression than did the mothers of the low-exposed group. It is reasonable to question how much the maternal depression influenced the report of the child's behavior problems.

In a cross-sectional study conducted in Denmark, a group of researchers examined the association between cognitive and motor functioning and lead exposure, as measured by dentine lead levels in 7-year-old children (Hansen et al., 1989). The population comprised 1,846 healthy first graders from six Danish municipalities. The shed deciduous teeth were collected from this group and analyzed for lead content. Subjects ($n = 110$) with the highest dentine lead levels (mean dentine level = 26.8 μg/g) were matched on the variables of sex and socioeconomic status with low dentine lead level (mean dentine lead level = 3.24 μg/g) controls ($n = 52$). The dentine lead levels were highly correlated ($r = .48$, $p < .001$) with the PbB levels in the two groups (PbB range = 1.6–14.1 μg/dL). Information about neonatal physiological jaundice also was obtained from both parent interview and review of medical records. Using data collectors blinded to group assignment, the subjects underwent a series of psychometric tests. Children determined to have high dentine lead levels scored significantly lower than children with low dentine lead levels on components of the Wechsler Intelligence Scale for Children (Wechsler, 1974) and on behavior rating scales. The researchers concluded that these findings were generalizable to the population, despite their selection bias and their lack of control for such variables as maternal IQ and parental education. What is especially notable about this study, however, was that mild neonatal physiological jaundice, identified as a confounding variable, was related to an increased risk of neurobehavioral deficit in the presence of increased dentine lead levels in the 162 children who made up the sample (Lyngbye, Hansen, & Grandjean, 1989, 1991).

In 1990, the Danish researchers conducted a follow-up study of

87.6% ($N = 142$) of the children who formed the original sample to explore the persistence of lead-related neurobehavioral effects and their association with mild neonatal jaundice (Damm, Grandjean, Lyngbye, Trillingsgaard, & Hansen, 1993). The attrition of subjects occurred primarily in the group originally identified with high dentine lead levels. Extensive interview data were obtained from subjects regarding their general health since the first study. Subjects with a history of any neurological trauma (e.g., head injury) were excluded from the study. At the time of the follow-up study, subjects were 15 years old, and they completed a battery of valid and reliable psychological tests (i.e., Wechsler Intelligence Scale for Children, Bender Visual Motor Gestalt Test, Trail Making Test, and Visual Gestalt Test) administered by a clinical psychologist who was blinded to all lead exposure data. The findings revealed that lead exposure continued to be negatively associated with neuropsychological performance; when confounding variables (e.g., neonatal jaundice, maternal education, gestational age, and maternal smoking) were controlled, the IQs of the high-level exposure children were lower than those of the low-level exposure group. However, the association was not statistically significant. Yet, in children with a history of neonatal jaundice, increased lead exposure was significantly associated with mild neuropsychological deficits, as evidenced by statistically significant lower verbal IQ scores and decreased visual-motor coordination (Damm et al., 1993). The researchers postulated that the two neurotoxins, lead and neonatal jaundice, may be synergistic in their effect on the developing nervous systems of children.

Several methodological problems appear in this study. For instance, the data were analyzed based on subject categorization (i.e., high or low lead) from 8 years previously. It is conceivable that some subjects' lead exposure could change over the 8-year period. Without reconfirming classification based on current PbB or dentine lead levels, one may assume that misclassification could have occurred. The researchers do provide data about the subjects' mean PbB levels obtained from the subjects when they were 9 years old. At that time, the mean PbB from the two groups were not significantly different (i.e., high-lead group mean = 5.7 μg/dL; low-lead group mean = 3.7 μg/dL). Three children in each group had PbB levels greater than 10.0 μg/dL; however, the actual values were not reported.

Longitudinal Studies

Longitudinal studies are particularly advantageous for determining the effects of lead exposure on children. Because lead is an accumulating poison, a longitudinal design has the potential to match more accurately the lead exposure and related health effects than is possible with a cross-sectional design.

Five prospective, longitudinal studies of low-level lead exposure have been conducted in the United States (Boston, Cleveland, and Cincinnati) and in Australia (Port Pirie and Sydney). As a group, the studies are methodologically strong because they employed (a) the same standardized instruments for assessing lead exposure and neurobehavioral outcome measures, facilitating direct comparison of the studies; (b) statistical controls for variables identified as confounders and covariates; (c) acceptable levels of statistical power to detect small effects; and (d) early lead exposure measurements (i.e., in utero or cord blood levels from birth). Data from these studies provide support for the relationship between low-level lead exposure and neurobehavioral deficits in children. Although many of the studies demonstrate some developmental deficit (i.e., outcome measure scores 2 to 9 points lower for every 10 μg/dL increment in PbB level) in children classified as high lead versus those classified as low lead, those classified as high lead had mean PbB levels in the low to moderate range (PbB = 10–44 μg/dL). Table 4.1 summarizes the five studies and includes the mean PbB levels of the samples, the instruments used to measure the outcome variables, as well as the major findings related to neurobehavioral outcomes.

The instruments used to measure the outcome variables in these studies have well-established validity and reliability (Bayley, 1969; Brazelton, 1984; Kaufman & Kaufman, 1983, 1985; McCarthy, 1972; Terman & Merrill, 1973; Wechsler, 1967, 1974). Furthermore, used as a group, they provide a comprehensive assessment of neurobehavioral functioning, including the ability to communicate and problem solve.

Boston Study. Bellinger and his colleagues (1984a) were the first of the five groups of researchers to report on the effects of prenatal lead exposure on child neurobehavioral development. Using a sample of 249 infants born to middle- and upper-middle-class women in Boston, Bellinger et al. (1984a) obtained specimens of umbilical cord blood from subjects at birth, and PbB determinations were made. This predominantly white socioeconomically advantaged sample was chosen to limit potential confounding variables, thus decreasing the possibility of errors from measurements of these confounders (e.g., socioeconomic status). Infants enrolled in the study were grouped into low (PbB < 3 μg/dL) and high (PbB > 10 μg/dL) lead-exposed groups, based on the cord PbB levels. At 6 months of age, infants' mental, motor, and emotional development were assessed by a psychologist, using the Bayley Scales of Infant Development (BSID) (Bayley, 1969) and blinded to the infant's lead exposure history and other aspects of the infant's development. Using multivariate regression analyses, statistically significant associations were found between cord PbB levels and infant performance on the BSID. A mean difference of 6 points on the mental development index of the BSID was seen between the low-lead-exposed (mean PbB = 1.8 μg/dL) and the high-lead-exposed (mean PbB = 14.6 μg/dL) groups.

Continued follow-up of these subjects at 12, 18, 24, and 57 months and at 10 years of age demonstrated the persistence of this pattern; the children in the high-lead-exposed group consistently scored lower on all neurobehavioral measures than the low-lead-exposed group. Interestingly, Bellinger, Leviton, and Waternaux (1987) reported that the Boston cohort of children at 57 months of age demonstrated cognitive deficits. However, the analysis revealed that prenatal lead exposure did not contribute to the deficits, but that PbB levels at 24 months of age were predictive of cognitive functioning at 57 months in this socially advantaged sample. Elevated blood lead levels (PbB = 10 μg/dL–25 μg/dL), still within the low range at 24 months of age also were significantly associated with poorer cognitive functioning and academic performance at 10 years of age (Bellinger, Stiles, & Needleman, 1992).

Although the studies conducted by Bellinger, Leviton, Needleman, Waternaux, and Rabinowitz (1986); Bellinger, Leviton, and Sloman (1990); Bellinger, Leviton, and Waternaux (1987); Bellinger, Needleman, Bromfield, and Mintz (1984); and Bellinger, Needleman, Leviton, Waternaux, Rabinowitz, and Nichols (1984) demonstrated statistical significance for neurobehavioral outcome measures between children classified with high PbB levels versus those classified with low PbB levels, subject mortality issues were not adequately addressed by the researchers. The original cohort consisted of 249 children; by the 57-month data collection point, 169 (68%) subjects remained in the study. By the time of the 10-year data collection point, 101 subjects were lost from the sample, leaving data from 148 (59%) subjects included in the final analysis. Significant differences between those subjects participating and not participating in the 10-year follow-up were reported for the important confounding variables (e.g., socioeconomic status and nature of home environment). The researchers stressed that their results were not generalizable to the population of lead exposed children; however, they speculated that the effects observed in their socially advantaged sample may be underestimated in populations of higher socioeconomic risk.

Cleveland Study. In a study conducted with children from inner-city Cleveland, Ernhart (1992a, 1992b); Ernhart et al. (1985); Ernhart et al. (1989); Ernhart et al. (1986); and Greene and Ernhart (1991, 1993) investigated the relationship between prenatal lead exposure and subse-

TABLE 4.1 Summary of Findings from Longitudinal Studies of Low-Level Lead Exposure

Mean PbB level of sample (μg/dL)	PbB measurement data points	Outcome measures	Developmental deficit size[a]	Sample site	References
6.5	Birth (cord blood)	N/A	N/A	Boston, MA	Bellinger et al. (1984a, 1984b, 1986, 1987, 1990)
6.7	6 months	BSID[b]	6 points		
7.7	12 moths	BSID	8 points		
7.8	18 months	BSID	Not reported		
6.5	24 months	BSID	4 points		
6.3	57 months	MISCA[c]	3 points		
2.9	10 years	WISC-R[d] KTEA[e]	6 points		
5.8	Birth (cord blood)	BNBAS[f]	Neurological Symptoms	Cleveland, OH	Ernhart et al. (1985, 1986, 1989); Ernhart (1992a, 1992b); Ernhart & Greene (1990); Greene & Ernhart (1991, 1993)
10.0	6 months	BSID			
N/A	12 months	BSID	None reported		
16.7	24 months	SBIS[g]	None		
16.7	36 months	WPPSI[h]	None		
N/A	58 months				
8.0	Prenatal (maternal)	N/A	N/A	Cincinnati, OH	Dietrich (1991); Dietrich et al. (1986, 1987, 1990, 1991, 1992, 1993a, 1993b)
6.2	3 months	BSID	Not reported		
N/A	6 month	BSID	8 points		

15.8	12 months	BSID	8 points		
17.5	24 months	BSID	None		
15.0	48 months	KABC[i]	2 points		
11.5	78 months	WISC-R	7 points		
9.1	Maternal (prenatal)	N/A	N/A	Sydney, Australia	Cooney et al. (1989)
8.1	Birth (cord blood)	N/A	N/A		
	6 months	BSID	None		
	12 months	BSID	None		
14.2	24 months	BSID	None		
10.1	36 months	MSCA	None		
14.0	Birth (cord blood)	BSID	2.0 points	Port Pirie, Australia	Vimpani et al. (1989); Wigg et al. (1988); McMichael et al. (1988); Baghurst, McMichael, et al. (1992); Baghurst, Tong, McMichael, Robertson, Wigg, & Vimpani (1992)
20.6	24 months	BSID	3.3 points		
18.8	36 months	BSID	4.4 points		
15.8	48 months	MSCA	7.2 points		
15.4	60 months	MSCA	5.3 points		
12.6	84 months	WISC-R	Not reported		

[a]Deficit per 10 μg/dL PbB. [b]Bayley Scales of Infant Development (1969). [c]McCarthy Scales of Children's Abilities (1972). [d]Wechsler Intelligence Scale for Children-Revised (1974). [e]Kaufman Test of Educational Achievement (1985). [f]Brazelton Neonatal Behavior Assessment Scales (1984). [g]Stanford-Binet Intelligence Scale (1973). [h]Wechsler Preschool and Primary Scale of Intelligence (1967). [i]Kaufman Assessment Battery for Children (1983).

CARL A. RUDISILL LIBRARY
LENOIR-RHYNE COLLEGE

quent infant/child development. Umbilical cord and maternal blood samples were obtained at delivery for 162 infants and 185 mothers to determine prenatal lead exposure. Using the Brazelton Neonatal Behavior Assessment Scale (Brazelton, 1984), infants were evaluated by examiners blinded to subjects' lead levels. Results indicated that abnormal reflexes, decreased muscle tone, and the presence of neurological soft signs (e.g., clumsiness, distractibility, irritability, etc.) were all associated with elevated infant lead levels.

Further analysis of this cohort at 12 months of age revealed significant differences in scores on the mental development index of the BSID between infants identified as low level, lead exposed and infants who were high level, lead exposed. However, no significant differences were detected at 24, 36, and 58 months of age (Ernhart et al., 1989; Greene & Ernhart, 1991). Interpretation of these studies is complicated somewhat by the sampling method used. The lead studies were conducted on a subset from a larger sample of women and children who were participating in a study of fetal alcohol exposure. Maternal alcohol use, measured by two different indexes, was statistically controlled for in the data analyses; however, most of the sample was prenatally exposed to the well-known neurobehavioral teratogen of alcohol. Sample selection bias in this study was not adequately addressed, nor were the generalizations of the study findings to the population of lead-exposed children justified. Furthermore, the study lacked adequate statistical power (.32) to detect a small effect.

Cincinnati Study. Another major prospective study has been conducted by Dietrich (1991); Dietrich, Berger, and Succop (1993); Dietrich, Berger, Succop, Hammond, and Bornschein (1993); Dietrich et al. (1986, 1987, 1990); Dietrich, Succop, Berger, Hammond, and Bornschein (1991); and Dietrich, Succop, Berger, and Keith (1992) among socioeconomically disadvantaged children in Cincinnati. These researchers measured blood lead levels (mean = 8.0 μg/dL) of 305 pregnant women during their first prenatal visit. The infants ($N = 280$) of these mothers had blood lead levels drawn on day 10 of life (mean = 4.5 μg/dL). Adjusting for covariates, such as maternal alcohol and tobacco use, the quality of the home environment, and socioeconomic status, the researchers, using regression analyses, found that prenatal lead levels were significantly inversely associated with male infants' scores on the BSID at 6 and 12 months of age. Furthermore, prenatal lead exposure was significantly related to lower gestational age and lower birthweight.

Prenatal lead exposure accounted for an 8-point deficit in the infants' BSID performance for every 10 μg/dL increase in PbB (Dietrich et

CARL A. RUDISILL LIBRARY
LENOIR-RHYNE COLLEGE

al., 1990). Because this relationship was demonstrated only in male infants, Dietrich et al. (1990) postulated that gender may be a significant modifier of the association between lead and infants' cognition. A similar finding has been reported by a group of researchers in Great Britain who reanalyzed data from a cross-sectional study conducted in Southampton (Smith, Delves, Lansdown, Clayton, & Graham, 1983), which examined the relationship between dentine lead levels and IQ in 6-year-olds (Pocock et al., 1987). These researchers found that in males, tooth lead levels were significantly inversely related to IQ level (a decline of 3 IQ points for each log unit increase in dentine lead), but in females, the relationship was nonsignificant.

In the Cincinnati cohort, postneonatal blood lead levels obtained from venous or capillary samples were not significantly associated with mental development of the infants at 3, 6, and 12 months of age (Dietrich et al., 1990). These results are consistent with those of Bellinger et al. (1984b) and demonstrate that prenatal rather than postnatal lead exposure had a significant influence on neurodevelopmental performance in young infants. However, Dietrich et al. (1991) also found that postnatal PbB levels were significantly and inversely related to the mental processing, simultaneous processing, and nonverbal standard scores on the Kaufman Assessment Battery for Children (Kaufman & Kaufman, 1983) at 48 months. At 6 years of age, this pattern was repeated. Postnatal PbB levels were inversely associated with full-scale IQ and performance IQ as measured by the Wechsler Intelligence Scale for Children–Revised (Wechsler, 1974). The study design would have been strengthened if only venous blood samples were obtained from subjects. It is well documented that procedures used to collect capillary samples introduce lead contaminants into the specimens, thus resulting in higher measurements of lead (CDC, 1991).

Researchers from the Cincinnati study investigated not only cognitive performance of cohort children but also neuromuscular performance. They hypothesized that measures of motor development would be less confounded by social and familial factors and, therefore, would be more sensitive indicators of the effect of lead on the developing central nervous system of children (Dietrich, Berger, & Succop, 1993). Results of evaluations at 6 years of age revealed that postnatal PbB concentrations were negatively associated with some elements of gross motor, fine motor, and visual-motor scales. These findings led the researchers to conclude that motor development as well as cognitive development are significantly impaired by prenatal and postnatal exposure to lead.

Sydney Study. Cooney, Bell, McBride, and Carter (1989) examined a cohort of 318 children in Sydney, Australia. In an attempt to control for confounding variables and to obtain a fairly homogenous sample, all healthy full-term babies born in 1982 to 1983 to married, English-speaking, and nonsubstance-abusing mothers from three maternity hospitals in Sydney were enrolled in the study. Maternal PbB levels were obtained just before birth, and cord PbB samples were obtained from infants during delivery; other blood samples were obtained from the infants every 6 months to age 4, and again at age 5. Neurobehavioral measures used to assess infant and child development included the BSID at 6, 12, and 24 months (Bayley, 1969), and the McCarthy Scales of Children's Abilities (1972) at 36 months. All assessments of subjects' development were obtained by psychologists who were blinded to PbB levels and developmental information on the subjects. Relationships between PbB levels and outcome measures were investigated by a series of multiple regressions using appropriate covariates and path analysis. At 6, 12, 24, and 36 months there was no significant relationship between cord PbB and neurobehavioral development. Therefore, the data were reanalyzed using the analysis scheme employed by Bellinger et al. (1986, 1987); subjects were divided into three groups, based on their PbB levels (low = 0–3 μg/dL; moderate = 4–9 μg/dL; high = 10–28 μg/dL), and group differences on the outcome variables were examined. Again, no statistically significant differences were found. Subject mortality was minimal in this study; attrition of only 19 subjects occurred during the first 3 years of the study. However, the validity of the findings is questionable given the sampling method, the design of the research instruments, and the data analysis techniques used. The researchers used self-report measures to determine substance abuse and excluded from the sample those individuals who responded positively to a question about drug use. Yet, 77% of the participating mothers consumed alcohol during their pregnancies, and 21% smoked (the quantities are unknown because the questions asked about alcohol and cigarette consumption were dichotomous and coded as 1 = yes, 2 = no). The researchers report the means of these categorical variables and entered them as coded into the regression equations.

Port Pirie Study. Begun in 1979, the Port Pirie cohort study followed an original sample of 723 infants, born in the lead-smelting community of Port Pirie, Australia, from birth to age 7 (Baghurst, McMichael et al., 1992; Baghurst, Tong et al., 1992; McMichael, Baghurst, & Wigg, 1988; Vimpani et al., 1989; Wigg et al., 1988), and investigated the relationship between early lead exposure and neurobehavioral development. The researchers determined lead exposure through lead levels obtained from venous antenatal (maternal), umbilical cord, and capillary blood samples. Both venous and capillary samples were used based on the results of a pilot study conducted with 147 subjects, where high correlations ($r = 0.97$) were found between PbB levels obtained from venous and capillary routes. To control for lead contamination of capillary samples, data collectors followed a strict protocol; however, the researchers do not report if reliability in using the protocol was calculated, nor do they report inter-rater reliability for the four data collectors. These are important research design issues, especially because the study period extended over 7 years. Developmental assessments using age appropriate, valid and reliable instruments (e.g., BSID, McCarthy Scales of Children's Abilities [MSCA], and Wechsler's Intelligence Scale for Children [WISC]) were conducted by a psychologist who was blinded to subjects' lead level information.

Over the course of the 7-year study, 207 (29%) subjects were lost to follow-up. The researchers reported that there were no differences in mean umbilical cord blood lead levels between those lost to follow-up and those who remained in the study. However, on several confounding variables, the two groups differed significantly.

PbB concentrations for the 516 remaining subjects ranged from 4.3 μg/dL to 34.4 μg/dL (low to moderate range) over the course of the 7 years. The PbB levels were highest at age 24 months; by the age of 7, the mean PbB level showed about a 40% decrease (Baghurst, McMichael et al., 1992).

Multiple regression analyses revealed that lead exposure was significantly related to decreased scores on the BSID (Bayley, 1969), as well as on the MSCA (McCarthy, 1972) and WISC (Wechsler, 1974). At 24 months, scores on the BSID dropped about 2 points for every 10 μg/dL increase in PbB level, which is consistent with findings from the studies conducted in Cincinnati and Boston. In simple regression analyses, all measures of PbB levels (antenatal, cord, and postnatal) were negatively associated with the outcome measures at 24, 48, 60, and 84 months. The strongest lead effect was observed when postnatal PbB concentrations, rather than antenatal or cord blood concentrations, were used in the multiple regression analyses. A shortcoming of this study was the use of 13 covariates in the multiple regression analyses. The use of numerous covariates may result in overcontrolling for the effect of lead and thus removing variance that belongs to the lead effect. Therefore, one could postulate that the lead effect demonstrated was underestimated.

In summary, the longitudinal studies reviewed here are fairly consistent in demonstrating an association between early childhood low-level lead exposure and later neurodevelopmental performance, as reflected in deficits on several neurobehavioral measurements. To demonstrate this relationship, researchers have performed extensive regression analyses with large samples and controlled for known confounding variables. The studies generally suggest that two critical points of exposure occur: one in the prenatal period, the effects of which are seen in early infant development; and the second during the first 24 months of life, the effects of which are observed in later childhood.

Lead effects have been demonstrated to be approximately 4 to 6 points (Baghurst, McMichael et al., 1992; Bellinger et al., 1986, 1990; Dietrich, 1991; Dietrich, Berger, & Succop, 1993; Dietrich et al., 1991; Dietrich et al., 1992; Needleman & Gatsonis, 1990). That is, for every 10 μg/dL increase in PbB, IQ level is likely to decrease 4 to 6 points. Some researchers may believe this effect size to be insignificant or minimal; however, Needleman and Bellinger (1991) have determined that this effect predicts a fourfold increase in the proportion of impaired children (i.e., IQ < 80). The effects of lead exposure, specifically decreased neurobehavioral functioning, are most probably permanent and are likely to be predictors of life success (Needleman & Bellinger, 1991).

RESEARCH DIRECTIONS

Although there are an impressive number of studies conducted on the neurodevelopmental effects of childhood low-level lead exposure, questions about the effects of lead exposure remain. For the most part, the longitudinal studies that have been conducted have focused on young children, although within the last 5 years, in utero lead exposure also has been measured. It is clear that the fetus is not immune to the effects of maternal lead exposure; lead easily crosses the placenta (Silbergeld, 1986, 1991). Researchers have speculated that because mobilization of lead from the long-term storage site of bone occurs during periods of altered mineral metabolism (specifically calcium metabolism), pregnancy, and lactation may precipitate toxic consequences for mothers and their developing fetuses (Borella, Picco, & Masellis, 1986; Thompson et al., 1985). Little attention has been paid to this, and it is clear that studies are needed to investigate the relationship between maternal bone lead levels, maternal blood lead levels, and fetal and infant development. Furthermore, researchers have not studied the relationship between paternal lead exposure and fetal/infant development, despite the evidence from animal studies that lead is a gametotoxin and, therefore, influences male reproductive function (Needleman & Bellinger, 1991).

The association of childhood lead exposure with intelligence has been the central issue of most investigations. Few researchers have studied the relationship of lead exposure to other psychosocial behaviors, such as aggressiveness and sociability. However, there is a growing body of evidence that deficits in attention and increased aggressiveness are associated with childhood lead exposure (Lansdown et al., 1986; Needleman et al., 1979); interestingly, these same attributes are strongly associated with antisocial behavior (Magnusson, Stottin, & Duner, 1983). Antisocial behavior also is associated with other factors that are related to lead exposure. For instance, the highest prevalence of PbB levels above the accepted criterion level of 10 μg/dL are found among inner-city, low-income children living in dilapidated housing (Crocetti, Mushak, & Schwartz, 1990). Epidemiological data reveal that antisocial behavior occurs most often among urban, poor individuals; criminals are more likely to have grown up in urban, low-income areas, and when young, to have had a history of developmental problems (Wilson & Herrnstein, 1985). Longitudinal, prospective, well-designed studies that control extraneous variables are required to investigate the relationship between childhood lead exposure and antisocial behavior.

Another area on which research efforts could focus is identifying mediators of lead exposure effects. More than 3 million children in the United States have blood lead levels high enough to affect their neurological and behavioral development (EPA, 1992), yet not all of these children develop neurobehavioral deficits. Are there socioenvironmental and physiological factors that modify lead-induced effects in children, or that protect some children from the effects of lead? Again, large-scale longitudinal prospective studies that control for confounding variables are needed to answer this question.

Few studies have investigated the effects of lowering PbB levels on the neurobehavioral outcomes of children with asymptomatic lead toxicity. Some animal studies suggest that performance deficits continue, despite pharmacological intervention (e.g., chelation) to decrease elevated lead levels (EPA, 1986). However, in a recent study, researchers have demonstrated long-term (6 months) positive changes in neurobehavioral performance in children who have received pharmacological and environmental (e.g., lead abatement of dwelling) interventions for elevated PbB (Ruff, Bijur, Markowitz, Ma, & Rosen, 1993). This suggests that lead associated cognitive deficits may be attenuated when exposure ends and blood lead levels decrease. More longitudinal studies are needed to investigate this.

Other needed studies could investigate if the current recommendations for decreasing lead in the child's environment proposed by the CDC (1991) will decrease PbB levels in children with low-level exposure

(PbB 10 to 20 μg/dL). Researchers have demonstrated that PbB in children with moderately elevated levels can be reduced by environmental interventions like controlling house dust (Charney, Kessler, Farfel, & Jackson, 1983; Kimbrough, LeVois, & Webb, 1994); however, no research has been conducted to see if this relationship exists in children with low-level exposure. Furthermore, future studies could be designed to investigate the effect of providing educational materials about reducing environmental lead exposure to families of low-level–exposed children.

Lead remains a significant hazard to the health of infants and children in this country. Data documenting the neurotoxicity of lead are abundant, yet many questions remain about the interaction of lead with such major functions as growth, development, and reproduction. Until these questions are answered, lead toxicity will continue to be a controversial health problem.

ACKNOWLEDGMENT

The author wishes to express appreciation to Elizabeth Tornquist for reviewing an early draft of this manuscript.

REFERENCES

Achenbach, T. M. (1986). *Manual for the Child Behavior Checklist*. Burlington, VT: University of Vermont Department of Psychiatry.

Agency for Toxic Substances and Disease Registry. (1988). *The nature and extent of lead poisoning in children in the United States: A report to congress*. Atlanta: Centers for Disease Control.

American Academy of Pediatrics. (1987). Statement on childhood lead poisoning. *Pediatrics, 79*, 457–465.

American Academy of Pediatrics. (1993). Lead poisoning: From screening to primary prevention (AAP policy summary). *AAP News, 9*, 9.

Annest, J. L., Pirkle, J. L., & Makuc, D. (1983). Chronological trend in blood-lead levels between 1976-1980. *New England Journal of Medicine, 308*, 1373–1376.

Baghurst, P. A., McMichael, A. J., Wigg, N. R., Vimpani, G. V., Robertson, E. F., Roberts, R. J., & Tong, S. (1992). Environmental exposure to lead and children's intelligence at the age of seven years: The Port Pirie cohort study. *New England Journal of Medicine, 327*, 1279–1284.

Baghurst, P. A., Tong, S. L., McMichael, A. J., Robertson, E. F., Wigg, N. R., & Vimpani, G. V. (1992). Determinants of blood lead concentrations to age 5 years in a big cohort study of children living in the lead smelting city of Port Pirie and surrounding areas. *Archives of Environmental Health, 47*, 203–210.

Bayley, N. (1969). *Bayley Scales of Infant Development*. New York: Psychological Corporation.

Bellinger, D., Leviton, A., Needleman, H. L., Waternaux, C., & Rabinowitz, M. (1986). Low-level lead exposure and infant development in the first year. *Neurobehavior, Toxicology, & Teratology, 8*, 151–161.

Bellinger, D., Leviton, A., & Sloman, J. (1990). Antecedents and correlates of improved cognitive performance in children exposed in utero to low levels of lead. *Environmental Health Perspectives, 89*, 5–11.

Bellinger, D., Leviton, A., & Waternaux, C. (1987). Longitudinal analysis of prenatal lead exposure and early cognitive development. *New England Journal of Medicine, 316*, 1037–1043.

Bellinger, D., & Needleman, H. L. (1992). Neurodevelopmental effects of low-level lead exposure in children. In H. L. Needleman (Ed.), *Human lead exposure* (pp. 191–208). Boca Raton, FL: CRC Press.

Bellinger, D., Needleman, H. L., Bromfield, R., & Mintz, M. (1984a). A follow-up study of the academic attainment and classroom behavior of children with elevated dentine lead levels. *Biology and Trace Elements Research, 6*, 207–223.

Bellinger, D., Needleman, H. L., Leviton, A., Waternaux, C., Rabinowitz, M. B., & Nichols, M. L. (1984b). Early sensory-motor development and prenatal exposure to lead. *Neurobehavior, Toxicology & Teratology, 6*, 387–402.

Bellinger, D., Stiles, K. M., & Needleman, H. L. (1992). Low-level lead exposure, intelligence, and academic achievement: A long-term follow-up study. *Pediatrics, 90*, 855–861.

Borella, P. Picco, P., & Masellis, G. (1986). Lead content in abortion material from urban women in early pregnancy. *International Archives of Occupational and Environmental Health, 57*, 93–99.

Brazelton, T. B. (1984). *Neonatal Behavior Assessment Scale*. Philadelphia, PA: Lippincott.

Byers, R. K., & Lord, E. E. (1943). Late effects of lead poisoning on mental development. *American Journal of Diseases in Children, 66*, 471–483.

Centers for Disease Control. (1991). *Preventing lead poisoning in young children: A statement from the Centers for Disease Control*. Atlanta, GA: Author.

Centers for Disease Control. (1992). Surveillance of children's blood lead-levels—United States, 1991. *Morbidity & Mortality Weekly Report, 41*, 620–622.

Charney, E., Kessler, B., Farfel, M., & Jackson, D. (1983). Childhood lead poisoning: A controlled trial on the effect of dust-control measures on blood lead levels. *New England Journal of Medicine, 309*, 1093–1098.

Chisolm, J. J. (1971). Lead poisoning. *Scientific American, 224*, 15–25.

Chisolm, J. J., & Harrison, H. E. (1956). The exposure of children to lead. *Pediatrics, 18*, 934–955.

Cooney, G. H., Bell, A., McBride, W., & Carter, C. (1989). Neurobehavioral consequences of prenatal low level exposure to lead. *Neurotoxicology and Teratology, 11*, 95–104.

Crocetti, A. F., Mushak, P., & Schwartz, J. (1990). Determination of numbers of lead-exposed U.S. children by areas of the United States: An integrated summary of a report to the U.S. Congress on childhood lead poisoning. *Environmental Health Perspectives, 89*, 109–120.

Damm, D., Grandjean, P., Lyngbye, T., Trillingsgaard, A., & Hansen, O. N. (1993). Early lead exposure and neonatal jaundice: Relation to neurobehavioral performance at 15 years of age. *Neurotoxicology and Teratology, 15*, 173–181.

David, O., Clark, J., & Voeller, K. (1972). Lead and hyperactivity. *Lancet, 2*, 900–903.

David, O., Hoffman, S. P., Sverd, J., Clark, J., & Voeller, K. (1976). Lead and hyperactivity. Behavioral response to chelation: A pilot study. *American Journal of Psychiatry, 113*, 1155–1158.

Dietrich, K. N. (1991). Human fetal lead exposure: Intrauterine growth, maturation, and postnatal neurobehavioral development. *Fundamental and Applied Toxicology, 16*, 17–19.

Dietrich, K. N., Berger, O. G., & Succop, P. A., (1993a). Lead exposure and the motor developmental status of urban six-year-old children in the Cincinnati Prospective Study. *Pediatrics, 91*, 301–307.

Dietrich, K. N., Berger, O. G., Succop, P. A., Hammond, P. B., & Bornschein, R. L. (1993b). The developmental consequences of low to moderate prenatal and postnatal lead exposure: Intellectual attainment in the Cincinnati Lead Study Cohort following school entry. *Neurotoxicology and Teratology, 15*, 37–44.

Dietrich, K. N., Kraft, K. M., Bier, M., Succop, P. A., Berger, O., & Bornschein, R. L. (1986). Early effects of fetal lead exposure: Neurobehavioral findings at 6 months. *International Journal of Biosocial Research, 8*, 151–168.

Dietrich, K. N., Krafft, K. M., Bornschein, R. L., Hammond, P. B., Berger, O., Succop, P. A., & Bier, M. (1987). Effects of low-level fetal lead exposure on neurobehavioral development in early infancy. *Pediatrics, 80*, 721–730.

Dietrich, K. N., Succop, P. A., Berger, O. G., Hammond, P. B., & Bornschein, R. L. (1991). Lead exposure and the cognitive development of urban preschool children: The Cincinnati Lead Study cohort at age 4 years. *Neurotoxicology and Teratology, 13*, 203–211.

Dietrich, K. N., Succop, P. A., Berger, O. G., & Keith, R. W. (1992). Lead exposure and the central auditory processing abilities and cognitive development of urban children: The Cincinnati Lead Study cohort at age 5 year. *Neurotoxicology and Teratology, 14*, 51–56.

Dietrich, K. N., Succop, P. A., Bornschein, R. L., Krafft, K. M., Berger, O. G., Hammond, P. B., & Buncher, C. R. (1990). Lead exposure and neurobehavioral development in later infancy. *Environmental Health Perspectives, 89*, 13–19.

Environmental Protection Agency. (1986). *Air quality criteria for lead*. Research Triangle Park, NC: Author.

Environmental Protection Agency. (1987). *Reducing lead in drinking water: A benefit analysis*. Research Triangle Park, NC: Author.

Environmental Protection Agency. (1992). *Strategies for reducing lead exposures*. Washington, DC: Author.

Ernhart, C. B. (1992a). A critical review of low-level prenatal lead exposure in the human: 1. Effects on the fetus and newborn. *Reproductive Toxicology, 6*, 9–19.

Ernhart, C. B. (1992b). A critical review of low-level prenatal lead exposure in the human: 2. Effects in the developing child. *Reproductive Toxicology, 6*, 21–40.

Ernhart, C. B., & Greene, T. (1990). Low-level lead exposure in the prenatal and early preschool periods: Language development. *Archives of Environmental Health, 45*, 342–354.

Ernhart, C. B., Landa, B., & Wolf, A. W. (1985). Subclinical lead level and developmental deficit: Reanalysis of data. *Journal of Learning Disabilities, 18*, 475–479.

Ernhart, C. B., Morrow-Tlucak, M., Wolf, A. W., Super, D., & Drotar, D. (1989). Low level lead exposure in the prenatal and early preschool periods: Intelligence prior to school entry. *Neurotoxicology and Teratology, 11*, 161–170.

Ernhart, C. B., Wolf, A. W., Kennard, M. J., Erhard, P., Filipovich, H. F., & Sokol, R. J. (1986). Intrauterine exposure to low levels of lead: The status of the neonate. *Archives of Environmental Health, 41*, 287–291.

Fergusson, D. M., Fergusson, J. E., Horwood, L. J., & Kinzett, N. G. (1988). A longitudinal study of dentine lead levels, intelligence, school performance and behavior: 3. Dentine lead levels and cognitive ability. *Journal of Child Psychology and Psychiatry, 29*, 793–809.

Fulton, M., Raab, G., Thomson, G., Laxen, D., Hunter, R., & Hepburn, W. (1987). Influence of blood lead on the ability and attainment of children in Edinburgh. *Lancet, 101*, 1221–1226.

Gatsonis, C. A., & Needleman, H. L. (1992). Recent epidemiologic studies of low-level lead exposure and the IQ of children: A meta-analytic review. In H. L. Needleman (Ed.), *Human lead exposure* (pp. 243–255). Boca Raton, FL: CRC Press.

Gibson, J. L. (1904). A plea for painted railings and painted walls of rooms as the source of lead poisoning among Queensland children. *Australia Medical Gazette, 23*, 149–153.

Gibson, J. L., Love, W., Hardie, D., Bancroft, P., & Turner, A. J. (1892). Notes on lead poisoning as observed among children in Brisbane. In L. Huxtable (Ed.), *Transactions from the Third Intercolonial Medical Congress of Australasia* (pp. 76–77). Sydney: Charles Potter.

Greene, T., & Ernhart, C. B. (1991). Prenatal and preschool age lead exposure: Relationship with size. *Neurotoxicology and Teratology, 13*, 417–427.

Greene, T., & Ernhart, C. B. (1993). Dentine lead and intelligence prior to school entry: A statistical sensitivity analysis. *Journal of Clinical Epidemiology, 46*, 323–339.

Hansen, O. N., Trillingsgaard, A., Beese, I., Lyngbye, T., & Grandjean, P. (1989). Neuropsychological study of children with elevated dentine lead level. *Neurotoxicology and Teratology, 11*, 205–213.

Hatzakis, A., Kokevi, A., & Katsouyanni, K. (1987). Psychometric intelligence and attentional performance deficits in lead exposed children. *International Conference on Heavy Metals in the Environment* (pp. 204–205). Edinburgh, UK: CEP Consultants.

Hayes, E. B., McElvaine, M. D., Orbach, H. G., Fernandez, A. M., Lyne, S., & Matte, T. D. (1994). Long-term trends in blood lead levels among children in Chicago: Relationship to air levels. *Pediatrics, 93*, 195–200.

Hedges, L V., & Okin, I. (1985). *Statistical methods for meta-analysis*. Orlando, FL: Academic Press.

Jelinek, C. F. (1982). Level of lead in the United States food supply. *Journal of the Association of Analytic Chemistry, 65*, 942–947.

Kaufman, A. S., & Kaufman, N. L. (1983). *Kaufman Assessment Battery for Children*. Circle Pines, MN: American Guidance Service.

Kaufman, A. S., & Kaufman, N. L. (1985). *Kaufman Test of Educational Achievement: Brief form Manual*. Circle Pines, MN: American Guidance Service.

Kimbrough, R. D., LeVois, M., & Webb, D. R. (1994). Management of children with slightly elevated blood lead levels. *Pediatrics, 93*, 188–191.

Lamm, S. H., & Rosen, J. F. (1974). Lead contamination in milk fed infants. *Pediatrics, 53*, 137–139.

Landrigan, P. J., Baker, E. L., & Himmelstein, J. S. (1982). Exposure to lead from the Mystic river bridge: The dilemma of deleading. *New England Journal of Medicine, 306*, 673–676.

Lansdown, R., Yule, W., Urbanowicz, M. A., & Hunter, J. (1986). The relationship between blood-lead concentrations, intelligence, attainment and behavior in a school population the second London study. *International Archives of Occupational and Environmental Health, 57*, 225–235.

Lin-Fu, J. S. (1992). Modern history of lead poisoning: A century of discovery and rediscovery. In H. L. Needleman (Ed.), *Human lead exposure* (pp. 23–43). Boca Raton, FL: CRC Press.

Lyngbye, T., Hansen, O. N., & Grandjean, P. (1989). Neurological deficits in children, medical risk factors and lead exposure. *Neurotoxicology and Teratology, 10*, 531–537.

Lyngbye, T., Hansen, O. N., & Grandjean, R. (1991). Low level lead absorption and neonatal jaundice: A synergistic effect? *Neurotoxicology, 12*, 810–815.

Magnusson, D., Stottin, H., & Duner, A. (1983). Aggression and criminality in a longitudinal perspectives. In K. T. VanDusen & S. A. Mednick (Eds.), *Antecedents of aggression and antisocial behavior* (pp. 210–219). Boston: Kluwer-Hijhoff.

Mahaffey, K. R. (1990). Environmental lead toxicity: Nutrition as a component of intervention. *Environmental Health Perspectives, 89*, 75–78.

McCarthy, D. (1972). *The McCarthy Scales of Children's Abilities*. New York: Psychological Corporation.

McKhann, C. F. (1933). Lead poisoning in children. *Journal of the American Medical Association, 101*, 1131–1135.

McLaughlin, M. C. (1956). Lead poisoning in children in New York City, 1950–1954: An epidemiologic study. *New York State Journal of Medicine, 56*, 3711–3714.

McMichael, A., Baghurst, P. A., & Wigg, N. R. (1988). Port Pirie cohort study: Environmental exposure to lead and children's abilities at the age of four years. *New England Journal of Medicine, 319*, 468–475.

Mitchell, D. G., & Aldous, K. M. (1979). Lead content of foodstuffs. *Environmental Health Perspectives, 7*, 59–65.

Moore, M. R. (1980). Lead in humans, In R. Lansdown & W. Yule (Eds.), *Lead toxicity: History and environmental impact* (pp. 54–95). Baltimore, MD: The Johns Hopkins University Press.

Mushak,P. (1992a). Defining lead as the premiere environmental health issue for children in America: Criteria and their quantitative application. *Environmental Research, 59*, 281–309.

Mushak, P. (1992b). The monitoring of human lead exposure. In H. L. Needleman (Ed.), *Human lead exposure* (pp. 45–64). Boca Raton, FL: CRC Press.

Needleman, H. L., & Bellinger, D. (1991). The health effects of low level exposure to lead. *Annual Review of Public Health, 12*, 111–140.

Needleman, H. L., & Gatsonis, C. A. (1990). Low level lead exposure and the IQ of children: A meta analysis of modern studies. *Journal of the American Medical Association, 263*, 673–678.

Needleman, H. L., Geiger, S. K., & Frank, R. (1985). Lead and IQ scores: A reanalysis. *Science, 227*, 701–704.

Needleman, H. L., Gunnoe, C., Leviton, A., Reed, R., Peresie, H., Maher, C., & Barrett, P. (1979). Deficits in psychologic and classroom performance of children and elevated dentine lead levels. *New England Journal of Medicine, 300*, 689–695.

Needleman, H. L., Schell, A., Bellinger, D., Leviton, A., & Allred, E. N. (1990). The long-term effects of exposure to low doses of lead in childhood: An 11 year follow-up report. *New England Journal of Medicine, 322*, 83–88.

Paterson, L. J., Raab, G. M., Hunter, R., Laxen, D. P. H., Fulton, M., Fell, G. S., Halls, D. J., & Sutcliffe, P. (1988). Factors influencing lead concentrations in shed deciduous teeth. *Science and the Total Environment, 74*, 219–224.

Perlstein, M. A., & Attala, R. (1966). Neurological sequelae of plumbism in children. *Clinical Pediatrics, 5*, 292–298.

Piomelli, S., Rosen, J. F., Chisolm, J. J., & Graef, J. W. (1984). Management of childhood lead poisoning. *Journal of Pediatrics, 105*, 523–531.

Pocock, S. J., Ashby, D., & Smith, V. (1987). Lead exposure and children's intelligence. *International Journal of Epidemiology, 16*, 57–67.

Rabin, R. (1989). Warnings unheeded: A history of child lead poisoning. *American Journal of Public Health, 79*, 1668–1674.

Rabinowitz, M. B., & Needleman, H. L. (1982). Temporal trends in the lead concentrations of umbilical cord blood. *Science, 216*, 1429–1431.

Rosenthal, R. (1984). *Meta-analytical procedures for social research*. Beverly Hills, CA: Sage.

Ruff, H. A., & Bijur, P. E. (1989). The effects of low to moderate lead levels on neurobehavioral functioning in children: Toward a conceptual model. *Journal of Developmental & Behavioral Pediatrics, 10*, 103–109.

Ruff, H. A., Bijur, P. E., Markowitz, M., Ma, Y. C., & Rosen, J. F. (1993). Declining blood lead levels and cognitive changes in moderately lead poisoned children. *Journal of the American Medical Association, 269*, 1641–1646.

Scanlon, J. (1971). Umbilical cord blood lead concentration: Relationship to urban or suburban residency during gestation. *American Journal of Diseases of Children, 121*, 325–326.

Schroeder, S. R., Hawk, B., Otto, D. A., Mushak, P., & Hicks, R. E. (1985). Separating the effects of lead and social factors on IQ. *Environmental Research, 91*, 178–183.

Sciarillo, W. G., Alexander, G., & Farrell, K. P. (1992). Lead exposure and child behavior. *American Journal of Public Health, 82*, 1356–1360.

Silbergeld, E. K. (1986). Maternally mediated exposure of the fetus: In utero exposure to lead and other toxins. *Neurotoxicology, 7*, 557–568.

Silbergeld, E. K. (1991). Lead in bones: Implications for toxicology during pregnancy and lactation. *Environmental Health Perspectives, 91*, 63–70.

Smith, M., Delves, T., Lansdown, R., Clayton, B., & Graham, P. (1983). The effects of lead exposure on urban children: The Institute of Child Health/Southampton study. *Developmental Medicine and Child Neurology, 25*(Suppl)., 47, 1–54.

Terman, L. M., & Merrill, M. A. (1973). *Stanford-Binet intelligence scale*. Boston: Houghton Mifflin.

Thurston, D. L., Middlekamp, J. N., & Mason, E. (1955). The late effects of lead poisoning. *Journal of Pediatrics, 47*, 413–423.

Thompson, G. N., Robertson, E. F., & Fitzgerald, S. (1985). Lead mobilization during pregnancy. *Medical Journal of Australia, 143*, 131–136.

Vimpani, G. V., Wigg, N. R., Robertson, E. F., McMichael, A. J., Baghurst, P. A., & Roberts, R. R. (1989). The Port Pirie cohort study: Cumulative lead exposure and neurodevelopmental status at age 2 years: Do HOME scores and maternal IQ reduce apparent effects of lead on Bayley mental scores? In M. Smith, L. Grant, & A. Sors (Eds.), *Lead exposure and children development: An international assessment* (pp. 161–178). Lancaster, UK: MTP Press.

Ward, N. I., Watson, R, & Bryce-Smith, D. (1987). Placental element levels in relation to fetal development for obstetrically normal births: A study of 37 elements. Evidence for the effects of cadmium, lead, and zinc on fetal growth, and for smoking as a source of cadmium. *International Journal of Biology Research, 9*, 63–81.

Wechsler, D. (1967). *Wechsler Preschool and Primary Scale of Intelligence*. New York: Psychological Corporation.

Wechsler, D. (1974). *Wechsler Intelligence Scale for Children—revised: A manual*. San Antonio: Psychological Corporation.

Wigg, N. R., Vimpani, G. V., McMichael, A. J., Baghurst, P. A., Robertson, E. F., & Roberts, R. J. (1988). Port Pirie cohort study: Childhood blood lead and neuropsychological development at age two years. *Journal of Epidemiologic and Community Health, 42*, 213–219.

Wilson, J., & Herrnstein, R. (1985). *Crime and human behavior*. New York: Simon & Schuster.

Winneke, G., Kramer, G., Brockhaus, A., Ewers, U., Kujanaek, G., Lechner, H., & Janke, W. (1983). Neuropsychological studies in children with elevated tooth lead concentration. *International Archives of Occupational and Environmental Health, 51*, 213–252.

Yule, W., & Lansdown, R. (1983). Lead and children's development: Recent findings. *International Conference: Heavy Metals in the Environment* (Vol. 2). Edinburgh, UK: CEP Consultants.

Yule, W., Lansdown, R., Millar, I., & Urbanowicz, M. (1981). The relationship between blood lead concentration, intelligence, and attainment in a school population: A pilot study. *Developmental Medicine and Child Neurology, 23*, 567–576.

PART II

Research on Nursing Care Delivery

Chapter 5

Case Management

Gerri S. Lamb
Carondelet St. Mary's Hospital

CONTENTS

For the past three decades, case management has been practiced by numerous professions with a variety of target populations, including individuals with chronic mental or physical illnesses, technology-dependent children and adults, and persons with catastrophic illnesses like cancer and AIDS. With the advent of managed care and the movement toward health care reform, the literature on case management has grown exponentially. The nursing profession, in particular, has taken a leadership role in the development of new models of case management; much of the descriptive literature has included the experience of nurses who are assuming case management roles in health care and workplace settings.

This chapter focuses on the evolution of nursing case management and examines (a) case management research conducted by health services researchers (outside the discipline of nursing) and its lessons for nursing case management; (b) the current state of nurse-conducted case management research; (c) gaps in knowledge; and (d) research priorities to advance the body of knowledge and justify the use of nurses as case managers in a restructured health care system. This review was limited to an analysis of the empirical literature on case management. Searches of CINAHL, MEDLINE, PsycInfo, and Sociofile databases for the years of 1984 to mid-1994 using the key word, case management, and other text word strategies, yielded several hundred references. Nonempirical anecdotal and narrative descriptions of case management practice were not systematically analyzed for this review. However, it is important to note that this extensive body of literature is a significant resource for explicating the processes and outcomes of nurse case management. In addition theses and dissertations about case management were not included.

HISTORY OF CASE MANAGEMENT RESEARCH

Contrary to popular belief, case management research did not begin with the advent of current nursing practice models. The history of case management research is extensive and rich with results of descriptive and experimental studies conducted in the fields of behavioral health, social work, and health services research beginning in the late 1970s and continuing to the present (Chamberlain & Rapp, 1991; Rubin, 1992). In the long-term care demonstrations of the late 1970s and 1980s, investigators used case management as a key intervention strategy to improve quality and cost outcomes for high-risk older adults in the community (Capitman, Haskins, & Bernstein, 1986; Kemper, Applebaum, & Harrigan, 1987). More recently, participants in the social health maintenance organization (S/HMO) demonstrations have published research exploring key processes of case management practice as they have attempted to create an integrated acute and long-term care system for Medicare beneficiaries (Abrahams, Capitman, Leutz, & Macko, 1989; Leutz, Abrahams, Greenlick, Kane, & Prottas, 1988).

Although current nurse case management models did not evolve directly from these earlier experiments with case management, the knowledge accumulated through these studies provides critical lessons for nursing research today. The following discussion summarizes the body of case management research outside of nursing science and highlights conclusions and recommendations relevant to developing nursing knowledge in this area. Studies of case management included in this review reflect the clusters of outcomes research: (a) case management research in behavioral health; (b) case management research in long-term care; and (c) case management research for special populations.

In the 1970s and 1980s, numerous studies were conducted to examine the impact of case management on outcomes of care for individuals with chronic mental illness. The impetus for this work came from the dramatic shift from acute care to community-based care for this population. Particular attention was focused on the effectiveness of case managers in increasing the use of community resources and reducing hospital admissions. As noted by Chamberlain and Rapp (1991), these studies were grounded in several different psychological and social frameworks, including the Program of Assertive Community Treatment Model (Bond, Miller, Krumwied, & Ward, 1988; Borland, McRae, & Lycan, 1989; Jerrell & Hu, 1989), the Generalist Model (Franklin, Solovitz, Mason, Clemons, & Miller, 1987), the Rehabilitation Model (Goering, Farkas, Wasylenki, Lancee, & Ballantyne, 1988a; Goering, Wasylenki, Farkas, Lancee, & Ballantyne, 1988b), and the Strengths Model (Modrcin, Rapp, & Poertner, 1988).

Although the body of work on case management in chronic mental illness most commonly has been associated with the disciplines of psychiatry and social work, it is important to note that nurses played major roles in these studies as principal investigators (Goering et al., 1988a, 1988b) and as the case managers who delivered the interventions. It was not unusual for investigators to use representatives of several different professions as case managers within the same study. For example, Goering et al. (1988a, 1988b) used nurses, social workers, and occupational therapists as case managers. Borland et al. (1989) used nurses and other unspecified professionals as case managers. The possible interaction between differing world views, values, and disciplinary perspectives and a generic case management intervention was not explored in any study. Although professional nurses functioned as case managers in many of these studies, the case management intervention was not identified explicitly as a nursing intervention.

In their separate reviews of case management in mental illness research, Chamberlain and Rapp (1991) and Rubin (1992) noted similar issues. They found few studies that were focused primarily on patient outcomes. In studies using quasi-experimental and experimental designs, the case management intervention often was poorly specified, study populations varied widely in demographic and disease characteristics, and few consistent outcome indicators were used across studies. Not surprisingly, the results showed little consistent influence of case management on quality or cost outcomes. However, Chamberlain and Rapp (1991) identified a trend of positive outcomes associated with the one or two outcome indicators most consistent with the theoretical model guiding the case management intervention. Thus, for example, studies in which researchers emphasized functionality of the mentally ill population in their conceptual framework were more likely to show a positive impact on functional outcomes (Goering et al., 1988a, 1988b; Modrcin et al., 1988). Perhaps the goal of functionality became embedded in the intervention of case management and that had an influence on outcomes.

In their reviews, Chamberlain and Rapp (1991) and Rubin (1992) concluded that priority must be given to conceptualization and measurement of outcomes if research is to demonstrate consistent impact of case management on quality and cost outcomes. In addition, Chamberlain and Rapp (1991) made a critical point that outcome measures need to be consistent with disciplinary perspectives and philosophy to demonstrate successful outcomes.

Also in the 1970s and 1980s, the Health Care Financing Administration (HCFA) funded a series of Medicare and Medicaid demonstrations on community-based long-term care of older adults. Researchers conducting high-profile demonstrations, including Channeling and On-Lok, provided case management and an expanded package of community services to assist older adults potentially at risk of nursing home placement to remain in the community (Kemper, Applebaum, & Harrigan, 1987).

In the late 1980s, critical reviews of the instances of the long-term care demonstrations (e.g., Channeling and On-Lok) were published (Capitman, Haskins, & Bernstein, 1986; Kemper, Applebaum, & Harrigan, 1987; Kemper, 1988; Weissert, 1988). Similar to the experience with chronic mental illness, the long-term care demonstrations, as a group, showed little consistent impact on quality or cost outcomes. Kemper (1988), Weissert (1988), and others criticized procedures that failed to target high-risk individuals as a significant deterrent to demonstrating positive outcomes, particularly in the areas of service use and cost savings. Few of the demonstration sites limited participation to individuals at measurable risk of nursing home placement; many of the individuals participating in these studies were not likely to be placed in a nursing home. Hence, the demonstrations suffered from a serious type II error; they lacked the power to detect differences even if they did exist because the study subjects consisted of many people who were not in the targeted risk pool.

In 1985, the S/HMO demonstration was funded by HCFA to examine the impact of an integrated acute and chronic health care continuum on quality and costs of health care for Medicare beneficiaries. In addition to traditional Medicare-covered services, the four S/HMOs offered expanded community care and nursing home services under a shared risk arrangement with HCFA (Leutz et al., 1988). Each of the participants in the S/HMOs received a comprehensive assessment on enrollment. Individuals identified at risk for adverse health outcomes and high service use were assigned to case managers who developed a plan of care and assisted them to get needed services. Nurses and social workers functioned as case managers with the nurses working primarily with individuals with "complex medical cases" and the social workers assigned to individuals with "complex social situations" (Abrahams et al., 1989, p. 726).

The S/HMO demonstrations have been extended and continue at the original four sites. Terminal outcomes of this project have not yet been reported. Interim reports have provided important new information about the costs of case management (Leutz, Malone, Kistner, O'Bar, Ripley, & Sandhaus, 1990) and key processes, like decisions about resource allocation (Abrahams, Capitman, Leutz, & Macko, 1989). In these studies, researchers discovered considerable variability in the costs and decision making of case managers.

Building on earlier trends discovered in the long-term–care demonstrations that case management decision making was influenced by nonclinical factors, Abrahams and colleagues (1989) conducted an exploratory study with case managers in the S/HMOs to look at the influence of organizational factors on the long-term–care allocation decisions. They asked case managers at each of the four S/HMO sites to make resource decisions and develop care plans for one or more of seven clinical case studies based on actual clients and a cross-section of risk factors commonly used in allocation decisions. Using record review and interview data, the researchers found differences by S/HMO site in eligibility determinations, care planning, and type and mix of allocated services. The discovery of the influence of nonclinical organizational factors on allocation decisions has important implications for the development of decision-making models for case management practice.

In several recent studies, researchers addressed aspects of case management not considered in earlier research. In contrast to the community-based models of case management explored in the long-term–care demonstrations, Warrick, Christianson, Williams, and Netting (1990) studied the development of hospital-based case management programs. They identified numerous organizational characteristics that were associated with successful implementation (Williams, Warrick, Christianson, & Netting, 1993). In 1991, Eggert, Zimmer, Hall, and Friedman reported the results of the first experimental study of case management for frail elderly in which the model of case management was the only difference between groups.

Eggert and colleagues (1991) compared the impact of two different models of case management, a centralized individual model and a neighborhood team model, on health service use and costs for community-dwelling older adults meeting skilled nursing-level criteria. Both models were implemented in the same service environment with services equally available to the two study groups. In the team model, the case managers had greater direct client contact and smaller caseloads than in the individual model. The group of clients cared for in the team model had lower annual health service costs, fewer hospital days, and lower use of home health services, but higher nursing home use than clients in the individual model. The authors suggested that the positive effects of the neighborhood team model were a result of continuity of providers, the availability of team support and expertise, smaller caseload size, and the potential for direct client contact through home visits.

Case management research has been expanded to new populations with catastrophic illnesses, like people with acquired immune deficiency syndrome (Fleishman, Mor, & Piette, 1991) and to new venues like the insurance industry (Collard, Bergman, & Henderson, 1990). Interest in client response to working with case managers has resulted in the development of new instruments to measure satisfaction and the introduction of quality improvement strategies for case management research and evaluation (Henderson & Collard, 1988).

Lessons from Case Management Research in Other Disciplines

Numerous studies have been conducted to examine the impact of case management on quality and cost outcomes for high-risk populations, including adults with chronic and severe mental illness, older adults with complex health problems, and individuals with catastrophic illnesses. Although these studies were not conducted within a nursing perspective or framework, nurses contributed to the development of this body of work by serving as investigators and case managers delivering the interventions.

In general, the development of a cumulative body of knowledge on case management outside of nursing has been limited by a nontheoretical task-oriented approach to case management definitions and interventions, limited monitoring of the content and intensity of the case management intervention, and lack of consistent quality and cost indicators across studies (Chamberlin & Rapp, 1991; Kemper, Applebaum, & Harrigan, 1987; Rubin, 1992; Weissert, 1988). In addition, it has been difficult to isolate the contribution of case management intervention to outcomes, because in most studies, case management was a part of a much larger intervention program.

There are, however, several excellent examples of studies within this body of literature that address the major limitations and provide a strong base for subsequent research. Studies conducted by Bond et al. (1988), Franklin et al. (1987), and Goering et al. (1988a, 1988b) in the field of chronic mental illness demonstrated effective integration of theoretical frameworks in case management research. Researchers studying the S/HMO demonstrations emphasized the importance of integrating well-designed descriptive research within the overall research plan to uncover the processes within case management practice (Abrahams et al., 1989; Leutz et al., 1988). Finally, Eggert and colleagues (1991) were among the first to isolate case management from other interventions and to examine its unique contribution to outcomes.

In this body of research that predates the recent emergence of nurse case management, researchers discovered numerous important lessons related to the design of case management research. Common research issues, like selection of appropriate theoretical models and outcomes, specification of interventions, sampling and measurement, required translation, and refinement for the study of case management. Several authors, including Kemper (1988) and Weissert (1988), asserted that lack of attention to identifying the special features of case management research has contributed to the development of a body of research with ambiguous findings. The lessons from studies conducted outside the discipline of nursing may be summarized as follows:

1. Case management interventions should be clearly linked to a theoretical framework. In the body of quasi-experimental and experimental research on case management for individuals with chronic and severe mental illness, researchers were more likely to show significant changes in outcomes linked to their underlying theoretical framework than outcomes included without theoretical support (Chamberlain & Rapp, 1991).

2. The case management intervention must be defined and specified. The ability to link positive outcomes to case management has been hampered by lack of clear definition of the intervention. Listing task activities, which has been the most common approach to defining case management, has provided a limited view of how and why case managers make a difference. Typically nested in a complex set of poorly defined and measured services, case management cannot be identified as

the sole source of change in most studies. As shown by Eggert et al. (1991), clearly defining, describing, and measuring the case management intervention provides better information to assess the contribution of case management to outcomes.

3. The sample should consist of a homogeneous group of individuals most likely to benefit from case management, that is, to have the potential to show a change in important outcomes. In critical analyses of the long-term-care demonstrations, reviewers have suggested that the ability of these projects to show consistent quality and cost savings was limited by the lack of targeting of individuals most likely to be affected by the intervention (Kemper, Applebaum, & Harrigan, 1987; Weissert, 1988). Many subjects who participated in these studies were not at significant risk for experiencing the key negative outcome of interest, namely, nursing home placement. Comparison of findings across demonstrations showed that only one of the six demonstrations that used randomized experimental designs and had complete data on nursing home use showed a statistically significant reduction in nursing home days in the treatment group compared with the control group. The one demonstration that had significant results was called the South Carolina Community Long-Term Care project. It was unique among the six studies because of its use of nursing home preadmission screening to limit participation to subjects at substantial risk of nursing home placement (Kemper et al., 1987). Thus, it targeted an appropriate group of recipients.

Achieving homogeneous samples may be a particular challenge in case management research. Several investigators have shown that several subtle factors, like source of referral (Warrick, Netting, Christianson, & Williams, 1992) and site of care (Fleishman, Mor, & Piette, 1991) may inadvertently contribute to substantial variability within samples. Warrick and colleagues (1992), for example, found distinctly different subgroups in a case management sample according to whether case management had been initiated in the hospital or community.

4. Researchers should strive for consistency in the selection of sensitive outcome indicators. The lack of consistent findings across studies may be attributed, in part, to the use of different instruments to measure the same or similar constructs. Support for sensitivity to the case management intervention has not been provided in most previous studies. Warrick and colleagues (1992) identified the use of a uniform set of instruments across study sites as a major strength of their study and one that contributed to their ability to detect important differences in subject characteristics, service use, and outcomes.

NURSE CASE MANAGEMENT: STATE OF THE ART

Current models of nurse case management evolved, in part, from community health nursing, primary nursing in acute care settings, and from clinical specialist care that bridges across service settings. Many authors noted the similarities between the present practice of case managers and public health nursing at the turn of the century (Erkel, 1993; Knollmueller, 1989; Mundinger, 1984).

The literature reflects considerable confusion about the purpose, scope, and functions of nurse case managers (Lyon, 1993). Not surprisingly, this confusion has been carried over into research on nurse case management practice. Like many of the studies conducted outside of nursing, research on nurse case management has been characterized by the absence of operational definitions of case management, lack of studies that control for the effects of extraneous variables, and a dearth of nursing-sensitive outcomes (Lamb, 1992). Unlike scientists in the field of behavioral health who have paid increasing attention to the role of theory in their research designs, researchers studying nursing case management have largely sidestepped nursing or social science theory as they rushed to document outcomes. A few authors have explored the applicability of various nursing theories to case management practice (Forchuk, Beaton, Crawford, Ide, & Voorberg, 1989; Wadas, 1993). However, theoretical frameworks have yet to be used as the underpinning for studies of nurse case management.

The literature on nursing case management practice is rich with description. In a large body of anecdotal stories about case management practice, authors have described the work of case managers and the individuals with whom they work. Zander (1988), Ethridge and Lamb (1989), and Rogers, Riordan, and Swindle (1991), for example, integrated case studies with their description of quantitative outcomes. Embedded in these case studies are details about client characteristics, their nursing problems and needs, and their response to nurse case management interventions.

Currently, qualitative descriptions of nurse case management practice are an untapped resource that nurse researchers might use to define operationally the nurse case management intervention. Case studies embedded in these descriptions point to common themes across all nurse case management practice. Nurse case managers appear to work with (a) individuals, families, and populations at high risk of adverse health outcomes; (b) they are responsible for applying the nursing process in ways that potentially enhance both quality and cost outcomes; and (c) they have access to individuals and families in more than one localized setting: case managers in hospital-based models work across units; case managers in continuum-based models work across multiple settings. The themes of coordination, integration, and advocacy figure prominently in many anecdotal reports. However, these themes have received limited theoretical attention within nursing.

Ideally, areas of substantive interest in nurse case management research would include the structure, process, and outcomes of case management. However, in current literature, the focus on outcomes dominates. In representative studies of both hospital-based and continuum-based nurse case management models, the major focus has been on the use and costs of acute care services. There has been little systematic study of either structure or process or the relationships among structure, process, and outcome. In the following section, the current state of knowledge in each of these areas is discussed.

Structure

Structural questions typically address issues related to preparation for practice, work-group composition, caseload size, and administrative support. There have been no investigations examining the influence of educational preparation or types of nursing experience on either process or outcomes of nurse case management practice. In fact, the educational preparation of nurse case managers was commonly omitted from published research reports. Several authors have suggested educational content necessary for case management practice (Bower, 1992; Redford, 1992; Wahlstedt & Blaser, 1987), and there appears to be a growing movement toward preparation of case managers at the graduate level in nursing. However, research support for graduate level preparation for nurse case managers was lacking in the literature.

Work-group or team composition of case management programs varied dramatically from study to study. The long-term–care demonstrations used social workers and individuals with a social science background as case managers, with nurses as supervisors or consultants (Kemper, 1988). In the S/HMO demonstrations, the case management department was composed of nurses and social workers who followed different populations according to health and social needs. The hospital-based case management demonstration reported by Warrick et al. (1990), used a variety of case management teams, but only one of six sites used an all nurse model. Although it makes intuitive sense that population characteristics might determine team assignments and composition, only Eggert and colleagues (1991) examined the relationship between patient assignment guidelines, case mix, and outcomes of care using an experimental design.

Appropriate caseload size is a topic of considerable conjecture in the case management literature. Ethridge and Lamb (1989) reported that nurse case managers in a continuum-based model typically follow 80 to 90 clients at any time, with approximately one half requiring face-to-face contact. Eggert et al. (1991) suggested that smaller caseload size was an incentive for a team case management model over an individual model. These authors and others indicated that a complex set of variables may determine caseload size, including patient acuity, team composition, and site of care. To date, there has been no published research linking caseload size and characteristics to outcomes. In addition, there are no published instruments that index patient acuity for case management practice.

Numerous organizational features have been associated with the successful implementation of case management (Williams, Warrick, Christianson, & Netting, 1993). Several authors have suggested that professional practice structures, including shared governance, credentialing systems, and professional practice committees, are particularly relevant to the development of nurse case management programs (Ethridge, 1991; McKenzie, Torkelson, & Holt, 1989). To date, there have been no studies examining whether specific support structures are prerequisites for successful case management outcomes.

In summary, there has been little study of structural features of nurse case management practice. Descriptions of common structural characteristics, such as organizational supports, educational and experiential preparation of case managers, and caseload size, are typically missing from published research. Although there are anecdotal reports about the possible role that structural variables may play in explaining variation in the outcomes of case management, empirical work in this area is lacking.

Process

As noted earlier, anecdotal reports of nurse case managers were rich with description of the work. These reports indicated that nurse case managers incorporated each of the steps of the nursing process in their care. Long-term caring relationships were emphasized as well as professional nursing functions of monitoring, pattern recognition, teaching, coordination, and advocacy. There has been little research that (a) operationalizes these central concepts and attempts to monitor their implementation, and (b) links nurse case management interventions to nursing or social science theory.

Newman, Lamb, and Michaels (1991) reported the results of interviews with 13 nurse case managers practicing in a continuum-based model in Arizona. The nurses emphasized themes consistent with Newman's nursing model of health as expanding consciousness (Newman, 1986), suggesting that Newman's model may be a useful source of concepts and hypotheses for future research.

Lamb and Stempel (1994) interviewed 16 clients of nurse case managers in the continuum-based practice in Arizona previously studied by Newman et al. (1991). They used grounded theory techniques to develop a model linking the process and outcomes of case management from the client's perspective. Their model suggested that it is through the relationship with the nurse case manager that clients are able to reframe their experience, think differently about their health problems and options, and then change their self-care behaviors.

Respondents in their study emphasized the interplay between two central aspects of the nurse case manager: the nurse as clinical expert in the management of complex illnesses and the nurse as a caring and accessible partner in their health experience. Both were integral to the achievement of outcomes. Lamb and Stempel (1994) indicated that current nursing and social science theories in the areas of mastery, self-care, caring, and cognition are relevant to nurse case management practice and may be used to operationalize the intervention, and predict and explain its outcomes.

In their survey of satisfaction with the care of psychiatric nurse case managers, Van Dongen and Jambunathan (1992) also found that clients emphasized their caring and supportive relationship with the nurse. There are striking similarities in the client's qualitative descriptions of the nurses between this study and Lamb and Stempel's (1994) study. In both instances, the nurses are described as genuine, caring, supportive, accessible, and clinically competent. In both studies, clients identified listening, counseling, problem solving, and teaching as central nurse case management interventions.

In summary, there has been little systematic study of the clinical process of nurse case management. The extensive body of anecdotal descriptions of nurse case management available in the literature is a fertile and as-yet untapped resource for content analysis. Research conducted by Newman and colleagues (1991), and Lamb and Stempel (1994) gives strong examples of the effective use of qualitative methods, such as phenomenology and grounded theory, for uncovering the process of case management.

Outcomes

There were few empirical studies of outcomes of nurse case management. Most of these studies addressed the impact of nurse case management on health service use and costs, particularly the use of hospitals and emergency departments, and their associated costs. There has been limited study of other relevant outcomes, such as nurse satisfaction, patient satisfaction, self-care, or functionality. In addition, there has been minimal exploration of the effect of case management on health care costs across the full continuum of care (Marschke & Nolan, 1993).

The emphasis on acute care service use and costs is consistent with the background and goals of the authors of most nurse case management studies. Most authors were administrators and clinicians in acute care settings who have conducted evaluative studies to support newly developed programs. It is only recently that nurse scientists have begun to develop proposals to study nurse case management, and it is too early for their findings to appear in the literature. In addition, the lack of outcome indicators sensitive to nurse case management interventions and integrated information systems that enable researchers to track outcomes across settings have limited the scope of outcome research (Lamb, 1992).

Outcome research emanating from service settings is largely concerned with two case management practice models: (a) hospital-based models in which nurse case managers coordinate care for high-risk individuals across nursing units using managed care tools, such as critical paths; and (b) continuum-based models in which nurse case managers work with clients and coordinate care across multiple settings. To date, most studies on both models use preexperimental designs using individuals receiving the case management intervention as their own controls or comparing them with a nonrandomly selected control group.

Health Service Use and Costs

There are several reports examining health service use and costs in hospital-based models of nurse case management. Typically, these reports emphasized the development and implementation of nurse case management programs. Results of program evaluation focused on findings with minimal information provided about research design or methods.

McKenzie et al. (1989) described the implementation of a case management program for patients undergoing coronary artery bypass surgery. They defined case management as a "set of logical steps and a process of interaction with service networks" (p. 30). As in many of the evolving hospital-based case management programs, nurse case managers were responsible for monitoring the implementation of a tool called a critical path, identifying deviations from the path, offering care alternatives, tracking outcomes, and planning discharge. The critical path is an interdisciplinary blueprint of key processes and outcomes to be accomplished within a specified time frame (Zander, 1988).

In comparison with 106 patients who did not receive nurse case management, the 84 case-managed patients in this study had a shorter hospital stay and lower pharmacy, laboratory, radiology, and overall charges. Sampling methods were not specified. The authors indicated that outcome audits and patient and satisfaction surveys were conducted, but neither measurement tools nor specific results were reported. Although the differences between groups were attributed to the nurse case management program, insufficient information about the evaluation design is provided to determine the extent to which the outcomes may be associated with the nurse case management intervention.

Mahn (1993) reported the results of a similar case management program for individuals undergoing coronary artery bypass procedures (diagnostic-related group [DRG] 107). As in the preceding study, the nurse case manager coordinated all of the preadmission phase, monitored the implementation and evaluation of a critical path, and participated in discharge planning. In the comparison of 25 case-managed patients with 25 noncase-managed patients, the case-managed patients had fewer hospital days, lower laboratory costs, and fewer hospital readmissions. In this study, an important effort is made to show comparability of the study groups on several demographic and severity indicators before conducting the analysis of outcomes. As in the previously cited study by McKenzie et al. (1989), however, limited information is provided about the satisfaction surveys and quality audits that were conducted.

Cohen (1991) compared hospital costs between women with cesarean sections on one hospital unit who received a nurse case management intervention and a control group on another hospital unit who did not. The case management intervention used a team nursing approach that consisted of the implementation of a critical path with consistent integration of early patient teaching and discharge planning. The results showed fewer hospital days and lower costs in the case-managed group. In addition, analysis of nursing activities on the two units showed that registered nurses and nursing assistants on the experimental unit spent more time in direct nursing care, particularly during the initial hospital days. Cohen suggested that the initial increase in direct nursing care hours contributed to reduced length of stay and associated cost savings.

In addition to bringing more sophisticated cost-accounting methods to the study of nurse case management, Cohen's dissertation research provided a good example of the potential for applying techniques of cross-level modeling and analysis to enhance case management outcome research. Cross-level research is concerned with phenomena that occur at different levels of the organization, and its methodology requires explicit attention to shifts in units of measurement and analysis for accurate interpretation of outcomes (Rousseau, 1985; Verran, Mark, & Lamb, 1992). In Cohen's research, for example, the nurse case management intervention was implemented at the unit level, yet outcomes are measured and analyzed at the individual level, suggesting that her theoretical framework was a downward cross-level model. Because much of case management research may involve shifting units of intervention, measurement, and analysis, the growing body of knowledge in cross-level research may be extremely useful in designing and interpreting case management studies.

Ethridge and Lamb (1989), and Rogers et al. (1991) reported the outcomes of pilot programs for continuum-based nurse case management models. Ethridge and Lamb described the development of an integrated system of nursing services in which nurse case managers provided continuity of care for high-risk adults with acute and chronic illnesses.

Case studies and limited comparisons of case-managed and non-case-managed patients were used to propose that nurse case management may reduce hospital length of stay through different mechanisms for patients with acute and chronic illness. For patients with time-limited acute illness episodes like total hip replacement, Ethridge and Lamb hypothesized nurse case managers may reduce total length of stay through facilitating earlier discharge. For patients with chronic, exacerbating illnesses, like chronic lung disease, they proposed that nurse case managers may reduce the high-cost and high-intensity days that occur at the beginning of hospitalization by facilitating early access to care when medical intervention is indicated. Insufficient data about sample selection and research methods were provided to judge the adequacy of support for their hypotheses. However, these authors pose important questions about how nurse case managers contribute to changes in health service use in different patient populations.

Rogers et al. (1991) described the implementation of a similar continuum-based model of nurse case management. Although they initially planned to match patients in a case-managed and noncase-managed comparison, they found that there were no patients of comparable acuity with the high-risk case-managed patients in their system. In a pretest posttest design in which they used 38 case-managed patients as their own controls, they found reduced hospital length of stay and admissions, and increased net reimbursement to the hospital following the case management intervention.

In summary, there has been a growing number of reports of the impact of nurse case management programs on health service use. Most of these reports have been published by clinicians in service settings whose primary intent has been to share the evolution of new nurse case management programs and preliminary support for the development of these programs.

Interpretation of findings from this body of research is severely limited by the omission of operational definitions of the case management intervention, the lack of clear specification and measurement of sample selection criteria, and the frequent use of weak preexperimental designs and unstandardized instruments. However, trends in the findings of these studies offer important hypotheses and methodological suggestions for future systematic research. McKenzie and colleagues (1989) identified groups of hospital charges, like pharmacy and radiology, that may be affected by the implementation of hospital-based nurse case management programs. Ethridge and Lamb (1989) proposed that nurse case managers may achieve cost savings through different interventions with populations with acute and chronic illnesses. Research by Mahn (1993) and Cohen (1991) introduced important improvements in the areas of establishing comparability between case-managed and comparison groups, and measuring cost outcomes.

Patient Satisfaction

There has been growing interest in consumer responses to nurse case management. In an influential article on quality assessment of case management programs, Collard, Bergman, and Henderson (1990) suggested that measurement of patient satisfaction is integral to any evaluation program.

Although anecdotal reports indicated consistently high patient satisfaction with nurse case management, nurse researchers have questioned whether current patient satisfaction instruments adequately capture the domain of satisfaction with nurse case management (Lamb, 1992; Van Dongen & Jambunathan, 1992). As a result, new satisfaction instruments are beginning to appear in the nursing literature.

Van Dongen and Jambunathan (1992) described several items on instruments they developed to measure client, nurse, and physician satisfaction with nurse case management. In the client instrument, the items address attributes of the case managers, including caring and availability, as well as nursing interventions. Unfortunately, the sample size

($n = 24$) was too small to permit any quantitative psychometric evaluation of the instrument. In future work, it will be important to compare and contrast systematically the dimensions of satisfaction addressed in newly evolving instruments with those of older instruments and their relationship to other outcome indicators.

CONCLUSIONS AND RECOMMENDATIONS

Case management researchers, particularly, nurse case management researchers and health services researchers, face critical challenges as health policy makers, administrators, and clinicians look for the data and information to support the use of case management as a central building block in a restructured health care system. The state of knowledge about case management has grown enormously in the past 30 years, but the demands for clear, consistent, and credible findings far exceed what researchers currently have to offer.

The task of researchers is complicated by the popularity and visibility of case management. As the number of professions and individuals with a stake in the future of case management expands, it is increasingly difficult to cut through the debate and rhetoric to get to some basic questions, such as: What is case management? Who needs it? Who provides it? For how long? What are its outcomes? What are its costs? Does it save money by keeping people from higher levels of care?

For nursing, the blueprint for the answers to these questions resides in the lessons of past case management research and the wealth of descriptive literature of nurse case management practice. To meet the demands and time frames of a rapidly changing health care system, nursing must identify a strategic plan and course of action to guide its research in this area. There are several strategies the nursing community might use to move ahead as expeditiously as possible.

- Create a team of researchers, theorists, and clinicians to analyze and synthesize current descriptions and definitions of case management and nurse case management to identify key components/processes of case management that can be used as a base for a consistent *disciplinary* approach to nurse case management research. This review needs to encompass and integrate recent studies of nurse case management practice with past studies whether conducted by nurse scientists or by others, but use nurses to provide the case management intervention. Critical analysis should help to identify important differences and similarities between case management models that are carried out under the conceptual label of nurse case management and those that are not explicitly labeled as nurse case management, but rely on nurses to offer the case management intervention.

This team must be composed of nurses and other key professionals who are able to apply their expertise to the task of expanding *nursing's* body of knowledge on case management. Experts from fields, such as health services research, health policy, health economics, psychology, psychometrics, and statistics, are integral to this work.

- Coordinate research programs that will bring together information on the relationship between nurse case management processes and outcomes. This program of research needs to be organized and targeted to (a) linking nurse case management practice to relevant theories; (b) expanding knowledge about processes that are considered core to practice, such as coordination and pattern recognition; and (c) developing and refining outcome instruments that are sensitive to nurse case management interventions.
- Encourage nurse researchers to incorporate consistent outcome indicators across nurse case management studies.

In contrast to many other areas of nursing research, the results of the studies of nurse case management are and will be explicitly linked to health policy decisions and opportunities for professional practice and reimbursement. Case management offers nursing a unique opportunity to develop a new collaborative and planned model of research to respond to the demands of a growing number of audiences for information that consistently supports the quality and cost-effectiveness of case management by nurses.

REFERENCES

Abrahams, R., Capitman, J., Leutz, W., & Macko, P. (1989). Variations in care planning practice in the Social/HMO: An exploratory study. *Gerontologist, 29*, 725–736.

Bond, G., Miller, L., Krumwied, R., & Ward, R. (1988). Assertive case management in 3 CMHCs: A controlled study. *Hospital and Community Psychiatry, 39*, 411–418.

Borland, A., McRae, J., & Lycan, C. (1989). Outcomes of five years of continuous intensive case management. *Hospital and Community Psychiatry, 40*, 369–376.

Bower, K. (1992). *Case management by nurses*. Washington, DC: American Nurses Publishing.

Capitman, J. A., Haskins, B., & Bernstein, J. (1986). Case management approaches in coordinated community-oriented long-term care demonstrations. *Gerontologist, 26*, 398–404.

Chamberlain, R., & Rapp, C. A. (1991). A decade of case management: A methodological review of outcome research. *Community Mental Health Journal, 27*, 171–188.

Cohen, E. (1991). Nurse case management: Does it pay? *Journal of Nursing Administration, 20*(4), 20–25.

Collard, A., Bergman, A., & Henderson, M. (1990). Two approaches to measuring quality in medical case management programs. *Quality Review Bulletin, 16*(1), 3–8.

Eggert, G. M., Zimmer, J. G., Hall, W. J., & Friedman, B. (1991). Case management: A randomized controlled study comparing a neighborhood team and a centralized individual model. *Health Services Research, 26*, 471–507.

Erkel, E. A. (1993). The impact of case management in preventive services. *Journal of Nursing Administration, 23*(1), 17–32.

Ethridge, P. 1991). A nursing HMO: Carondelet St. Mary's experience. *Nursing Management, 22*(7), 22–29.

Ethridge, P., & Lamb, G. S. (1989). Professional nurse case management improves quality, access and costs. *Nursing Management, 20*(3), 26–29.

Fleishman, J. A., Mor, V., & Piette, J. (1991). AIDs case management: The client's perspective. *Health Services Research, 26*, 447–470.

Forchuk, C., Beaton, S., Crawford, L., Ide, L., & Voorberg, N. (1989). Incorporating Peplau's theory and care management. *Journal of Psychosocial Nursing, 27*(2), 35–38.

Franklin, J., Solovitz, B., Mason, M., Clemons, J., & Miller, G. (1987). An evaluation of case management. *American Journal of Public Health, 77*, 674–678.

Goering, P. N., Farkas, M., Wasylenki, D. A., Lancee, W., & Ballantyne, R. (1988a). Improved functioning for case management clients. *Psychosocial Rehabilitation Journal, 12*(1), 3–17.

Goering, P. N., Wasylenki, D. A., Farkas, M., Lancee, W., & Ballantyne, R. (1988b). What difference does case management make? *Hospital and Community Psychiatry, 39*, 272–276.

Jerrell, J. M., & Hu, T. (1989). Cost-effectiveness of intensive clinical and case management compared with an existing system of care. *Inquiry, 26*, 224–234.

Kemper, P. (1988). The evaluation of the national long term care demonstration: Overview of the findings. *Health Services Research, 23*, 161–174.

Kemper, P., Applebaum, R., & Harrigan, M. (1987). Community demonstrations: What have we learned? *Health Care Financing Review, 8*, 87–100.

Knollmueller, R. N. (1989). Case management: What's in a name? *Nursing Management, 20*(10), 38–42.

Lamb, G. S. (1992). Conceptual and methodological issues in nurse case management research. *Advances in Nursing Science, 15*(2), 16–24.

Lamb, G. S., & Stempel, J. E. (1994). Nurse case management from the client's view: Growing as insider-expert. *Nursing Outlook, 42*, 7–14.

Leutz, W., Abrahams, R., Greenlick, M., Kane, R., & Prottas, J. (1988). Targeting expanded care to the aged: Early SHMO experience. *Gerontologist, 28*, 4–17.

Leutz, W., Malone, J., Kistner, M., O'Bar, T., Ripley, J. M., & Sandhaus, M.

(1990). Financial performance of the social health maintenance organization: 1985–1988. *Health Care Financing Review, 12*, 9–18.

Lyon, J. C. (1993). Models of nursing care delivery and case management: Clarification of terms. *Nursing Economics, 11*, 163–169.

Mahn, V. (1993). Clinical nurse case management: A service line approach. *Nursing Management, 24*(9), 48–50.

Marschke, P., & Nolan, M. T. (1993). Research related to case management. *Nursing Administration Quarterly, 17*(3), 16–21.

McKenzie, C. B., Torkelson, N. G., & Holt, M. A. (1989). Care and cost: Case management improves both. *Nursing Management, 20*(10), 30–34.

Modrcin, M., Rapp, C., & Poertner, J. (1988). The evaluation of case management services with the chronically mentally ill. *Evaluation and Program Planning, 11*, 307–314.

Mundinger, M. O. (1984). Community based care: Who will be the case managers? *Nursing Outlook, 32*, 294–295.

Newman, M. A. (1986). *Health as expanding consciousness*. St. Louis: Mosby.

Newman, M. A., Lamb, G. S., & Michaels, C. (1991). Nursing case management: The coming together of theory and practice. *Nursing & Health Care, 12*, 404–408.

Redford, L. (1992). Case management: The wave of the future. *Journal of Case Management, 1*(1), 5–8.

Rogers, M., Riordan, J., & Swindle, D. (1991). Community based nurse case management pays off. *Nursing Management, 22*(3), 30–37.

Rousseau, D. (1985). Issues of level in organizational research: Multi-level and cross-level perspectives. *Research in Organizational Behavior, 7*, 1–37.

Rubin, A. (1992). Is case management effective for people with serious mental illness: A research review. *Health and Social Work, 17*, 138–150.

Van Dongen, C. J., & Jambunathan, J. (1992). Pilot study results: The psychiatric RN case manager. *Journal of Psychosocial Nursing, 30*(11), 11–14.

Verran, J. A., Mark, B. A., & Lamb, G. S. (1992). Psychometric examination of instruments using aggregated data. *Research in Nursing & Health, 15*, 237–240.

Wadas, T. M. (1993). Case management and caring behavior. *Nursing Management, 24*(9), 40–42.

Wahlstedt, P. & Blaser, W. (1987). Nurse case management for the frail elderly: A curriculum to prepare nurses for that role. *Home Healthcare Nurse, 4*(2), 30–35.

Warrick, L., Christianson, J., Williams, F., & Netting, F. E. (1990). The design and implementation of hospital-based coordinated care programs. *Hospital and Health Services Administration, 18*, 503–524.

Warrick, L. H., Netting, F. E., Christianson, J. B., & Williams, F. G. (1992). Hospital-based case management: Results from a demonstration. *Gerontologist, 32*, 781–788.

Weissert, W. G. (1988). Seven reasons why it is so difficult to make community based long-term care cost-effective. *Health Services Research, 20*, 423–433.

Williams, F. G., Warrick, L. H., Christianson, J. B., & Netting, F. E. (1993). Critical factors for successful hospital-based case management. *Health Care Management Review, 18*, 63–70.

Zander, K. (1988). Nursing case management: Strategic management of cost and quality outcomes. *Journal of Nursing Administration, 18*(5), 23–30.

Chapter 6

Technology and Home Care

CAROL E. SMITH
SCHOOL OF NURSING
UNIVERSITY OF KANSAS

CONTENTS

Advances in the treatment of illnesses, development of reliable technology, expansion of home care services, reimbursement patterns, cost containment, and growth in public or consumer demands for technological care have resulted in a growing population of technologically dependent individuals being cared for in their homes. Technological home care has been described as a sociotechnological system resembling a miniature intensive care unit or small clinic where ventilation, oxygen, nutrition support, dialysis, venous or intraspinal infusions, and cardiopulmonary monitoring are managed by a family in their homes (Andre, 1986; Copeman & Weigel, 1987; Lange, 1986). This chapter provides a review of research on technologies used in the home. Historical endeavors that have influenced research in the area, such as consensus conferences, demonstration projects, and international reports, are cited.

Persons are technology-dependent when they need both a medical device to compensate for the loss of a vital body function and ongoing nursing care to avert death or further disability (U.S. Congress, Office of Technology Assessment, 1987a). Nurses need research-generated knowledge about the mechanisms by which the devices interact with patient physiological states to produce outcomes. Nurses need to understand patient and family responses to machine dependency. The goal of this chapter is to review critically the current state of the art and stimulate further research related to technological dependence across the life span.

Research cited herein was identified through computerized searches that included MEDLINE, Psycholiterature, and CINAHL, using the terms home care, technology, devices, rehabilitation, home care guidelines/standards, and the names of the various technologies. The technologies selected for the literature review were based on extent of use as reported in recent government and home care industry reports. Studies included in this review came from multiple disciplines, but were all germane to human response to technological dependency and home nursing care. The literature review revealed a common pattern in the problems studied within each area of technology. The pattern begins with the early studies testing efficacy of the technical equipment and home care procedures; then, a wave of cost-effectiveness studies follow. The third wave is research on patient quality of life, followed by or paralleled with problems experienced by family caregivers. Lastly, after home care technology was well entrenched, a few studies addressing ethical issues, patient education, or health care delivery were conducted.

This chapter contains a review of studies on the efficacy, cost-effectiveness, and delivery of home services of the six most commonly used homecare technologies. A companion chapter in a future volume will contain a critique of research on quality of life, family caregivers, patient education, and ethical issues surrounding technology home care. In this chapter, findings from selected studies are presented in detail to more clearly depict the human experiences of technology dependence and the challenges to researchers in this area.

HOME CARE TECHNOLOGIES

Mechanical Ventilation at Home

Annually there are approximately 4,000 to 7,000 adults and 2,000 to 3,000 children dependent on long-term, home, mechanical ventilation (U.S. Congress, Office of Technology Assessment, 1987a). Health care industry reimbursement figures indicate that up to 25,000 new cases of short-term home ventilation care occur yearly (National Association for Home Care, 1991). Total costs of all home respiratory therapies were projected to be $2 billion in 1994 (National Association for Home Care, 1992). In retrospective studies, researchers have verified the efficacy and cost-effectiveness of home care for ventilator-dependent adults and children (Burr, Guyer, Todres, Abrahams, & Chiodo, 1983; Feldman & Tuteur, 1982; Fischer, 1989; Gilmartin & Make, 1983; Goldberg & Frownfelter, 1990; Kopacz & Moriarty-Wright, 1984; Make, Gilmartin, Brody, & Snider, 1984; Schreiner, Donar, & Kettrick, 1987; Splaingard, Frates, Harrison, Carter, & Jefferson, 1983; Splaingard, Frates, Jefferson, Rosen, & Harrison, 1985).

Adults Depend on Ventilation. Motwani and Herring (1988) reported that home care for severely disabled adults requiring ventilators was satisfactory to families, did not incur malpractice suits, and, even when housing was subsidized, saved millions of dollars over institutionalization. Advantages of home care over institutional care for the ventilated patient include decreased nosocomial infections (Lehner, Ballard, Figueroa, & Woodruff, 1980), increased mobility (Sivak, Cordasco, & Gipson, 1983), and improved nutritional status (Banaszak, Travers, Frazier, & Vinz, 1981). A greater sense of control and higher morale have been reported by both family members and patients because of resumption of more normal interactions and routines of daily living (Frace, 1986; Gipson, Sivak, & Gulledge, 1987; Goldberg, 1983, 1986; Smith, Mayer, Parkhurst, Perkins, & Pingleton, 1991).

Disadvantages to home ventilation included increased long-term family stress related to changes in family members' responsibilities and financial strain because of costs not covered by third-party payers, such as electrical bills, supplies, portable ventilators, and special transportation needs for patients (Lobosco, Eron, Bob, Kril, & Chalanick, 1991; Plummer, O'Donohue, & Petty, 1989). Through the Katie-Beckett waiver of 1984 (funding allowable for home care under Medicaid) families have obtained funds without required copayments that would have reduced them to the poverty level (Foundation for Hospice and Homecare, 1987; U.S. Congress, Office of Technology Assessment, 1987b). Other issues raised in consensus groups and research were withdrawal from the technology when quality of life deteriorates and nurses' ambivalence about discontinuing the technology (Bayer, 1987; Daly, Newlon, Montenegro, & Langdon, 1993).

Ventilator-Dependent Children. For children, thorough family preparation as well as proper patient selection; characteristics, including cardiopulmonary stability growth and weight gain; and "stamina to play while ventilated" were described as essential to successful home care (Schreiner et al., 1987). Most families have no outside assistance in caring for the child (Frates, Splaingard, Smith, & Harrison, 1985). Focus group interview technique, ethnographic, and content analysis revealed several strong recurrent themes from 80 parents who managed daily home technology care (Diehl, Moffitt, & Wade, 1991). Providing medication, pain relief, and daily physical care were problematic, but financial strain and rehospitalizations were more stressful for these parents. Counseling, support groups, respite care, and school mainstreaming were desired but either not consistently available or, if available, not consistently of high quality. Parents wanted more timely information about the child's growth, emotional development, schooling, and communication needs. The available medical and support services were described as satisfactory but the lack of coordination among them consistently led to fragmented care.

Delivery of Technology Home Care Services. In terms of delivery of health care services, a 1991 survey conducted in the state of New York identified 210 medically stable technologically dependent children who were in hospitals because of shortages of skilled home care nursing services (Millner, 1991). Investigators evaluated systems that coordinate home care for technology-dependent children. They found a dearth of professionally trained personnel for technology home care. In particular, there was a lack of reliable sources of registered nurses for nighttime care when the child first came home (Copeman & Weigel, 1987; Fields, Coble, Pollack, & Kaufman, 1991; Lobosco, Eron, Bobo, Kril, & Chalanick, 1991; Zahr & Montijo, 1993). The home ventilation studies of both adults and children identified that most families had no help in the home; used nurses on an on-call basis; had limited visits from respiratory, occupational, or physical therapists; and used the services of attendants more often than registered nurses (Lobosco et al., 1991). However, few cases were reported of patients being rehospitalized because of the family's inability to cope, although rehospitalization for pneumonia or other medical problems was reported.

Data Collection in the Home. Conducting research with technology-dependent persons, especially those on ventilators, is challenging for many reasons. Using technological measurements with data being carried across telephone lines, as a method of monitoring home care, is currently being evaluated in a study of 18 adult lung transplant patients (Snyder, Finkelstein, Edin, & Hertz, 1993). Most patients ($n = 14$) consistently transmitted data. The authors reported that changes in the spirometer measures and diary recordings of coughing, shortness of breath, and decreased well-being allowed for detection of impending problems in several patients. This type of technological monitoring has also been used successfully to measure length of time on and amount of oxygen used with home ventilation equipment to evaluate compliance (Millman, Kipp, Beadles, & Braman, 1988). Being able to obtain specific physiological data in prospective research designs will increase the usefulness of home care studies. Obtaining reliable data from patients who have compromised verbal communication skills is a concern as well. In most studies, the instruments have been limited to self-report by the family caregiver with little direct information from patients. The use of structured telephone interviews for measuring home care outcomes of technology-dependent children was documented as acceptable in a study by Kun and Warburton (1987). Data from telephone interviewers with 60 parents were interpreted to indicate that parents had an adequate understanding of symptomology and appropriately could seek hospitalization when necessary. Rarely reported in study findings were difficulties in reaching subjects by telephone or procedures used to contact families who do not have telephones (Ponferrada et al., 1993; Rundle, 1988). A study of direct observation in the home was conducted by Martin (1988); however, in this approach, the Hawthorn effect must be considered.

Overall, researchers concluded that family members, even with the wide ranges of age, education, and income, adequately managed home technology. In addition, families were satisfied with having the ventilated patient at home. Implications drawn by authors from these studies were that financing mechanisms need to be more comprehensive and less punitive toward family home care and that coordination of resources through a nurse case manager would improve the situation (Wegener & Aday, 1989). The emphases in the efficacy and cost-effectiveness studies were on physiological complications and direct costs of health care delivery in the home. When study aims were expanded to include psychological complications and indirect costs of loss of income because of family caregiving responsibilities, the findings were more difficult to interpret.

The major limitation of the studies on home ventilation is that outcomes have been defined from a health care (third-party) payer's perspective emphasizing cost control. Thus data were analyzed by comparing acute versus home care services bills. Hospital bills typically are larger than home care charges where fewer services are given because families provide their own 24-hour care. Indirect costs, such as loss of income because of caregiving responsibilities or out-of-pocket expenses paid by the family rarely were considered. More extensive investigations of costs to the family members need to be undertaken.

Few researchers have compared the differential costs of groups receiving differing health care delivery systems in the home. If cost-effectiveness for families is the goal then alternative mechanisms of care delivery need to be tested and compared (Fields, Coble, Pollack, & Kaufman, 1991; Weinstein, 1983).

Apnea Detection and Oxygen-Assist Device Technologies

The office of Technology Assessment (1987) estimated that 7,000 to 45,000 children are dependent on apnea monitoring per year, some for as long as 2 years. There have been recent descriptions of sleep apnea as life threatening in adults (National Commission on Sleep Disorders Research,1993; Young et al., 1993); therefore, apnea in children is of concern.

Apnea-Monitored Infants and Children. Investigators have verified parents' ability to manage infants that are sent home with electronic apnea monitoring, supplemental oxygen, and bilirubin phototherapy resulting from prolonged sleep apnea, bronchopneumonary dysplasia, low birthweight, apnea during feeding, or those at risk for sudden infant death syndrome (Bakke & Dougherty, 1981; Parlett & Spitzer, 1986; Roeder & Williams, 1985; Splaingard, Frates, Harrison, Carter, & Jefferson, 1983; Steinschneider, Weinstein, & Diamond, 1982; Valdes-Dapena, 1980). Retrospective study results indicated mothers were bonding with their technology-dependent infants (Black, Hersher, & Steinschneider, 1978; Cain, Kelly, & Shannon, 1980; Nuttall, 1988). Researchers suggested that mothers of monitored babies have high but not abnormally high levels of situation anxiety, and should be taught how to adjust their lifestyle. They might learn to realistically limit household responsibilities and obtain support from intimates, friends, and neighbors (Kruger & Rawlins, 1984; McElroy, Steinschneider, & Weinstein, 1986; Steele & Harrison, 1986; Vohr, Chen, Coll, & Oh, 1988). Concerns of mothers caring for an infant on an apnea monitor at home were related to monitor and cardiopulmonary resuscitation (CPR), infant care, mother's rest and sleep, and lifestyle changes including emotional tension, sibling, and household demands, or feeling tied down 24 hours a day (DiMaggio & Sheetz, 1983). The most frequently reported difficulties were home respiratory companies' billing procedures and stress related to length of time needed to wean the infant from oxygen (Thilo, Comito, & McCullis, 1987; Wasserman, 1984). Difficulty in finding baby-sitters and the inconvenience of traveling with monitors were identified as stressful factors (Cabin, 1985; Donn, 1982; Klijanowicz, 1984). Few parents reported problems with faulty equipment, running out of oxygen, or infant cyanosis. However, a common complaint reported by parents was keeping the oxygen cannula in place.

Williams and Williams (1990) identified a lack of prospective research about the influence of the caregiver and family interaction on the developmental status of the apnea-monitored infant. To decrease this gap in knowledge, a conceptual framework based on child development was used to guide their study of the primary family caregivers of 25 apnea-monitored infants. Assessments of mother-infant interactions in the home were obtained. The results of the study indicated that family cohesion, caregiver self-esteem, and social support were related to positive family coping strategies, child-caregiver interactions, and higher expressive language development in the children (Williams & Williams, 1990; Williams, Williams, & Griggs, 1990).

Weaknesses of the research included the lack of organizing conceptual frameworks, few prospective longitudinal studies, and dependence on telephone follow-up surveys. No home observations were made to verify results of even a small sample of the telephone surveys. Obtaining valid and reliable data in home care settings may be difficult but can be achieved. The most commonly used data collection procedures in children with apnea monitors has been telephone interviews and retrospective chart audits. Both these techniques have several limitations. Telephone interviews have advantages (Howard, Meade, Booth, & Whall, 1988), but researchers need to assess reliability and validity (Dillman, 1978). Geary (1989) found no differences in quality of information from audiotaped versus face-to-face telephone interviews of 20 caregivers of apnea-monitored infants.

Apnea-Monitored Adults. Adults also live at home while dependent on apnea-hypoapnea devices for life-threatening sleep-related breathing disorders. These symptoms increase during sleep by 10% to 28% (National Commission on Sleep Disorders Research, 1993; Young et al., 1993). Sleep apnea syndrome or sleep-disordered breathing leads to sleep deprivation and decreased oxyhemoglobin saturation, complete airway collapse, and has been associated with myocardial infarction in men (Hung, Whitford, Parsons, & Hillman, 1990; Partinen & Guilleminault, 1990; Winegard & Berkman, 1983). Sleep apnea also has been associated with respiratory failure in adults with neuromuscular disease (Dye, 1983; Guilleminault, Quera-Salva, Partinen, & Jamieson, 1988; Orr, 1983). Continuous positive airway pressure (CPAP) for sleep apnea requires use of a face mask breathing device, but some patients do not comply with the procedures of this treatment (Kerby, Mayer, & Pingleton, 1987; Kerr, Shoenut, Millar, Buckle, & Kryger, 1992). Cost comparisons of types of CPAP systems have been reported (Henry, West, & Wilson, 1983). Nurses have programs of research in sleep deprivation, sleep-wake cycles, and fatigue (Ashley, 1989; Shaver & Giblin, 1988) that could be expanded to study home care of the technology-dependent sleep apnea patient. Research on noncompliance with CPAP, the major treatment, has rarely been attempted. Cummings and colleagues (1981, 1982, 1984), in a series of studies, determined that predictors of compliance varied depending on the measurement method used. In addition, the conceptual meaning of compliance and any operational definitions selected need to coincide.

Nutrition Support Technologies

Almost 1.5 million persons use enteral or total parenteral nutrition (TPN) yearly (U.S. Congress, 1987a). Annual growth rates of 10% to 30% are projected per year (National Association for Home Care, 1992).

Total Parenteral Nutrition. Investigators have verified the cost-effectiveness of home-based total parenteral nutrition (Jeejeehbouy, Zohrab, Langner, Phillips, Huhns, & Anderson, 1983; Howard & Michalek, 1984; Twomey & Patching, 1985). Most patients (70%–80%) require lifelong parenteral nutrition resulting from benign bowel disorder, radiation enteritis, or malnutrition. Currently, home TPN therapy costs from \$90,000 to \$120,000 per year per patient (Howard, Heaphy, Fleming, Lininger, & Steiger, 1991). In reviewing studies of the costs of home TPN, Goel (1990) concluded that home care costs are 60% to 70% lower than hospital costs. He noted, however, that wide variability in costs are probably attributed to differences in accounting methods, reimbursement mechanisms, agency type, and lack of information on indirect costs and out-of-pocket expenses.

Home TPN patients reported frustration over their inability to eat normally (MacRitchie, 1978), distorted body image, and disturbed sexual relations (Parrish, Mitallo, & Fabri, 1982; Perl, Peterson, Dudrick, & Benson, 1981), social stigma (Perl, Hall, & Dudrick, 1980; Price & Levine, 1979), and financial burden (Smith, 1993). Other problems include maintaining asepsis and appropriate storage for solutions (Englert & Dudrick, 1978). Fatigue from pump alarms or infusion dysfunction during the night is frequent (Payne & Ball, 1991). Issues of decreased control; loss of independence, relationship, or role changes within the family; and developmental level of the family also influence adaptation to home TPN (Gulledge, 1985; Gulledge, Gipson, Steiger, Hooley, & Sep, 1980; Robinovitch, 1981). Data from several cross-sectional studies revealed that after 3 to 4 months of some TPN therapy, patients experience depressive reactions related to the complexity of long-term or lifelong therapy and the constant presence of technology (Hall & Beresford,

1987; Malcolm, Robson, & Vanderveen, 1980; Perl et al., 1981; Robb et al., 1983).

Physiological complications in home TPN patients have been related to the length of time on therapy. Patients were at risk to experience fluid and electrolyte imbalances, glucose intolerance, and unresolved fatigue in the 1st year and catheter-related complications (insertion site or line infection, thrombus, and breakage) during the 2nd year of home TPN (Oley Foundation, 1989). The first episode of septicemia most often occurred between the 2nd and 4th year of TPN therapy (Herfindal, Bernstein, Wong, Hogue, & Darbinian, 1992). Animal studies indicated that parenterally fed rats are predisposed to immunodeficiency because of decreased serum-immunoglobulin A and subsequent transfer of *Escherichia coli* and bacteria to mesenteric lymph nodes (Alverdy, Aoys, & Moss, 1988; Alverdy, Chi, & Sheldon, 1985; Berg, 1981).

In 1990 a panel of experts reported the current state of knowledge regarding use of TPN in various clinical populations, discussed cost control strategies, debated legal/ethical issues, and developed practice guidelines for clinical decision making. The consensus panel called for prospective studies to be done (Fry, 1990; Pillar & Perry, 1990). Multisite studies used to control geographical variation in medical practice, medical expenses, and nursing service delivery systems would decrease error variance from inappropriately compared samples in future prospective studies. The initiation of the National Registry database for parenteral and enteral nutrition is a valuable source, although nursing data are currently not being entered into that registry.

Enteral Nutrition. Enteral nutrition is the most extensively used nutrition technology in home care (U.S. Congress, 1987a). Nurses singly and in collaboration with others are lauded as adding to the knowledge of enteral feeding tolerance, delivery, nutrition assessment (Moore, Guenter, & Bender, 1986), and nutritional care of cancer patients (Dixon, 1984). Nurses have developed advances in enteral formula and infusion systems, feeding schedules/procedures, and identification of adverse effects, such as nausea, vomiting, diarrhea, and pulmonary aspiration (Ciocon, Galindo-Ciocon, Tiessen, & Galindo, 1992; Heitkemper, Martin, Hansen, Hanson, & Vanderburg, 1980; Padilla et al., 1979; Smith, Faust-Wilson, Lohr, Kallenberger, & Marien, 1992; Smith et al., 1990; Walike et al., 1974; Zimmaro et al., 1988). No studies on potential problems or patient education for home nasogastric feedings were identified, although clinical care plans and articles abound. Researchers have challenged others to identify characteristics such as home environmental risk factors, that predispose individuals to have adverse outcomes (Bergstrom, 1986; Winkler, 1987). Heitkemper and Shaver (1989) provided a conceptual framework for guiding such studies. External validity will continue to be a problem as long as heterogeneous samples contain subjects with enteral feedings of different calorie amounts and comparisons are made among subjects with varying characteristics, such as age and medical disorder.

Hemodialysis and Peritoneal Dialysis

The earliest home technology treatment was hemodialysis, thus the research and writings in this area provide a rich historical literature. Persons working with any technology-dependent population are encouraged to read the classic studies (Downs, 1966; Hoffart, 1989; Levy, 1974; O'Brien, 1983; Schmeck, 1965; Warshofsky, 1965; Watkins, 1966). The United States Renal Data system (1993) report indicated that approximately 16.11% of the 190,000 end-stage patients manage dialysis (hemodialysis or peritoneal) treatments in their homes.

Hemodialysis. Investigators have substantiated the efficacy of home hemodialysis for patients (George, 1983; Goodenough, Lutz, & Gregory, 1988; Gutman & Amara, 1978; Johnson et al., 1984; Kurtz & Johnson, 1984, Mailloux et al., 1988; Roberts, 1976; Roberts, Maxwell, & Gross, 1980; Whalen & Freeman, 1978). Advantages of home hemodialysis are reported to be reduced travel time to centers for dialysis and ease of return to work (Gutman, Stead, & Robinson, 1981; O'Brien, 1983; Soskolne & De Nour, 1987). Christensen and colleagues (1990) identified an association between higher levels of patient involvement with treatment (home dialysis) and greater dietary adherence (outcome measures of lower serum potassium and lower interdialytic weight). However, in a more recent study, home hemodialysis patients' adherence to dietary restrictions were not associated with the level of perceived family support; rather it was associated with adherence to fluid restrictions (Christensen, Smith, Turner, Holman, Gregory, & Rich, 1992). Stressors for hemodialysis and continuous ambulatory peritoneal dialysis (CAPD) patients have been identified to be fatigue; sleep disturbances (Eichel, 1986; Srivastava, 1988); limited physical activity (Baldree, Murphy, & Powers, 1982; Gurklis & Minke, 1988; Stevenson, 1984); financial problems (Ferrans & Powers, 1985); feelings of helplessness (Rydholm & Pauling, 1991); disease-related issues, such as itching and muscle cramps (Fuchs & Schreiber, 1988); and difficulty adhering to the diet (Bollin & Hart, 1982; Cummings, Becker, Kirscht, & Levine, 1982; O'Brien, 1980). The HCFA has encouraged home dialysis as a less expensive method of treatment compared with in-center treatment (Goodspeed & Sylvester, 1985). Early studies indicated that patients and caregivers managed home hemodialysis, regardless of personality characteristics, as long as the family was effectively educated to communicate about technical problems and any distress they encountered (Maurin & Schenkel, 1976; Pentecost, Zwerenz, & Manuel, 1976; Wiegmann et al., 1983).

Accusations of using race or socioeconomic level to determine modes of treatment (in-center, home dialysis, or renal transplant) have been made (Rettig & Levinsky, 1991). However, variation in the treatment modalities of 419 patients at four treatment centers was similarly distributed across age, sex, race, marital and employment status, presence of diabetes mellitus, and travel time to the centers (Smith, Hang, Michelman, & Robson, 1983). Suicide by patient-initiated withdrawal of hemodialysis has been reported. Roberts and Kjellstrand (1988) identified 26 home dialysis patients, where no technical or medical complication occurred, indicating these patients died because they stopped dialysis. Recommendations were made for more realistic descriptions of home care, improved training, and better psychological support to reduce the stress of home dialysis procedures. Questions of health providers not offering alternatives or pressuring patients to continue unwanted treatment and other ethical issues were raised in a report issued by the National Institute of Medicine (Rettig & Levinsky, 1991).

Continuous Ambulatory Peritoneal Dialysis. CAPD is the technology whereby solution is infused through an indwelling abdominal catheter, and the peritoneum serves as the dialyzing membrane. In the United States, there are approximately 3,800 patients on CAPD annually, with most children using this method of dialysis (Nolph, 1990). The procedures for CAPD are complex, not fully automated, and time-consuming. CAPD patients require 4 to 6 or more infusion/drainage cycles daily. Consalves-Ebrahim, Gulledge, and Miga (1990) studied 49 adult patients and suggested that those with compulsive tendencies to repeat behaviors specifically might be the best candidates to train for this tedious continuous technology. In patients treated for 3 years or longer, peritonitis, the most frequent complication, occurred on the average at 11.7 months, although this infection can occur at any time (Nolph, 1990). In a prospective study, the probability of needing a catheter replaced during the first year of CAPD was determined to be twice as high for pediatric patients as for adults. A significant inverse correlation existed between the number of children treated at a center and peritonitis risk, indicating a possible relationship between treatment experience and reduced patient side effects (Alexander, Lindblad, Nolph, & Novak, 1990). Dekeyser (1990) identified a weak relationship between peritoneal immune function and psychosocial measures of stress, anxiety, and depression in 32 CAPD patients.

Home CAPD is described as offering several advantages, such as maintenance of steady biochemical/fluid control, reduced dietary restrictions, freedom from needle punctures, and ability to receive treatment in the familiar home environment (Alexander et al., 1990). In assessing return to work or school, no differences were found between those treated with hemodialysis versus peritoneal dialysis when elderly and debilitated patients were excluded from the comparison groups (Rubin, Case, & Bower, 1990; Soskolne & De-Nour, 1987). Scribner (1985) suggested that nighttime peritoneal dialysis may be the optimum alternative when a fully automated peritoneal dialysis machine becomes affordable. Key factors noted for success with CAPD were adequate cognitive function, good body image, tolerance for environmental stresses, effective patient education, and support and acceptance of relatives who can provide care. Unfortunately, researchers rarely described issues related to validity of psychological testing. They also did not discuss limitations of their data nor the problem of missing data. Yet, limitations of psychological testing in technology-dependent populations were described (Yanagida & Streltzer, 1979), and Kaplan-DeNour (1982) developed a scale with good psychometric properties for determining psychosocial adjustment to hemodialysis.

Infusion Therapies in the Home

A 1991 survey of the staff of certified homecare agencies identified intravenous therapy as one of the top 10 concerns for home care (McAbee, Grupp, & Horn, 1991). Specific issues raised were inadequate discharge planning, overregulation, and insufficiently trained home care staff. They also listed a lack of guidelines for use, caregiver assessment parameters, standards of care, and legal-ethical concerns. Chemotherapy, blood, and blood component infusions were listed as the most problematic technologies. Annual growth in home antibiotic and chemotherapy infusion is reported to be 31.5% (National Association for Home Care, 1991).

Home Antibiotic Infusions. Home antibiotic therapy was found to be efficacious in that infections resolved, and adverse occurrences did not differ from hospital infusion complications (Corby, Schad, & Fudge, 1986; Eisenberg & Kitz, 1986; Kind, Williams, & Gibson, 1984; Poretz et al., 1984; Rehm, 1985; Stiver, Trosky, Cote, & Oruck, 1982; Swenson, 1981). Most of these studies had small samples and used strict selection protocols so that subjects were alert, well educated, cooperative, and afebrile. Subjects also had insurance coverage and a supportive caregiver at home (Antoniskis, Anderson, Van Volkinburg, Jackson, & Gilbert, (1978; Kind & Williams, 1979, 1982; Poretz et al., 1982; Ricker & Harrison, 1974; Stiver et al., 1978). Generalizing efficacy of home infusions to symptomatic, unsupported patients requiring triple antibiotic therapy is cautioned. Balinsky and Nesbitt (1989), in a review of home antibiotic infusion research, emphasized that early cost analyses were limited to data on direct costs of therapy. More recent studies (Rehm & Weinstein, 1983; Rehm, 1985) considered indirect costs to the family (such as loss of caregiver income and nonreimbursable costs, such as transportation for laboratory blood draws and tests).

Other Infusion Therapies. Studies of home immunoglobulin infusions, with small samples ranging from 1 to 13 subjects, for a total of 23 (five subjects were children) have been reported. After 3 weeks of extensive in-hospital training, family members performed the weekly vena punctures and infused intravenous immunoglobulin at home (Ashida & Saxon, 1986; Ochs et al., 1987; Ryan, Thomson, & Webster, 1988; Sorensen, Kallick, & Berger, 1987). In these studies data were collected in the home by one or two trained observers using rating scales that had established interrater reliability. Researchers concluded that patients and family members were able to identify phlebitis or superinfection and treat anaphylactic shock; and did desire home therapy. The frequency of adverse effects (drug reactions and intravenous site problems) were comparable with hospital treatments. Nevertheless, costs of the medications and extensive training, as well as problems with multiple vena punctures and the fact that immune therapy is lifelong, undergird the need for longitudinal research (Brennan, 1991).

Infusing chemotherapy at home was studied in a stratified, randomly assigned trial of home care versus hospitalization of 422 cancer patients who required 4 to 8 hours of chemotherapy infusion daily (Mor et al. 1988). Over a 60-day period there were no statistically significant differences in medical or psychosocial outcomes; costs were one third less in the home care group. In another study of 629 patients with advanced cancer receiving chemotherapy at home, two thirds indicated they did not have enough help (Mor, Allen, Siegel, & Houts, 1992). Concerns included adult children not living nearby and lack of resiliency in family helpers. Six months after completion of treatment, response from 434 of the 629 patients indicated that unmet needs were most strongly associated with patients' immobility, and the inability of an informal support system to provide care (Mor, Masterson-Allen, Houts, & Siegel, 1992). Only one instrument was reported (McCusker, 1984) that measures satisfaction with long-term, home care and physician-family involvement in treatment decisions. Cronbach's alphas ranged from .10 to .87; only one dimension (preference for home care) satisfied the discriminant validity criterion (McCusker, 1984).

St. Marie (1989) observed 18 patients receiving long-term epidural analgesia via an intraspinal catheter, where various combinations of medications were infused. The investigator concluded that epidural access was managed without complications and patients remained alert and maintained adequate pain control. For the past decade in the Netherlands clinical outcomes have verified successful home care of 229 terminally ill cancer patients using spinal infusion to control pain (Boersma, Bosma, Giezen, & Theuvenet, 1992). The model of delivery included home care provided by the district nurse, anesthesiologist, and general practice physician. The United States Cancer Pain Relief Committee has adopted this model (Boersma et al., 1992). Ethical-legal concerns about infusions of addictive medications in the home have been raised but not studied. Internal validity of studies could be improved by developing more objective measurements of the patient's status and family members' needs.

Care of Venous Access. Care of venous access devices is a grave responsibility for any type of infusion therapy at home. Catheter-related infections, either local site irritation or catheter colonization, are estimated to occur in 3% to 12% of central venous lines, many escalating to fatal septicemia (Conly, Grieves, & Peters, 1989; Curtas & Tramposch, 1991; Faubion, Wesley, Khalidi, & Silva, 1986; Jarrard, Olson, & Freeman, 1980; Maki & Ringer, 1987; Maki, Ringer, & Alvarado, 1991). Maki and colleagues (1988, 1991) have shown reduced incidence of infection by using catheters designed with antiseptic coating, silver-impregnated collagen, or Dacron cuffs. In reviewing the research on septicemia, thrombosis, and occlusion of central venous catheters, Orr and Ryder (1993) called for continuing research on mechanisms to reduce skin and touch contamination of catheters. In a review of 48 articles on preventing infection in invasive lines, consistent findings were gauze dressings are preferred, good hand-washing techniques are essential, and iodophor ointment is recommended for site care of central lines (Riegel et al., 1993). More research is needed on the length of time that tubing can be kept in one site. Single-study findings and meta-analyses have shown that heparin flushes in intravenous lines do not enhance patency and may lead to osteoporosis (Bern et al., 1990; Goode et al., 1991). Studies of home infusion site care and therapy outcomes are limited because patient populations are small in number and often geographically dispersed. Quasi-experimental comparison group designs with randomization were used in a few home care studies. Selecting cogent comparison samples is difficult because within-group differences of technology-dependent patients and their caregivers are often extreme. Longitudinal studies assessing patient and family members' physical, social-spiritual, and technical adaptation are warranted.

Automatic External Defibrillation in the Home

Automatic external defibrillation (AED) is done with a device that is placed over the chest to deliver electrical impulses for cardioversion. Cummins and colleagues (1984, 1985); Eisenberg and Cummins (1985), and Moore and colleagues (1987) conducted a series of studies that verified family members can be trained successfully to use AED with cardiopulmonary resuscitation for patients who have cardiac arrest at home. In these prospective, controlled studies, only 3% of subjects initially gave unsatisfactory AED-CPR demonstrations, but all skill levels of all subjects declined over time. Caregivers reported feeling more confident because AED was available, only 10% reported feeling strain in their interpersonal relationships with the care recipient, and no changes were reported in anxiety or obsessiveness about AED. However, no data were presented on actual use of AED by caregivers, sleep pattern alterations, availability of services for defibrillator maintenance, or third-party and out-of-pocket costs. The researchers concluded that frequent caregiver retraining is required, but there were no common adverse psychological sequelae to the training or presence of AED. Using odds ratios, better AED survival rates were associated with the younger patient who had higher fibrillation amplitude waves, a witnessed collapse, and a short period before defibrillation (Weaver et al., 1988). No clinical studies monitoring the effect of interruption of CPR to deliver AED countershock have been reported (Cummins et al., 1985). Eisenberg and Cummins (1985) called for further research and refinement of the defibrillator design to reduce operator error.

Researchers raised questions about a layperson's ability to verify a cardiac arrest before using this technology in the home. However, new technology of implantable automatic defibrillators may make this a mute issue. Unfortunately none of the AED studies was extended beyond 3 months, a considerable limitation in light of the recommendations that retraining be instituted every 6 weeks. Authors raised important ethical questions about the difficulty and expense of making this lifesaving technology available to all candidates (Shepherd, Gardynik, & Cleary, 1990).

CONCLUSIONS AND RECOMMENDATIONS FOR FUTURE RESEARCH

Studies to date have described the prevalence of technology in the home, clinical outcomes of therapy, desire of families to have the patient at home, and cost savings when compared with institutional care. Prevalence of technology in home care is increasing, and clinical outcomes have been positive. However, studies rarely provided detailed information on negative outcomes, untoward effects, or maladaptation of patient or family. Longitudinal studies are needed to follow patients and families over time. Data on untoward events would be helpful in making judgments about technology effectiveness and for developing future interventions. Generally, it is acknowledged that costs are shifted to families who provide home nursing care. Ample data document the economic and emotional strain resulting from the nonreimbursed costs, insurance coverage regulations, and loss of income resulting from caregiving responsibilities for home technology care (Smith, Fernengel, Workowitch & Holcroft, 1992). Studies are needed that compare families' use of home care resources under different funding mechanisms (federal versus private payers) and different service delivery systems. Conclusions from this review are consistent with those of Barkauskas (1990) who indicated that the predominate interest in cost-containment research (i.e., costs) limited study of quality of life, and patient or family caregivers needs. A chapter reviewing studies of these issues will be included in a future volume. Qualitative studies are needed on the individuals' experience of technology dependency, that is, how it feels to live connected to a machine (Gries & Fernsler, 1988). Reactions of families to home technology have been addressed superficially by comparing their preference for home care or institutionalization. However, more sensitive research on social isolation, family functional dysfunction, and long-term lived experiences and outcomes are needed.

Health professionals consistently affirm through consensus conferences, guidelines, position papers, and textbooks that an experienced multidisciplinary team is essential for assisting families to manage home technology. Further, some data indicated that improvement in patient condition (e.g., lower infections) occurred when an experienced multidisciplinary team guided home care. The research reviewed herein, however, documented that few families had access to skilled multidisciplinary teams. Family members served as their own nursing care team working around the clock. Studying families as nearly self-contained systems of health care may help delineate sets of variables predictive of successful home care outcomes.

Most of the research reviewed has been descriptive, narrow in focus, and cross-sectional rather than longitudinal. Few studies have been conceptually or theoretically based, although the combination of quantitative and qualitative methods has strengthened many research designs. Research based on Brooten and colleagues' (1986, 1988) conceptualization of transitional care or McConnell (1989) and others' (Christman et al., 1988) framework of man-machine interface have guided research in home care and technology dependence, respectively. Clinical models of comprehensive or family-centered approaches for delivering technology home care services might also be fruitful in guiding research (Kaufman & Hardy-Ribakow, 1987; Smith, Giefer, & Bieker, 1991). Ingersoll, Hoffart, and Schultz (1990) applied Toulmin's Model of Knowledge Development in their review of nursing health services research and concluded that the most conspicuously absent studies pertained to health care technology, information systems, and ethical decision making.

Research on technology in the home also should include issues that are germane to the elderly and to culturally diverse populations (King, Figge, & Jarman 1986; Roy, Flynn, & Atcherson, 1980). Although ethnicity and gender were reported in a few studies, most samples did not analyze or discuss data relative to these perspectives or characteristics (Guilleminault et al., 1988). Nurses will need to determine if the findings from research on caregiving of frail elderly in the home (e.g., restructuring caregiving routines to decrease fatigue) or from research on acute care (e.g., promoting sleep, preventing infection) can be applied reliably in the home. Evaluations are also needed of mainstreaming technologically dependent children into schools and returning adults to work.

Nurse educators are faced with testing curricula that adequately educate nurses for community-based health care systems where technology treatments are managed by families (Hegyvary, 1993; Jacox, 1992). Nurse administrators will need to evaluate case management or clinical pathway approaches that guide implementation of nursing intervention taxonomies for home care (Bulechek & McCloskey, 1992; Saba, O'Hare, Boondas, Levine, & Oatway, 1992). Mechanisms for quality assurance, easing transition to home care, and cost savings for families need study (Lalonde, 1986). The clinical competence and caring attitudes of professionals and nonprofessionals who work with technology-dependent individuals (Carnevali, 1985; Braun et al., 1984; Luker & Box, 1986) and ethical problems in home technology care should be described (Haddad, 1992). Nurse clinicians can lead in the development of the technology itself by providing databased input into mechanical device design that will increase ease of use, reuse cost savings, and enhance fail-safe mechanisms (Lindeman, 1992; Prowant & Ryan, 1989). Improved technical equipment is needed, but with limited numbers of patients using technology, little incentive exists for manufacturers to expand funds to develop and then test new equipment. As with all home environments, contamination during technical procedures or a social environment lacking in support for the patient are potential nursing problems needing study (Winkler 1987).

The areas of highest priority for research include continuing study of the impact of technology in the home, identifying and treating problems of technology dependence, evaluating the caregiving effectiveness of families, and coordinating services for efficient use and access to resources. Lastly, because most home technology studies to date have been conducted by other health professionals, nurses should be encouraged to collaborate but also develop programs of research in areas of human response to technology dependence and home care.

ACKNOWLEDGMENTS

Roma Lee Taunton, RN, PhD, is acknowledged for her review of this chapter and for her ongoing encouragement. Thank you to colleagues Nancy Hoffart, Janet Pierce, and Phoebe Williams for their helpful comments.

REFERENCES

Alexander, S. R., Lindblad, A. S., Nolph, K. D., & Novak, J. W. (1990). Pediatric CAPD/CCPD in the United States. In J. H. Stein (Ed.), *Peritoneal dialysis* (pp. 231–255). New York: Churchill Livingstone.

Alverdy, J. A., Chi, H. S., & Sheldon, G. S. (1985). The effect of parenteral nutrition on gastrointestinal immunity: The importance of enteral stimulation. *Annals of Surgery, 202*, 681–684.

Alverdy, J. C., Aoys, E., & Moss, G. S. (1988). Total parenteral nutrition promotes bacterial translocation from the gut. *Surgery, 104*, 185–190.

Andre, J. (1986). Home health care and high-tech medical equipment. *Caring, 5*, 9–12.

Antoniskis, A., Anderson, B. C., Van Volkinburg, E. J., Jackson, J. M., & Gilbert, D. N. (1978). Feasibility of outpatient self-administration of parenteral antibiotics. *The Western Journal of Medicine, 128*, 203–206.

Ashida, E. R., & Saxon, A. (1986). Home intravenous immunoglobulin therapy by self-administration. *Journal of Clinical Immunology, 6*, 306–309.

Ashley, M. J. (1989). Concerns of sleep apnea patients. *Western Journal of Nursing Research, 11*, 600–608.

Bakke, K., & Dougherty, J. (1981). Sudden infant death syndrome and infant apnea: Current questions, clinical management and research directions. *Issues in Comprehensive Pediatric Nursing, 5*, 77–78.

Baldree, K., Murphy, S., & Powers, M. (1982). Stress identification and coping patterns in patients on hemodialysis. *Nursing Research, 31*, 107–112.

Balinsky, W., & Nesbitt, S. (1989). Cost-effectiveness of outpatient parenteral antibiotics: A review of the literature. *American Journal of Medicine, 87*, 301–305.

Banaszak, E., Travers, H., Frazier, M., & Vinz, T. (1981). Home ventilator care. *Respiratory Care, 26*, 1266–1268.

Barkauskas, V. (1990). Home health care. In J. V. Fitzpatrick, R. L. Taunton, & J. Q. Benoliel (Eds.), *Annual review of nursing research*. (Vol. 8, pp. 103–132). New York: Springer Publishing.

Bayer, R. (1987). Ethical challenges in the movement for home health care. *Generations, 27*, 44–46.

Berg, R. D. (1981). Promotion of the translocation of enteric bacteria from the gastrointestinal tracts of mice by oral treatment with penicillin, clindamycin, or metroidazole. *Infection and Immunity, 33*, 854–861.

Bergstrom, N. (1986). Selecting methods to measure nutrition outcomes. *Oncology Nursing Forum, 13*(1), 96–98, 102–103.

Bern, M. M., Lokich, J. J., Wallach, S. R., Bothe, A., Jr., Benotti, P. N., Arkin, C. F., Greco, F. A., Huberman, M., & Moore, C. (1990). Very low doses of Warfarin can prevent thrombosis in central venous catheters: A randomized prospective trial. *Annals of Internal Medicine, 112*, 423–428.

Black, L,. Hersher, L., & Steinschneider, A. (1978). Impact of the apnea monitor on family life. *Pediatrics, 62*, 681–685.

Boersma, F. P., Bosma, E. S., Giezen, L. M., & Theuvenet, P. J. (1992). Cancer pain control by infusion techniques in the home situation in the northern Netherlands: An innovative project on the use of medical technology in the home situation. *Journal of Pain and Symptom Management, 7*(3), 155–159.

Bollin, B. W., & Hart, L. K. (1982). The relationship of health belief motivations, health locus of control and health valuing to dietary compliance of hemodialysis patients. *American Association of Nephrology Nurses and Technicians, 9*(5), 41–47.

Braun, J. L., Baines, S. L., Olson, N. G., Scruby, L. S., Manteuffel, C. A., & Cretilli, P. K. (1984). The future of nursing: Combining humanistic and technological values. *Health Values: Achieving High Level Wellness, 8*(3), 12–15.

Brennan, V. (1991). Home self-infusion of I. V. immunoglobulin. *Nursing Standard, 5*, 37–39.

Brooten, D., Brown, L. P., Hazard-Munro, B., York, R., Cohen, S. M., Roncoli, M., & Hollingsworth, A. (1988). Early discharge and specialist transitional care. *Image: The Journal of Nursing Scholarship, 20*, 64–68.

Brooten, D., Kumar, S., Brown, L., Buitts, P., Finkler, S., Bakewell-Sachs, S., Gibbens, A., & Delivoria-Papadopoulos, M. (1986). A randomized clinical trial of early hospital discharge and home follow-up of very-low-birth-weight infants. *The New England Journal of Medicine, 315*, 934–938.

Bulecheck, G. M., & McCloskey, J. C. (1992). Future directions in nursing. In Bulechek & McCloskey (Eds.), *Nursing interventions: Essential nursing treatments* (2nd ed., pp. 602–609). Philadelphia: Saunders.

Burr, B. H., Guyer, B., Todres, I. D., Abrahams, B., & Chiodo, T. (1983). Home care for children on respirators. *New England Journal of Medicine, 309*, 1319–1323.

Cabin, B. (1985). Cost-effectiveness of pediatric home care. *Caring, 4*, 48–49.

Cain, L. P., Kelly, D. H., & Shannon, D. C. (1980). Parents' perceptions of the psychological and social impact of home monitoring. *Pediatrics, 66*, 37–41.

Carnevali, D. L. (1985). Nursing perspectives in health care technology. *Nursing Administration Quarterly, 9*(4), 10–18.

Christensen, A. J., Smith, T. W., Turner, C. W., Holman, J. M., Jr., & Gregory, M. C. (1990). Type of hemodialysis and preference for behavioral involvement: Interactive effects on adherence in end-stage renal disease. *Health Psychology, 9*(2), 225–236.

Christensen, A. J., Smith, T. W., Turner, C. W., Holman, J. M., Jr., Gregory, M. C., & Rich, M. A. (1992). Family support, physical impairment, and adherence in hemodialysis: An investigation of main and buffering effects. *Journal of Behavioral Medicine, 15*, 313–325.

Christman, N. J., McConnell, E. A., Pfeiffer, C., Webster, K. K., Schmitt, M., & Ries, J. (1988). Uncertainty, coping, and distress following myocardial infarction: Transition from hospital to home. *Research in Nursing & Health, 11*, 71–82.

Ciocon, J. O., Galindo-Ciocon, G., Tiessen, C., & Galindo, D. (1992). Continuous compared with intermittent tube feeding in the elderly. *Journal of Parenteral and Enteral Nutrition, 16*, 525–528.

Conly, J. M., Grieves, K., & Peters, B. (1989). A prospective randomized study comparing transparent and dry gauze dressing for central venous catheters. *Journal of Infectious Diseases, 159*, 310–319.

Copeman, E., & Weigel, L. (1987). Training homemaker-home health aides for high-tech home care. *Caring, 6*, 34–37.

Corby, D., Schad, R. F., & Fudge, J. P. (1986). Intravenous antibiotic therapy: Hospital to home. *Nursing Management, 17*(8), 52–61.

Cummings, K. M., Becker, M. H., Kirscht, J. P., & Levine, N. W. (1981). Intervention strategies to improve compliance with medical regimens by ambulatory hemodialysis patients. *Journal of Behavioral Medicine, 4*, 111–127.

Cummings, K. M., Becker, M. H., Kirscht, J. P., & Levine, N. W (1982). Psychosocial factors affecting adherence to medical regiments in a group of hemodialysis patients. *Medical Care, 20*, 567–580.

Cummings, K. M., Kirscht, J. P., Becker, M. H., & Levine, N. W. (1984). Construct validity comparisons of three methods for measuring patient compliance. *Health Services Research, 19*, 103–116.

Cummins, R. O., Eisenberg, M. S., Bergner, L., Hallstrom, A., Hearne, T., & Murray, J. A. (1984). Automatic external defibrillation:Evaluations of its role in the home and in emergency medical services. *Annals of Emergency Medicine, 13*, 798–801.

Cummins, R. O., Eisenberg, M. S., Moore, J. E., Hearne, T. R., Andersen, E., & Wendt, R. (1985). Automatic external defibrillators: Clinical, training, psychological, and public health issues. *Annals of Emergency Medicine, 14*, 755–760.

Curtas, S., & Tramposch, K. (1991). Culture methods to evaluate central venous catheter sepsis. *Nutrition in Clinical Practice, 6*, 43–48.

Daly, B. J., Newlon, B., Montenegro, H. D., & Langdon, T. (1993). Withdrawal of mechanical ventilation: Ethical principles and guidelines for terminal weaning. *American Journal of Critical Care, 2*(3), 217–223.

Dekeyser, F. G. (1990). *Psychosocial factors and peritoneal immune function in CAPD patients*. Baltimore, MD: University of Maryland.

Diehl, S. F., Moffitt, K. A., & Wade, S. M. (1991). Focus group interview with parents of children with medically complex needs: An intimate look at their perceptions and feelings. *Children's Health Care, 20*, 170–178.

Dillman, D. A. (1978). *Fail and Telephone Surveys: The Total Design Method*. New York: Wiley.

DiMaggio, G., & Sheetz, A. (1983). The concerns of mothers caring for an infant on an apnea monitor. *MCN: The American Journal of Maternal/Child Nursing, 8*, 294–297.

Dixon, J. (1984). Effect of nursing interventions on nutritional and performance status in cancer patients. *Nursing Research, 33*, 330–334.

Donn, S (1982). Cost-effectiveness of home management of bronchopulmonary dysplasia. *Pediatrics, 70*, 330–331.

Downs, F. S. (1966). Technical innovation and the future of the nurse–patient relationship. In *American Nurses Association clinical sessions* (pp. 232–237). New York: Appleton-Century-Crofts.

Dye, J. P. (1983). Living with a tracheostomy for sleep apnea. *New England Journal of Medicine, 308*, 1167.

Eichel, C. J. (1986). Stress and coping in patients on CAPD compared to hemodialysis patients. *American Nephrology Nurses' Association Journal, 13*, 9–13.

Eisenberg, J. M., & Kitz, D. S. (1986). Savings from outpatient antibiotic therapy for osteomyelitis. *Journal of the American Medical Association, 255*, 1584–1588.

Eisenberg, M. S., & Cummins, R. O. (1985). Automatic external defibrillation: Bringing it home [Editorial]. *The American Journal of Emergency Medicine, 3*, 568–569.

Englert, D. M., & Dudrick, S. J. (1978). Principles of ambulatory home hyperalimentation. *American Journal of Intravenous Therapy, 5*(5), 11–28.

Faubion, W. C., Wesley, J. R., Khalidi, N. & Silva, J. (1986). Total parenteral nutrition catheter sepsis: Impact of the team approach. *Journal of Parenteral and Enteral Nutrition, 10*, 642.

Feldman, J., & Tuteur, P. (1982). Mechanical ventilation: From intensive care to home. *Heart & Lung, 11*, 162–165.

Ferrans, C. E., & Powers, M. J. (1985). The employment potential of hemodialysis patients. *Nursing Research, 34*, 273–277.

Fields, A. I., Coble, D. H., Pollack, M. M., & Kaufman, J. (1991). Outcome of home care for technology-dependent children: Success of an independent, community-based case management model. *Pediatric Pulmonology, 11*, 310–317.

Fischer, D. A. (1989). Long-term management of the ventilator-dependent patient: Levels of disability and resocialization. *The European Respiratory Journal Supplementary, 7*(Suppl.), 651S–654S.

Foundation for Hospice and Homecare. (March 23, 1987). Crisis of chronically ill children in America:Triumph of technology—failure in policy. Paper presented to U.S.Congress, Washington, DC.

Frace, R. (1986). Home ventilation: An alternative to institutionalization. *Focus on Critical Care, 13*(6), 28–34.

Frates, R. C., Splaingard, M. L., Smith, E. O., & Harrison, G. M. (1985). Outcome of home mechanical ventilation for children. *The Journal of Pediatrics, 106*, 850–856.

Fry, S. T. (1990). Ethical issues in total parenteral nutrition. *Nutrition, 6*, 329–331.

Fuchs, J., & Schreiber, M. (1988). Patients' perceptions of CAPD and hemodialysis stressors. *American Nephrology Nurses' Association Journal, 15*, 282–285.

Geary, P. A. (1989). Stress and social support in the experience of monitoring apneic infants. *Clinical Nurse Specialist, 3*, 119–125.

George, C. R. (1983). Feasibility of universal home hemodialysis with simplified techniques. *Lancet, 2*, 895–897.

Gilmartin, M., & Make, B. (1983). Home care of the ventilator-dependent person. *Respiratory Care, 28*, 365–366.

Gipson, W. T., Sivak, E. D., & Gulledge, A. D. (1987). Psychological aspects of ventilator dependency. *Psychiatric Medicine, 5*, 213–245.

Goel, V. (1990). Economics of total parenteral nutrition. *Nutrition, 6*, 332–335.

Goldberg, A. I. (1983). Home care for a better life for ventilator-dependent people. *Chest, 84*, 365–366.

Goldberg, A. I. (1986). Home care for life-supported persons: Is a national approach the answer? *Chest, 90*, 744–748.

Goldberg, A. I., & Frownfelter, D. (1990). The ventilator-assisted individuals study. *Chest, 98*, 428–433.

Gonsalves-Ebrahim, L., Gulledge, A. D., & Miga, S. (1990). Continuous ambulatory peritoneal dialysis: Psychological factors. *Psychosomatics, 23*, 944–949.

Goode, C. J., Titler, M., Rakel, B., Ones, D. S., Kleiber, C., Small, S., & Triolo, P. (1991). A meta-analysis of effects of heparin flush and saline flush: Quality and cost implications. *Nursing Research, 40*, 324–330.

Goodenough, G. K., Lutz, L. J., Gregory, M. C. (1988). Home-based renal dialysis. *American Family Physician, 37*, 203–214.

Goodspeed, N. B., & Sylvester, B. S. (1985). New technology and economic incentives will spur the growth of dialysis at home. *Caring, 4*, 28–34.

Gries, M. L., & Fernsler, J. F. (1988). Patient perceptions of the mechanical ventilation experience. *Focus on Critical Care, 15*(2), 52–59.

Guilleminault, C., Quera-Salva, M. A., Partinen, M., & Jamieson, A. (1988). Women and the obstructive sleep apnea syndrome. *Chest, 93*, 104–109.

Gulledge, A. D. (1985). Common psychiatric concerns in home parenteral nutrition. *Cleveland Clinic Quarterly, 52*, 329–332.

Gulledge, A. D., Gipson, W. T., Steiger, E., Hooley, R.,& Sep, F. (1980). Home parenteral nutrition for the short bowel syndrome psychological issues. *General Hospital Psychiatry, 2*, 271–281.

Gurklis, J. A., & Menke, E. M. (1988). Identification of stressors and use of coping methods in chronic hemodialysis patients. *Nursing Research, 37*, 236–239.

Gutman, R. A., & Amara, A. H. (1978). Outcome of therapy for end-stage uremia: An informed prediction of survival rate and degree of rehabilitation. *Postgraduate Medicine, 64*, 183–194.

Gutman, R. A., Stead, W. W., & Robinson, R. (1981). Physical activity and employment status of patients on maintenance dialysis. *New England Journal of Medicine, 304*, 309-313.

Haddad, A.M. (1992). Ethical problems in home health care. *Journal of Nursing Administration, 22*(3), 46–51.

Hall, R., & Beresford, T. P. (1987). Psychiatric factors in the management of long-term hyperalimentation patients. *Psychiatric Medicine, 5*, 211-216.

Hegyvary (1993). *A vision for nursing education*. New York: National League for Nursing.

Heitkemper, M. M., Martin, D. L., Hansen, B. C., Hanson, R., & Vanderburg, V. (1980). Rate and volume of intermittent enteral feeding. *Journal of Parenteral and Enteral Nutrition, 5*, 125–129.

Heitkemper, M. M., & Shaver, J. F. (1989). Nursing research opportunities in enteral nutrition. *Nursing Clinics of North America, 24*, 415–427.

Henry, W. C., West, G. A., & Wilson, R. S. (1983). A comparison of the oxygen cost of breathing between a continuous-flow CPAP system and a demand-flow CPAP system. *Respiratory Care, 28*, 1273-1281.

Herfindal, E. T., Bernstein, L R., Wong, A. G., Hogue, V. W., & Darbinian, J. A. (1992). Complications of home parenteral nutrition. *Clinical Pharmacy, 11*, 543-548.

Hoffart, N. (1989). Nephrology nursing 1915-1970: A historical study of the integration of technology and care. *American Nephrology Nurses' Association Journal, 16*, 169-178.

Howard, B. J., Meade, P. A., Booth, D., & Whall, A. (1988). The telephone interview. *Applied Nursing Research, 1*, 45–46.

Howard, L., Heaphey, L., Fleming, C. R., Lininger, L., & Steiger, E. (1991). Four years of North American registry home parenteral nutrition outcome data and their implications for patient management. *Journal of Parenteral and Enteral Nutrition, 15*, 384–393.

Howard, L., & Michalek, A. V. (1984). Home parenteral nutrition. *Annual Review of Nutrition, 4*, 69–99.

Hung, J., Whitford, E. G., Parsons, R. W., & Hillman D. R. (1990). Association of sleep apnea with myocardial infarction in men. *Lancet, 336*, 261-264.

Ingersoll, G. L., Hoffart, N., & Schultz, A.W. (1990). Health services research in nursing: Current status and future directions. *Nursing Economics, 8*, 229-238.

Jacox, A. (1992). Health care technology and its assessment: Where nursing fits in. In L. Aiken & C. Fagin (Eds.), *Charting nursing's future: Agenda for the 1990s* (pp. 70-84). Philadelphia: Lippincott.

Jarrard, M. M., Olson, C. M., & Freeman, J. B. (1980). Daily dressing change effects on skin flora beneath sub-clavian catheter dressings during total parenteral nutrition. *Journal of Parenteral and Enteral Nutrition, 4*, 391-392.

Jeejeebhoy, K. N., Zohrab, W. J., Langer, B., Phillips, H. J., Kukis, A., & Anderson, G. H. (1973). Total parenteral nutrition at home for 23 months, without complications, and with good rehabilitation. *Gastroenterology, 65*, 811-820.

Johnson, W. J., Kurtz, S. B., Anderson, C. F., Mitchell, J. C., Zincke, H., & O'Fallon W. M. (1984). Results of treatment of renal failure by means of home hemodialysis. *Mayo Clinic Proceedings, 59*, 663-668.

Kaplan-DeNour, A. (1982). Psychosocial adjustment to illness scale (PAIS): A study of chronic hemodialysis patients. *Journal of Psychosomatic Research, 26*, 11–22.

Kaufman, J., & Hardy-Ribakow, D. (1987). Home care: A model of a comprehensive approach for technology-assisted chronically ill children. *Journal of Pediatric Nursing, 2*, 244–249.

Kerby, G., Mayer, L., & Pingleton, S. (1987, March). Nocturnal positive pressure ventilation via nasal mask. *American Review of Respiratory Disease, 135*, 738–740.

Kerr, P., Shoenut, J. P., Millar, T., Buckle, P., & Kryger, M. H. (1992). Nasal CPAP reduces gastroesophageal reflux in obstructive sleep apnea syndrome. *Chest, 101*, 1539–1544.

Kind, A. C., & Williams, D. N. (1979). Intravenous antibiotic therapy at home. *Archives of Internal Medicine, 139*, 413–415.

Kind, A. C., & Williams, D. N. (1982, March). Outpatient intravenous antibiotic experience with 65 patients. *American Journal of Intravenous Therapy and Clinical Nutrition, 9*,(3), 33–40.

Kind, A. C., Williams, D. N., & Gibson, J. (1984). Outpatient intravenous antibiotic therapy: Ten years' experience. *Postgraduate Medicine, 77*, 105–111.

King, F. E., Figge, J., & Jarman, P. (1986). The elderly coping at home: A study of continuity of nursing care. *Journal of Advanced Nursing, 11*, 41–46.

Klijanowicz, A. S. (1984). Psychosocial aspects of home apnea monitoring. *Perinatology-Neonatology, 8*(5), 28–36.

Kopacz, M., & Moriarty-Wright, R. (1984). Multidisciplinary approach for the patient on a home ventilator. *Heart & Lung, 13*, 255–262.

Kruger, S., & Rawlins, P. (1984). Pediatric dismissal protocol to aid the transition from hospital care to home care. *Image: The Journal of Nursing Scholarship, 16*, 120–125.

Kun, S., & Warburton, D. (1987). Telephone assessment of parents' knowledge of home-care treatments and readmission outcomes for high-risk infants and toddlers. *American Journal of Diseases of Children, 141*, 888–892.

Kurtz, S. B., & Johnson, W. J. (1984). A four-year comparison of continuous ambulatory peritoneal dialysis and home hemodialysis: A preliminary report. *Mayo Clinic Proceedings, 59*, 659–662.

Lalonde, B. (1986). *Quality assurance manual of the Home Care Association of Washington*. Edmonds, WA: Home Care Association of Washington.

Lange, M. H. (1986). Managing Blue Cross & Blue Shield benefits for high-tech home care. *Caring, 5*, 58–60.

Lehner, W., Ballard, I., Figueroa, W., &Woodruff, D. (1980). Home care utilizing a ventilator in a patient with amyotrophic lateral sclerosis. *Journal of Family Practice, 10*, 39–42.

Levy, N. B. (Ed.). (1974). *Living or dying: Adaptation to hemodialysis*. Springfield, IL: Charles C Thomas.

Lindeman, C. A. (1992). Nursing & technology: Moving into the 21st century. *Caring, 11*(5), 7–10.

Lobosco, A. F., Eron, N. B., Bobo, T., Kril, L., & Chalanick, K.(1991). Local coalitions for coordinating services to children dependent on technology and their families. *Children's Health Care, 20*, 75–86.

Luker, K. A., & Box, D. (1986). The response of nurses towards the management and teaching of patients on continuous ambulatory peritoneal dialysis (CAPD). *International Journal of Nursing Studies, 23*, 51–59.

MacRitchie, K. J. (1978). Life without eating or drinking: Total parenteral nutrition outside hospital. *Canadian Psychiatric Association Journal, 23*, 373–379.

Mailloux, L. U., Bellucci, A. G., Mossey, R. T., Napolitano, B., Moore, T., Wilkes, B. M., & Bluestone, P. A. (1988). Predictors of survival in patients undergoing dialysis. *American Journal of Medicine, 84*, 855–862.

Make, B., Gilmartin, M., Brody, J. S., & Snider, G. L. (1984). Rehabilitation of ventilator-dependent subjects with lung diseases—the concept and initial experience. *Chest, 86*, 358–365.

Maki, D. G., Cobb, L., Garman, J. K., Shapiro, J. M., Ringer, M., & Helgerson, R. B. (1988). An attachable silver impregnated cuff for prevention of infection with central venous catheters: A prospective randomized multicenter trial. *The American Journal of Medicine, 85*, 307–314.

Maki, D. G., & Ringer, M. (1987). Evaluation of dressing regimens for prevention of infection with peripheral intravenous catheters. *Journal of the American Medical Association, 258*, 2396–2403.

Maki, D. G., Ringer, M., & Alvarado, C. J. (1991). Prospective randomized trial of povidone-iodine, alcohol, and chlorhexidine for prevention of infection associated with central venous and arterial catheters. *Lancet, 338*, 339–343.

Malcolm, R., Robson, J. R., Vanderveen, T. W., & O'Neil, P. M. (1980). Psychosocial aspects of total parenteral nutrition. *Psychosomatics, 21*, 115–125.

Martin, K. (1988). Research in home care. *Nursing Clinics of North America, 23*, 373–385.

Maurin, J., & Schenkel, J. (1976). A study of the family unit's response to hemodialysis. *Journal of Psychosomatic Research, 20*, 163–168.

McAbee, R. R., Grupp, K., & Horn, B. (1991). Home intravenous therapy: Issues: 1. *Home Health Care Services Quarterly, 12*(3), 59–108.

McConnell, E. A. (1989). The nurse: Liaison between patient and machine. *Plant, Technology & Safety Management Series, 10*, 5–10.

McCusker, J. (1984). Development of scales to measure satisfaction and preferences regarding long-term and terminal care. *Medical Care, 22*, 476–493.

McElroy, E., Steinschneider, A., & Weinstein, S. (1986). Emotional health impact of home monitoring on mothers: A controlled prospective study. *Pediatrics, 78*, 780–786.

Millman, R. P., Kipp, G. J., Beadles, S. C., & Braman, S. S. (1988). A home monitoring system for nasal CPAP. *Chest, 93*, 730–733.

Millner, B. N. (1991). Technology-dependent children in New York State. *Bulletin of New York Academy of Medicine, 67*, 131–142.

Moore, J. E., Eisenberg, M. S., Cummins, R. O., Hallstrom, A., Litwin, P., & Carter, W. (1987). Lay person use of automatic external defibrillation. *Annals of Emergency Medicine, 16*, 669–672.

Moore, M. C., Guenter, P. A., & Bender, J. H. (1986). Nutrition-related nursing research. *Image: The Journal of Nursing Scholarship, 18*, 18–21.

Mor, V., Allen, S. M., Siegel, K., & Houts, P. (1992). Determinants of need and unmet need among cancer patients residing at home. *Health Services Research, 27*, 337–360.

Mor, V., Masterson-Allen, S., Houts, P., & Siegel, K. (1992). The changing needs of patients with cancer at home: A longitudinal view. *Cancer, 69*, 829–838.

Mor, V., Stalker, M. Z., Gralla, R., Scher, H. I., Cimma, C., Park, D., Flaherty, A. M., Kiss, M., Nelson, P., Laliberte, L., Schwartz, R., Marks, S. P., & Oehgen, H. (1988). Day hospital as an alternative to inpatient care for cancer patients: A random assignment trial. *Journal of Clinical Epidemiology, 41*, 771–785.

Motwani, J. K., & Herring, G. M. (1988). Home care for ventilator-dependent persons: A cost-effective, humane, public policy. *Health and Social Work, 13*(1), 20–24.

National Association for Home Care. (1991). Basic statistics about homecare—1991. Washington, DC: Author.

National Association for Home Care. (1992). Basic statistics about home care—1992. Washington, DC: Author.

National Commission on Sleep Disorders Research. (1993). *Wake-up America: A national sleep alert*. (Vol. 1., Executive summary, No. 4969350). Bethesda: MD: National Institutes of Health.

Nolph, K. D. (1990). Clinical results with peritoneal dialysis—registry experiences. In J. H. Stein (Ed.), *Peritoneal dialysis* (pp. 127–144). New York: Churchill Livingstone.

Nuttall, P. (1988). Maternal responses to home apnea monitoring of infants. *Nursing Research, 37*, 354–357.

O'Brien, M. E. (1980). Hemodialysis regimen: Compliance and social environment. *Nursing Research, 29*, 250–255.

O'Brien, M. E. (1983). *The courage to survive: The life career of the chronic dialysis patient*. New York: Grune & Stratton.

Ochs, H. D., Lee, M. L., Fischer, S. H., Delson, E. S., Chang, B. J., & Wedgwood, R. J. (1987). Self-infusion of intravenous immunoglobulin by immunodeficient patients at home. *Journal of Infectious Diseases, 156*, 652–654.

Oley Foundation. (1989). *OASIS Home nutrition support patient registry: Annual reports, 1985–1986, 1987*. Albany, NY: Author.

Orr, M. E., & Ryder, M. A. (1993). Vascular access devices: Perspectives on designs, complications, and management. *Nutrition in Clinical Practice, 8*(4), 145–152.

Orr, W C. (1983). Sleep-related breathing disorders—an update. *Chest, 84*, 475–480.

Padilla, G. V., Grant, M. M., Wong, H., Hansen, B. W., Hanson, R. L., & Bergstrom, N. (1979). Subjective distresses of nasogastric tube feeding. *Journal of Parenteral and Enteral Nutrition, 3*, 53–57.

Parlett, C. H., & Spitzer, A. (1986). Home phototherapy: Keeping baby home. *Caring, 5*, 50–60.

Parrish, R. H., Mitallo, J. M., & Fabri, P. J. (1982). Behavioral management concepts with application for home parenteral nutrition patients. *Drug Intelligence Clinical Pharmacy, 16*, 581–586.

Partinen, M., & Guilleminault, C. (1990). Daytime sleepiness and vascular morbidity at seven-year follow-up in obstructive sleep apnea patients. *Chest, 97*, 27–32.

Payne, J. J., & Ball, P. (1991). Support group for patients receiving home nutritional support. *British Journal of Hospital Medicine, 46*, 269.

Pentecost, R. L., Zwerenz, B., & Manuel, J. W. (1976). Intrafamily identity and home dialysis success. *Nephronology, 17*, 88–103.

Perl, M., Hall, R. C., & Dudrick, S. J. (1980). Psychological aspects of long-term home hyperalimentation. *Journal of Parenteral and Enteral Nutrition, 4*, 554-560.

Perl, M., Peterson, L. G., Dudrick, S. J., & Benson, D. M. (1981). Psychiatric effects of long-term home hyperalimentation. *Psychosomatics, 22*, 1047-1048.

Pillar, B., & Perry, S. (1990). Evaluating total parental nutrition. *Nutrition, 6*, 314–318.

Plummer, A. L., O'Donohue, W. J., & Petty, T. L. (1989). Consensus conference on problems in home mechanical ventilation. *The American Review of Respiratory Disease, 140*, 555-560.

Ponferrada, L., Burrows, L. M., Prowant, B., Satalowich, R. J., Schmidt, L. M., & Bartelt, C. (1993). Home visit effectiveness for peritoneal dialysis patients. *American Nephrology Nurses' Association Journal, 20*, 333-336.

Poretz, D. M., Eron, L. J., Goldenberg, R. I., Gilbert, A. F., Rising, J., Sparks, S., & Horn, C. E. (1982). Intravenous antibiotic therapy in an outpatient setting. *Journal of the American Medical Association, 248*, 336–339.

Poretz, D. M., Woolard, D., Eron, L. J., Goldenberg, R. I., Rising, J., & Sparks, S. (1984). Outpatient use of ceftriaxone: A cost-benefit analysis. *American Journal of Medicine, 77*, 77–83.

Price, B. S., & Levine, E. L. (1979). Permanent total parenteral nutrition: Psychology and social responses of the elderly stages. *Journal of Parenteral and Enteral Nutrition, 3*, 48–52.

Prowant, B. F., & Ryan, L. P.(1989). Peritoneal dialysis transfer set change procedures study. *American Nephrology Nurses' Association Journal, 16*, 23–26.

Rehm, S. J. (1985). Home intravenous antibiotic therapy. *Cleveland Clinic Quarterly, 52*, 333–338.

Rehm, S. J., & Weinstein, A. J. (1983). Home intravenous antibiotic therapy: A team approach. *Annals of Internal Medicine, 99*, 388–392.

Rettig, R. A., & Levinsky, N. G. (Eds.). (1991). *Committee for the Study of the Medicare ESRD Program Division of Health Care Services*. Washington, DC: National Academy Press.

Riegel, B., Banasik, J., Barnsteiner, J., Beecroft, P., Kern, L., Lindquist, R., Prevost, S., & Titler, M. (1993). Reviews and summaries of research related to AACN 1980 priorities. *American Journal of Critical Care, 2*, 413–425.

Robb, R. A., Bradebill, J. I., Ivey, M. F., Christensen, D. B., Young, J. H., & Scribner, B. H. (1983). Subjective assessment of patient outcomes of home parenteral nutrition. *American Journal of Hospital Pharmacy, 40*, 1646–1650.

Roberts, J. C., & Kjellstrand, C. M. (1988). Choosing death: Withdrawal from chronic dialysis without medical reason. *ACTA Medical Scandinavica, 223*, 181–186.

Roberts, J. L. (1976). Analysis and outcome of 1,068 patients trained for home hemodialysis. *Kidney International, 9*, 363–374.

Roberts, S. D., Maxwell, D. R., & Gross, T. L. (1980). Cost-effective care of end-

stage renal disease: A billion dollar question. *Annals of Internal Medicine, 92*, 243–248.
Robinovitch, A. E. (1981). Home total parenteral nutrition: A psychosocial viewpoint. *Journal of Parenteral and Enteral Nutrition, 5*, 522–525.
Roeder, B. J., & Williams, D. N. (1985). Diagnosis-specific home care. *Postgraduate Medicine, 77*, 79–88.
Roy, C., Flynn, E., & Atcherson, E. (1980). Home hemodialysis and the older patient. *American Association of Nephrology Nurses' and Technicians Journal, 7*, 317–324.
Rubin, J., Case, G., & Bower, J. (1990). Comparison of rehabilitation in patients undergoing home dialysis: Continuous ambulatory or cyclic peritoneal dialysis vs. home dialysis. *Archives of Internal Medicine, 150*, 1429–1431.
Rucker, R. W., & Harrison, G. W. (1974). Outpatient intravenous medications in the management of cystic fibrosis. *Pediatrics, 54*, 358–360.
Rundle, R. L. (1988, August 10). Phone-linked medical devices are giving a new meaning to the words "house call." *Wall Street Journal*, p. 19.
Ryan, A., Thomson, B., & Webster, A. (1988). Home intravenous immunoglobulin therapy for patients with primary hypogammaglobulinaemia. *Lancet, 2*, 793.
Rydholm, L., & Pauling, J. (1991). Contrasting feelings of helplessness in peritoneal and hemodialysis patients: A pilot study. *American Nephrology Nurses' Association Journal, 18*, 183–186.
Saba, V., O'Hare, P., Boondas, J., Levine, E., & Oatway, D. (1992). A nursing intervention taxonomy for home health care. *Nursing Scan in Research, 12*, 296–299.
Schmeck, H. M. (1965). *The semi-artificial man*. New York: Walker.
Schreiner, M. S., Donar, M. E., & Kettrick, R. G. (1987). Pediatric home mechanical ventilation. *Pediatric Clinics of North America, 34*, 47–60.
Scribner, B. H. (1985). Forward. In K. D. Nolph (Ed.), *Peritoneal dialysis* (2nd ed., p. 15). Boston: Martinus Nijhoff.
Shaver, J. L., & Giblin, E. C. (1989). Sleep. In J. J. Fitzpatrick, R. L. Taunton, & J. Q. Bensoliel (Eds.), *Annual Review of Nursing Research*. (Vol. 7, pp. 71–93). New York: Springer Publishing.
Shepherd, R. C., Gardynik, J., & Cleary, J. M. (1990). The challenge of disseminating new medical technologies: Treatment of cardiac arrhythmias. *Quality Review Bulletin, 16*, 229–233.
Sivak, E., Cordasco, E., & Gipson, W. (1983). Pulmonary alternative. *Respiratory Care, 28*, 42–49.
Smith, C. E. (1993). Quality of life in long-term total parenteral nutrition patients and their family caregivers. *Journal of Parenteral and Enteral Nutrition, 17*, 501–506.
Smith, C. E., Faust-Wilson, P., Lohr, G., Kallenberger, S., & Marien, L. (1992). A measure of distress reaction to diarrhea in ventilated tube-fed patients. *Nursing Research, 41*, 312–313.
Smith, C. E., Fernengel, K., Werkowitch, M., & Holcroft, C. (1992). Financial and psychological costs of high technology home care. *Nursing Economics, 10*, 369–372.
Smith, C. E., Giefer, C. K., & Bieker, L.(1991). Technological dependency: A preliminary model and pilot of home total parenteral nutrition. *Journal of Community Health Nursing, 8*, 245–254.

Smith, C. E., Marien, L., Brogdon, C., Faust-Wilson, P., Lohr, G., Gerald, K., & Pingleton, S. (1990). Diarrhea associated with tube feeding in mechanically ventilated critically ill patients. *Nursing Research, 39*, 148–152.

Smith, C. E., Mayer, L., Parkhurst, C., Perkins, S., & Pingleton, S. (1991). Adaptation in families with a member requiring mechanical ventilation at home. *Heart & Lung, 20*, 349–356.

Smith, M., Hang, B. A., Michelman, J. E., & Robson, A. M. (1983). Treatment bias in the management of end-stage renal disease. *American Journal of Kidney Diseases, 3*, 21–26.

Snyder, M., Finkelstein, S., Edin, C., & Hertz, M. (1993, April). *Use of a computerized home-monitoring diary program for lung transplant patients*. Unpublished manuscript, University of Minnesota. Minneapolis.

Sorensen, R. U., Kallick, M. D., & Berger, M. (1987). Home treatment of antibody-deficiency syndromes with intravenous immune globulin. *The Journal of Allergy Clinical Immunology, 80*, 810–815.

Soskolne, V., & De Nour, A. K. (1987). Psychosocial adjustment of home hemodialysis, continuous ambulatory peritoneal dialysis, and hospital dialysis patients and their spouses. *Nephronology, 47*, 266–273.

Splaingard, M. L., Frates, R. C., Jr., Harrison, G. M., Carter, R. I., & Jefferson, L. S. (1983). Home positive-pressure ventilation: Twenty years' experience. *Chest, 84*, 376–382.

Splaingard, M. L., Frates, R. C., Jr., Jefferson, L. S., Rosen, C. L., & Harrison, G. M. (1985). Home negative-pressure ventilation: Report of 20 years of experience in patients with neuromuscular disease. *Archives of Physical Medicine and Rehabilitation, 66*, 239–242.

Srivastava, R. H. (1938). Coping strategies used by spouses of CAPD patients. *American Nephrology Nurses' Association Journal, 15*, 174–179.

St. Marie, B. (1989). Administration of intraspinal analgesia in the home care setting. *Journal of Intravenous Nursing, 12*, 164–168.

Steele, N., & Harrison, B. (1986). Technology-assisted children: Assessing discharge preparation. *Journal of Pediatric Nursing, 1*, 150–158.

Steinschneider, A., Weinstein, S., & Diamond, E. (1982). The sudden infant death syndrome and apnea/obstruction during neonatal sleep and feeding. *Pediatrics, 70*, 858–863.

Stevenson, J. A. (1984). Health-related problems of patients on hemodialysis. *Journal of Nephrology Nursing, 1*, 101–105.

Stiver, H. G., Telford, G. O., Mossey, J. M., Cote, D. D., Van-Middlesworth, E. J., Trosky, S. K., McKay, N. L., & Mossey, W. L. (1978). Intravenous antibiotic therapy at home. *Annuals of Internal Medicine, 89*, 690–693.

Stiver, H. G., Trosky, S. K., Cote, D. D., & Oruck, J. L. (1982). Self-administration of intravenous antibiotics: An efficient, cost-effective home care program. *Canadian Medical Association, 127*, 207–211.

Swenson, J. P. (1981). Training patients to administer intravenous antibiotics at home. *American Journal of Hospital Pharmacy, 38*, 1480–1483.

Thilo, E. H., Comito, J., & McCullis, D. (1987). Home oxygen therapy in the newborn: Costs and parental acceptance. *American Journal of Diseases of Children, 141*, 766–768.

Twomey, P. L., & Patching, S. C. (1985). Cost-effectiveness of nutritional support. *Journal of Parenteral and Enteral Nutrition, 9*, 3.

U.S. Congress, Office of Technology Assessment (1987a). Mechanical ventilation. In *Life sustaining technology and the elderly* (Publication No. OTA-BA-306). Washington, DC: U.S. Government Printing Office.

U.S. Congress, Office of Technology Assessment (1987b, May). *Technology-dependent children: Hospital vs. home care—a technical memorandum* (Publication No. OTA-TM-H-38). Washington, DC: U.S. Government Printing Office.

U.S. Renal Data System (1993). *USRDS 1993 annual data report* (Publication No. IOH-91-06). Bethesda, MD: The National Institutes of Health.

Valdes-Dapena, M. (1980). Sudden infant death syndrome: A review of the medical literature, 1974–1979. *Pediatrics, 66*, 597–614.

Vohr, B., Chen, A., Coll, C. G., & Oh, W. (1988). Mothers of preterm and full-term infants on home apnea monitors. *American Journal of Diseases of Children, 142*, 229-231.

Walike, B. C., Padilla, G., Bergstrom, N., Hanson, R. I., Kubo, W., Grant, M., & Wong, H. I. (1974). Patient problems related to tube feeding. *Communicating Nursing Research, 7*, 89–111.

Warshofsky, F. (1965). *The rebuilt man.* New York: Thomas Y. Crowell.

Wasserman, A. L. (1984). A prospective study of the impact of home monitoring on the family. *Pediatrics, 74*, 323-329.

Watkins, F. L. (1966). The patient who has peritoneal dialysis: Long-term considerations. *American Journal of Nursing, 66*, 1572-1577.

Weaver, W. D., Hill, D., Fahrenbruch, C. E., Copass, M. K., Martin, J. S., Cobb, L. A., & Hallstrom, A. P. (1988). Use of the automatic external defibrillator in the management of out-of-hospital cardiac arrest. *New England Journal of Medicine, 319*, 661-666.

Wegener, D. H., & Aday, L. A. (1989). Home care for ventilator-assisted children: Predicting family stress. *Pediatric Nursing, 15*, 371–376.

Weinstein, M. C. (1983). Economic assessments of medical practices and technologies. *Medical Decision Making, 1*, 309–330.

Whalen, J. E., & Freeman, R. M. (1978). Home hemodialysis review in Iowa, 1970-1977. *Archives of Internal Medicine, 138*, 1787-1790.

Wiegmann, T. B., Blumenkrantz, M., Layard, M., Schmidt, R. W., Shen, F., & Stead, W. (1983). Home dialysis and dialysis treatment modalities in the VA system. *American Journal of Kidney Disease, 3*, 32-36.

Williams, A. R., & Williams, P. D. (1990). Home caregivers and children on apnea monitors. *Family Systems Medicine, 8*, 151-158.

Williams, P.D., Williams, A. R., & Griggs, C. (1990). Children at home on mechanical assistive devices and their families: A retrospective study. *Maternal-Child Nursing Journal, 19*, 297-311.

Winegard, D. L., & Berkman, L. F. (1983). Mortality risk associated with sleeping patterns among adults. *Sleep, 6*, 102-107.

Winkler, H. R. (1987). Home enteral nutrition in practice. *Nutrition Supplement Services, 7*(12), 27-29.

Yanagida, E., & Streltzer, J. (1979). Limitations of psychological tests in a dialysis population. *Psychosomatic Medicine, 41*, 557-566.

Young, T., Palta, M., Dempsey, J., Skatrud, J., Weber, S., & Badr, S. (1993). The occurrence of sleep-disordered breathing among middle-aged adults. *The New England Journal of Medicine, 328*, 1230-1235, 1279.

Zahr, L. K., & Montijo, J. (1993). The benefits of home care for sick premature infants. *Neonatal Network, 12*, (1), 33–37.

Zimmaro, D., Rolandelli, R., Koruda, M., Settle, R. G., Stein, T. P., & Rombeau, J. L. (1989). Isotonic tube feeding formula induces liquid stool in normal subjects: Reversal by Pectin. *Journal of Parenteral and Enteral Nutrition, 3*, 117–123.

Chapter 7

Nursing Minimum Data Set

POLLY RYAN
JOHN L. DOYNE HOSPITAL AND CLINICS

CONNIE DELANEY
COLLEGE OF NURSING
THE UNIVERSITY OF IOWA

CONTENTS

Since the introduction of the Nursing Minimum Data Set (NMDS) at the 1985 NMDS Conference (Werley, 1986; Werley, Devine, Westlake, & Manternach, 1986; Werley, Lang, & Westlake, 1986), there have been numerous publications further describing the elements and purposes of this data set (Werley, 1987; Werley & Devine, 1987; Werley, Devine, & Zorn, 1988a, 1988b, 1989a, 1989b, 1990, 1992; Werley, Devine, Zorn, Ryan, & Westra, 1991; Werley & Lang, 1988; Werley, Ryan, & Zorn, in press; Werley, Ryan, Zorn, & Devine, 1994; Werley & Zorn, 1989). In addition, dissemination of information related to the NMDS has occurred through paper presentations at professional conferences locally, regionally, nationally, and internationally. Although the history, definitions, elements, benefits, and potential for research of the NMDS are readily available, research using the NMDS has begun to emerge only recently. The purposes of this chapter are twofold: (a) to identify research in which the NMDS has been tested, and (b) to provide a stimulus for future research on or including the use of the NMDS.

SELECTION OF STUDIES

Studies relative to the NMDS were identified through several methods. A computerized search of the Cumulative Index to Nursing and Allied Health Literature (CINAHL) and MEDLINE was conducted using the following search words: (a) the term NMDS; (b) a combination of two or more of the nursing care elements of the NMDS (diagnosis, intervention, outcome, or intensity), or (c) the phrase "nursing care." A search of the works that referenced H. H. Werley also was conducted. The thesis and dissertation titles from all accredited masters' and doctoral programs were searched. Additional sources of articles included conference proceedings and personal communication with researchers or other colleagues. A request for works using the NMDS also was sent through Internet.

BACKGROUND

The concept of the Uniform Minimum Health Data Set (UMHDS) was developed in 1969 from efforts to identify national health data standards and guidelines (Murnaghan, 1973, 1976; Murnaghan & White, 1970). A UMHDS has been defined by the United States Health Information Policy Council (1983) as "a minimum set of items of information with uniform definitions and categories, concerning a specific aspect or dimen-

TABLE 7.1 Elements of the Nursing Minimum Data Set

Nursing care elements	
1.	Nursing diagnosis
2.	Nursing intervention
3.	Nursing outcome
4.	Intensity of nursing care
Patient or client demographic elements	
5.	Personal identification[a]
6.	Date of birth[a]
7.	Sex[a]
8.	Race and ethnicity[a]
9.	Residence[a]
Service elements	
10.	Unique facility or service agency number[a]
11.	Unique health record number of patient or client
12.	Unique number of principal registered nurse provider
13.	Episode admission or encounter date[a]
14.	Discharge or termination date[a]
15.	Disposition of patient or client[a]
16.	Expected payer for most of this bill (anticipated financial guarantor for services)[a]

[a]Elements comparable with those in the Uniform Hospital Discharge Data Set.

sion of the health care system which meets the essential needs of multiple data users" (p. 3). Under the auspice of the National Committee on Vital and Health Statistics (NCVHS) three patient-focused health data sets were developed. These data sets include (a) the Uniform Hospital Discharge Data Set, (b) the Long-Term Health Care Minimum Data Set, and (c) the Uniform Ambulatory Medical Care Minimum Data Set (NCVHS, 1980a, 1980b, 1981). However, none of these data sets contains essential nursing data. Therefore, a minimum data set for nursing was needed. The NMDS was built on the concept of the UMHDS and contains the common, core data elements to be collected for all patients receiving nursing care. The NMDS is a standardized approach that facilitates the abstraction of a minimum, common, essential core of data to describe nursing practice (Werley & Lang, 1988). It is appropriate and intended for use in any setting where nursing care is provided.

The NMDS (see Table 7.1) was conceptualized through small group work at the Nursing Information Systems conference held in 1977 at the University of Illinois College of Nursing as discussed by Newcomb (1981) in the book edited by Werley and Grier (1981). In 1985 Werley and colleagues provided the leadership for the NMDS Conference at the University of Wisconsin-Milwaukee School of Nursing. During this conference the NMDS was formalized. The NMDS was developed consensually through the efforts of a multidisciplinary group of 64 experts, who participated in this 3-day invitational conference. In 1991, the American Nurses Association (ANA) recognized the NMDS as the minimum data elements to be included in any nursing data set or clinical record. In addition, ANA Resolution No. 24 was passed unanimously by the 1986 House of Delegates. This resolution supported research and development of computerized nursing information systems (NISs). In 1990, the American Nurses Association Steering Committee on Data Bases to Support Clinical Nursing Practice accepted the NMDS as a framework to guide their work (McCormick et al., 1994).

INTERNATIONAL WORK ON MINIMUM DATA SETS FOR NURSING

Efforts to define a minimum data set for nursing are not limited to the United States. Nursing minimum data sets from places throughout the world have been or are being developed (see Table 7.2). Although similarities and differences exist among these data sets in terms of data elements and their definitions, most of them include several of the nursing care elements of the NMDS. The Australian data set (Australian Council of Community Nursing Services, 1991; Gliddon & Weaver, 1994) has been constructed for use by nurses in community settings. Although this data set continues to be refined and tested, widespread use will occur as implementation of the data set is mandated federally for the continent of Australia. Likewise, the Canadian data set (Canadian Nurses Association, 1993) is mandated federally; however, work on this database has not yet been finalized. The Belgium data set has been used since 1987 (Sermeus, 1988). Data for this data set are collected over a 15-day period, 4 times per year. The World Health Organization-European data set has not yet been used for widespread data collection (International Council of Nurses, 1993).

Although it is important to recognize the international context of the work on minimum data sets that incorporate nursing care data, in this chapter the focus is on the research related to the NMDS as developed by Werley and colleagues (Werley & Lang, 1988). The NMDS developed by Werley and colleagues has been in existence since 1985, the elements of the data set have been integrated into several nursing information systems throughout the United States, and data are available for testing the efficacy of the NMDS. It is anticipated that research using other national data sets in concert with the NMDS will emerge so that in the not too distant future nursing practice can be compared internationally.

OVERVIEW OF THE NURSING MINIMUM DATA SET

Data Set Elements

The NMDS includes three broad categories of elements: (a) nursing care, (b) patient or client demographics, and (c) service elements (see Table 7.1). When data are used for the purposes of research, approval from committees for the protection of the rights of human subjects should be obtained before abstraction of these elements from patient records. Elements being collected already need not be recollected if they can be obtained through existing relational database management systems.

Purposes of the Nursing Minimum Data Set

The purposes of the NMDS are to (a) establish comparability of nursing data across clinical populations, settings, geographical areas, and time; (b) describe the nursing care of patients or clients and their families in a variety of settings, both institutional and noninstitutional; (c) demonstrate or project trends regarding nursing care provided and allocation of nursing resources to patients or clients according to their health problems or nursing diagnoses; (d) stimulate nursing research, using the NMDS elements alone or through links to the detailed data existing in nursing information systems (NIS) and other health care information systems; and (e) provide data about nursing care to facilitate and influence clinical, administrative, and health policy decision making (Werley & Lang, 1988).

EVALUATING DATA FOR USE WITH THE NMDS

For data to be used for research with the NMDS, the data must meet certain criteria. That is, the elements must be (a) available within the patient record, (b) retrievable, (c) linked, and (d) the data must be reliable and valid.

Availability and Retrievability

Data for research on the NMDS are abstracted from patient records. Some of the studies cited in this chapter took place at sites that had in-

TABLE 7.2 Comparison of Nursing Minimum Data Sets

NMDS[a] (Werley, US)	NMDS (Belgium)	WHO-EURO[b]	Canadian (Recommendations)	CNMDSA[c] (Australia)
Care items	Care items	Care items		Care items
	Medical care items			*Medical care items*
	Main diagnosis			Medical diagnosis
	Complications			Career availability
	Medical procedures and operations			
Nursing care items	*Nursing care items*	*Nursing care items*	*Nursing care items*	*Nursing care items*
Nursing diagnosis	23 Nursing activities	Assessment	Client status (nursing diagnosis)	Client dependency
Nursing intervention	Activities of daily living	Patient need/problems	Nursing interventions	Nursing diagnosis
Nursing outcome		Nursing interventions	Nursing intensity	Nursing interventions
Intensity/nursing care		Patient outcome	Client outcomes	Nursing resource utilization
Patient demographics	*Patient demographics*		*Patient demographics*	*Patient demographics*
Personal identification	Patient number		Racial/ethnic	Birth date of client
Date of birth	Year of birth		Unique geographical location	Sex of client
Sex	Sex		Unique lifetime identifier	Ethnicity—country of birth

Race, ethnicity		Language	Ethnicity—Language spoken at home
Residence		Occupation	Location of client
		Living arrangement	
		Home environment including physical structure	
		Responsible caregiver on discharge	
		Functional health status	
		Burden on care provider	
		Education level	
		Literacy level	
		Work environment	
		Lifestyle data	
		Income level	
Services items	*Services items*	*Services items*	*Services items*
Facility/agency	Code of the hospital	Unique nurse identifier	Agency identifier
Health record	Code of the department	Principal nurse provider	Client identifier
			Admission date
Principal nurse	Code of the nursing unit		
Provider identification	Day of admission		Referral source
Admission date	Day of stay		Discharge date
Discharge date	Day of discharge		Discharge destination (also a nursing element)
Disposition of patient	Nursing hours available on the nursing unit		Other support services
Expected principal source of payment	Number of nurses available		
	Number of beds		
	Nurse qualification mix		

[a]Nursing minimum data set. [b]World Health Organization, Europe. [c]Community Nursing Minimum Data Set Australia.

formation systems designed to include the elements of the NMDS, other sites did not. Initial studies were needed to determine the extent to which elements of the NMDS were both available in the patient record and retrievable from the information system. Studies were conducted to determine the availability of the elements of the NMDS in the patient records in sites that were not computerized and did not have the elements of the NMDS present in the NIS. Conversely, some sites had elements present in their information system, used this information for day-to-day activities, but had not abstracted these data for the purposes of testing the NMDS.

Five studies were found in which the availability and retrievability of the elements of the NMDS were reported (Androwich, 1992; Delaney, Mehmert, Prophet, & Crossley, 1994; Devine & Werley, 1988; Grier, Grier, Greiner, & Stanhope, 1991; Tillman, 1990). Devine and Werley (1988) determined the availability of the elements of the NMDS in four clinical sites: a hospital, nursing home, home health care agency, and two clinics affiliated with a teaching hospital. Four instruments, one for each type of setting, were designed to collect manually data from a sample of 116 health records. Most of the NMDS elements were available for more than 90% of the cases. The exceptions were the unique number of principal registered nurse provider, which was never available; ethnicity, which was available only 9% of the time; race, which was available for 71% of the subjects; resolution status, which was available for 79% of the documented nursing diagnoses (nursing outcome measure); and personal identification number of the client, which was available for 86% of the subjects.

Androwich (1992) reported on a study in which 50 charts of patients who were provided nursing services in an ambulatory care setting were reviewed. The instrument used to collect the data was identical to that used in the Devine and Werley (1988) study, and data collection was manual. Race and ethnicity were not well documented, and the codes used for race and ethnicity were not used consistently. The unique number of principal registered nurse provider was not available. Eight-four percent of the charts had no nursing diagnosis recorded, as the nursing records for many services are not kept with the patient's chart. Forty-two percent of the charts had nursing interventions recorded, but because there were no nursing diagnoses, these interventions could not be linked to any nursing diagnoses. Intensity of nursing care was available 20% of the time.

Grier, Grier, Greiner, and Stanhope (1991) determined the availability of elements of the NMDS in the existing database from an ambulatory care clinic for indigent people. Of the 16 NMDS elements, 10 were documented in 83% to 100% of the records. Those items that were never documented included outcomes, client residence, unique facility number, unique number of registered nurse provider, discharge date, and expected payer. Outcomes may not have been documented, in part, because the indigent population served did not return frequently for follow-up care. However, even when clients returned for follow-up care outcomes were not documented. The authors concluded that a framework, such as the NMDS, would facilitate both the documentation and collection of appropriate data.

Tillman (1990) examined the availability of the NMDS elements in a community-based, academic nursing center. The health care records of 60 randomly selected clients were examined. The instrument used to collect the data was identical to that used in the Devine and Werley (1988) study, and data collection was manual. Five elements (unique facility number, expected payer, unique number of principal registered nurse provider, discharge date, and disposition) were never available, the residence element was available 10% of the time, and all other elements were available 90% of the time.

Delaney et al. (1994) reported on the availability and retrievability of elements of the NMDS in five databases from two hospitals, one private and one public. Data were downloaded from the hospital computerized information systems. The size of the data sets ranged from 26 to 4,248 patient records. Elements were available 95.5 to 100% of the time with the exception of the unique number of registered nurse provider number, which is not widely used in the United States.

The extent to which the elements of the NMDS were available and could be retrieved differed from study to study. There are several possible factors that could contribute to the discrepancy in availability and retrievability of data elements. One factor could be the site in which the study was conducted. Studies conducted in hospitals tended to have a higher percentage of elements available. It is federally mandated that hospitals providing care to Medicare patients collect elements of the UHDDS. Ten of the 16 elements of the NMDS are included in the UHDDS. Therefore, at least 10 of the elements of the NMDS would be available in the data from hospital settings. An additional factor that could help explain the differences in availability is the presence of computerized information systems. One of the advantages of using a computerized information system is that practitioners are prompted to enter data, thus increasing the likelihood of documentation of an item in the patient record.

The results of these studies demonstrate the need to ascertain the availability and retrievability of the elements of the NMDS in the patient record as the first phase of a minimum data-set project. Missing data threaten the reliability of the information as an accurate representation of the sample is not obtained. Computerized systems constructed to include the elements of the NMDS provided researchers with more complete databases.

Ability to Link the NMDS Elements

A second step in initial research with the NMDS was a determination of the linkages among the elements of the NMDS. All elements must be linked with each other so that the relationship among the elements can be determined. Researchers must be able to determine from the database the interventions, outcomes, and intensity that are related to specific diagnoses for each patient.

Grier, Grier, Hickman, and Berry (1991) reported problems experienced when they tried to link the elements of the NMDS from data collected in a nurse managed community-based health care clinic for the indigent. The database initially developed for this clinic was not relational, that is, interventions could not be linked directly with the diagnoses for each patient. As a result, it was not possible to describe the nursing care provided to a patient with a specific diagnosis. Likewise, outcomes and intensity of nursing care could not be examined in relation to other nursing care elements. Although establishing linkages among the elements may appear obvious from a conceptual standpoint, the actual coding of data requires an in-depth understanding of the intended uses of the NMDS.

Data Retrieval: Manual or Electronic

Data have been retrieved manually (Androwich, 1992; Devine & Werley, 1988; Helberg, 1993a; Marek, 1992; Rios, Delaney, Kruckeberg, Chung, & Mehmert, 1991; Tillman, 1990) or electronically (Delaney & Mehmert, 1991; Hays, 1992; Lundeen, Coenen, & Marek, 1993; Rios et al., 1991; Sheil & Wierenga, 1994). Manual retrieval was associated with small samples. Typically, availability of elements included in the patient record was not known so that preliminary work was required to determine availability of data. In manual retrieval, it was necessary to train data coders to abstract the data, obtain measures of intrarater and interrater reliability, enter data into a computer, and determine the accuracy of the data entry. In several studies (Androwich, 1992; Devine & Werley, 1988; Tillman, 1990) the *NMDS Data Collection Manual* (Werley, Devine, & Zorn, 1992) was used to collect the data.

Electronically retrieved data were obtained from computerized NISs. Although the data elements in the system were known, preliminary work was necessary to determine whether or not the data elements could be retrieved and linked. In general, electronically retrieved data were downloaded from a NIS and transferred to a university computer for analysis. Electronic data were retrieved for specified medical diagnoses, surgical procedures, nursing diagnoses, or for a specific time frame. Retrieval of all NMDS elements and medical diagnoses for a specific time frame provided the least restrictive databases, enabling the researcher to examine multiple research questions. In addition, retrieval over a specified period allowed the researcher to study the characteristics of persons with and without a select nursing or medical diagnosis for comparative analysis.

Cost. Karpiuk (1995) and Delaney et al. (1994) were concerned with identifying costs associated with manual and electronic retrieval of data. Karpiuk was funded in 1993 by the American Nurses' Foundation to describe nursing resource use and patient outcomes for patients with a fractured hip with pinning, across seven hospitals in South Dakota. The time for manual data collection ranged from 0.25 hours to 3.77 hours with a mean of 1.65 hours. Findings will be available during 1994. Delaney et al. (1994) used five databases from two hospitals to compare the cost associated with manual and electronic retrieval. The costs associated with manual retrieval of one data set from each site ranged from $20.20 to $82.50 per patient record. The costs associated with electronic retrieval of data from established computerized NISs, one database from one of the hospitals, and two other databases from the other hospital ranged from $0.05 to $0.50 per patient record.

Although manual retrieval is possible, it is costly and increases the potential for error associated with data abstraction and entry. Electronic retrieval requires a computerized NIS from which data elements can be both retrieved and linked. However, once a computerized NIS is in place data retrieval is much less time-consuming, less expensive, facilitates work with large databases, and increases the feasibility of multisite comparison.

Reliability and Validity

The issues of reliability and validity are complex. Reliability and validity of a database are often confused with the reliability and validity of a classification system used to describe nursing practice. Although the reliability and validity of the data used for research with the NMDS will be affected by the reliability and validity of the classification system, it is the reliability and validity of the actual data that must be determined. It is essential the data be obtained from sites that (a) use a standardized classification system of nursing practice and (b) regularly monitor the reliability of their data.

The usefulness of clinical data may be limited by incomplete records, unreliable or invalid coding, or missing variables (Kaplan & Berry, 1990; Rubin & Schenker, 1991; Tierney & McDonald, 1991). Missing or incomplete data, resulting from lack of initial collection or loss in transmission, must be determined. Data must be inspected and the frequency of each element determined. Small databases can be visually inspected, whereas large data sets need to be checked using a computerized coding system. The data inspection provides an estimate of validity. Data elements need to be consistent or have a logical relationship among certain data elements. For example, a specific admission date restricts the discharge date, or a total sample size of 200 necessarily precludes a subsample of greater than 200. The reliability of the database also needs to be estimated. Coding errors need to be identified. For example, an age of 201 is an obvious coding error. Interrater and intrarater reliability needs to be determined for all manually collected data. Data that has been electronically retrieved from computerized systems should match exactly the data in the patient record. A few cases in the database should be checked against actual patient records. Frequency counts also provide a method of determining the availability of each data element.

REVIEW AND RESEARCH ON THE NMDS

According to Werley and Lang (1988), the purposes of the NMDS were to describe nursing practice, establish comparability of nursing data, project trends, stimulate research, and influence decision making. Evaluation of the effectiveness of the NMDS to achieve these purposes can be determined, in part, by an integration of the research testing the NMDS. Those studies that contribute to the ability of the NMDS to achieve a specific purpose were retrieved. There was no attempt to make the categories mutually exclusive as studies related to more than one of the purposes of the NMDS.

Purpose 1: Description of Nursing Practice

One of the purposes of the NMDS is to describe the nursing care of patients, or clients, and their families in a variety of settings, both institutional and noninstitutional. Researchers described nursing care using the

NMDS in hospitals (Delaney & Mehmert, 1990, 1991; Delaney et al., 1994; Karpiuk, 1995; Mehmert & Delaney, 1991; Rios et al., 1991; Ryan et al., 1994; Sheil & Wierenga, 1994); in nursing centers (Coenen, 1993; Lundeen et al., 1993; Tillman, 1990); and in home health care agencies (Marek, 1992).

Hospitals. The NMDS has been used in hospital studies to create demographic profiles of patients with specific nursing diagnoses (Delaney et al., 1994). Five databases from two sites were combined. Demographic profiles were established for all nursing diagnostic categories for all of the databases. Examples of patient profiles for three of the nursing diagnoses were provided in reports of these studies. Among their findings it was noted that while nursing diagnostic groups were not significantly different in terms of sex, race, or discharge disposition, they were significantly different in terms of age and length of stay.

Ryan et al. (1994), Sheil and Wierenga (1994), and Karpiuk (1995) examined the prevalence and relationship among the elements of the NMDS in hospitalized patients, specifically, diagnoses, interventions, outcomes, and intensity. The sample in the study by Ryan and colleagues (1994) included all patients admitted to a public acute care facility during 1991 with the five most common medical diagnoses, surgical procedures, and the six most common nursing diagnoses. They concluded that there was more variance among the types of nursing diagnoses used with medical patients than surgical patients, related factors as well as diagnostic labels were determinate of interventions for specific nursing diagnoses, and intensity of nursing care was a more sensitive measure when examined daily than when examined over length of hospital stay. Although the nursing diagnoses of potential for injury and pain were identified for a percentage of the patients in all of the selected medical and surgical procedures, different clusters of nursing diagnoses occurred within each of the selected medical and surgical diagnoses, providing evidence of variance in nursing diagnosis associated with medical diagnoses and surgical procedures.

Sheil and Wierenga (1994) reported on all patients admitted to a hospital in 1991 with the medical diagnosis of diabetes and all women with normal vaginal delivery. They found that patients in both groups had nursing diagnoses of pain and anxiety; although they had some similar interventions at least 50% of the interventions differed between the groups. The purpose of the study by Karpiuk (1995) was to describe the nursing elements of the NMDS for 50 patients with fractured hip with pinning, in each of eight hospitals in South Dakota. The most frequent nursing diagnoses were acute pain (57%) and impaired physical mobility (46%). Only 25% of the nursing interventions were related to nursing diagnoses. And the intervention categories of monitoring and/or surveillance and teaching were used most frequently. The results of this study will be available during 1994. These are the first studies that contain descriptions of and relationships among all of the nursing elements in an acute care setting.

Use of the NMDS has provided descriptions of nursing practice for select patient groups in hospitals. Additionally, the results of these studies have made contributions to the development and refinement of the nursing diagnosis classification systems, provided empirical evidence attesting to the importance of the related factors in the selection of nursing interventions, and provided evidence of the contribution of nursing diagnoses and interventions to the prediction of resource use and length of stay.

Community Nursing Centers. In a study in an academic nursing center Lundeen et al. (1993) found that nursing diagnoses were the stronger predictors of primary care use when compared with client demographics of age, gender, and ethnicity. When nursing diagnoses and client demographics were examined as predictors of use, 13 nursing diagnoses alone accounted for 55% of the variance in use. In a follow-up study, Coenen (1993) examined the nature of case management at a community nursing center and found that the complexity of health care needs, increased nursing intensity, and complexity of nursing interventions were predictors of case management.

In these studies, investigators used several of the nursing elements of the NMDS to provide descriptions of advanced practice nursing in nursing centers. In addition, data on use of nursing resources at one center are available for comparison with other settings.

Home Health Care. Marek (1992) analyzed the relationships among patient characteristics (including nursing and medical diagnoses), home health care resource use (including nursing intensity and number of nursing interventions), and home health care outcomes. Nursing diagnoses were the only patient characteristics that were identified as significant predictor variables for each utilization measure tested and were consistently more useful than medical diagnoses in explaining variance in the utilization measures. Research, in which the NMDS was used to describe nursing practice in nursing homes or in ambulatory care, was not found.

Purpose 2: Comparability of Nursing Data

The second purpose of the NMDS is to establish comparability of nursing data across clinical populations, settings, geographical areas, and time. Two studies were identified in which NMDS data from multiple sites were used. Karpiuk (1995) used the NMDS to describe the nursing care of patients with open reduction and internal fixation of a hip fracture across seven sites. These seven sites are all hospitals but represent both large and small as well as urban and rural facilities. The results of Karpiuk's study will be available in 1994. She will describe the similarities and differences of the nursing care provided to patients across multiple sites. Delaney et al. (1994) compared seven databases from two hospitals. These researchers aggregated data from the seven databases, enabling them to have a broad, multisite description of demographic characteristics and defining characteristics for select nursing diagnoses.

Cross-site comparison of nursing practice is restricted by the use of multiple classification systems. Three classification systems were used in NMDS research identified for this chapter; specifically (a) the North American Nursing Diagnosis Association (NANDA) classification system, (b) the Omaha System (OS) (Martin, Scheet, & Stegman, 1993; Visiting Nurses Association of Omaha, 1986) and (c) the classification system for interventions developed by the Task Force of the NMDS Conference Group (Werley & Lang, 1988). In general, the NANDA classification system was used most frequently in hospital studies, and the OS was used exclusively in home health care and community nursing center studies.

Although the use of multiple classification systems is an issue with ramifications much broader than comparability of NMDS data collected across sites, until the comparability data can be established, all of the benefits of the NMDS cannot be realized. However, progress is under way to establish the comparability of data among classification systems. The Unified Medical Language System (UMLS) was designed from several sources including but not limited to biomedical clinical records, literature, and data banks (National Library of Medicine, 1992). The UMLS was built on the assumption that numerous classifications and vocabularies will continue to be used in the health sciences and conceptual links are needed. The UMLS consists of three knowledge sources to facilitate such bridging. First, biomedical concepts, their various names, and relationships among them are contained within the metathesaurus. Second, the Semantic Network links the concepts within the metathesaurus to semantic types. And, third, the Information Sources Map contains human and computer information about sources of information and facilitates the links (National Library of Medicine, 1992).

At this time, two of the nursing classification systems have been included in the UMLS, namely, NANDA and Nursing Intervention Classification (NIC) (McCloskey & Bulechek, 1992). However, it is anticipated that the Omaha System and the Home Health Care Classification system will soon be included in the UMLS. Thus, the UMLS will assist in determining the comparability among the classification systems used in nursing practice.

Purpose 3: Projection of Trends in Nursing Care

The third purpose of the NMDS is to demonstrate or project trends regarding nursing care provided and allocation of nursing resources to patients or clients according to their health problems or nursing diagnoses. Delaney et al. (1994) compared nursing care requirements for patients with a specific diagnostic related group (DRG) over a 4-year period. They found that between 1988 and 1992, patients with DRG 209, major joint and limb reattachment procedures, had a significantly shorter hospital stay with higher acuity. Although this is the first and only study of this nature identified, the results of this study provide evidence for the potential for use of NMDS data to project trends for patients with specific problems.

Purpose 4: Stimulation of Nursing Research

The fourth purpose of the NMDS is to stimulate nursing research through links to the detailed data existing in nursing information systems and other health care information systems. The research previously discussed under description of nursing care in hospitals as reported by Delaney and Mehmert (1990, 1991), Mehmert and Delaney (1991), and Rios et al. (1991) provides an example of linkage of the data from the NMDS with other data existing in information systems. The purpose of this area of research was to provide estimates of the validity of the 10 most frequently used nursing diagnoses. The NIS contained both the elements of the NMDS and the defining characteristics for each nursing diagnosis, elements not included in the NMDS. The etiology or related factor for each nursing diagnosis was linked with defining characteristics. The prevalence of defining characteristics was determined for each etiology as a method of validating specific nursing diagnoses.

Purpose 5: Influencing Health Policy

The final purpose of the NMDS is to provide data about nursing care to influence health policy decision making. As research using the NMDS is just beginning to emerge, it is premature to expect examples of the results of NMDS research influencing national policy decisions. However, implications for policy are beginning to emerge. The results of this early research have demonstrated that nursing diagnoses have accounted for a greater percentage of variance in resource use than medical diagnoses or sociodemographic characteristics. Clearly, nursing data, once available, will play a major role in determining the cost of health care and resource allocation.

The ability to influence national health care policy will require the replication of studies across sites and settings. In addition, large, multisite studies need to be conducted to compare nursing practice across geographical locations. This type of research will require support from agencies such as the National Institute for Nursing Research and the Agency for Health Care Policy and Research.

OTHER RELATED WORK

Although actual research testing or using the NMDS are just beginning to emerge, there are several research projects that, if linked to the NMDS, could strengthen the research program of the NMDS. Likewise, linkage of a study to the NMDS would strengthen the results of the individual study as the results of the study could be compared across clinical populations, settings, and time. What is needed to link a study to the NMDS is use of the elements of the NMDS. Examples of studies in which the elements of the NMDS could have potentially been added to the study or linked to the NMDS have been provided so that the reader can begin to understand the richness of such linkages.

There are several studies in which two or more of the nursing elements of the NMDS were used in the study, but the study was not conceptually linked with the NMDS. Holzemer and Henry (1992) used the NMDS elements of nursing diagnoses, nursing interventions, and outcomes in a study in which they compared patient problems, nursing interventions, and outcomes on computer-supported versus manually generated nursing care plans. Lutjens (1991) conducted a study to determine the explanatory power of medical condition, nursing condition, nursing intensity, and medical severity for length of stay for hospitalized patients. She found that nursing intensity accounted for the largest amount of variance and explained 14% of the variance in length of hospital stay.

Sociodemographic factors, medical conditions, and nursing dependency were examined as predictors of nursing problems and nursing care provided (Helberg, 1993a, 1993b). Helberg found that nursing dependency was the strongest predictor of the nursing problems and nursing care provided in home health care patients. Hays (1992) found that nursing intensity and nursing diagnoses explained significant variation in nursing resource consumption in home health care.

A large ($N = 2,403$), multisite, descriptive study of home health clients was reported by Martin et al. (1993). They provided a description of the persons served by home care and identified the number and type of nursing problems, interventions, and outcomes. The sample for this study was drawn from four states and consisted of both urban and rural settings. Changes in the clients' knowledge, behavior, and status from admission to discharge provided evidence of the effectiveness of nursing care provided to persons in this sample.

Although some individuals have accepted the concept of a minimum data set for nursing they have altered the elements of the NMDS. The Pascucci, Adams, Jacobson, Holtzen, and Knickerbocker (1993) study provides an example of research based on the concept of a minimum data set that did not use the elements of the NMDS. The nursing records from the nontechnical medical care program, a statewide Medicaid long-term community care program, were used to develop a minimum data set for that practice setting. Rather than collecting the elements of the NMDS, this group reviewed records to ascertain common data elements and developed a classification system specific to their setting. The authors did identify those items common between the NMDS and their data set (case number, date of birth, sex, race, county, date services began, services continuous/intermittent, responsible person and client problems). Although this effort will provide them with a database to describe their practice, comparison between sites using the NMDS is not possible as data elements are different.

DISCUSSION

Elements of the NMDS are available and retrievable in a relational format for analysis. Computerization enables rapid collection of large data sets at low costs once the computer system and retrieval program are in place. Several classification systems for nursing care are being used currently, and the number of systems used will increase with the development of new systems: specifically, the Home Health Care Classification system (Saba, 1992; Saba et al., 1991; Saba & Zuckerman, 1992), the Nursing Intervention Classification (McCloskey & Bulechek, 1992; McCloskey et al., 1990; Moorhead, McCloskey, & Bulechek, 1993), and the nursing intervention lexicon and taxonomy developed by Grobe (1990). Although the development of these systems will enable the profession of nursing to begin to "name" its phenomena of concern (Clark & Lang, 1992), the use of multiple classification systems results in data that are not comparable. Efforts are in progress to develop a universal language for nursing. The International Council of Nurses is providing the leadership to develop an International Classification of Nursing Practice (Clark & Lang, 1992). The primary components of this classification system are (a) patient needs, (b) nursing actions, and (c) patient outcomes. This International Classification for Nursing Practice will contain three of the four nursing elements of the NMDS. The only nursing element not included in this classification is intensity. These efforts to standardize language for nursing practice will enable a description nursing practice that is comparable across sites and settings. Once this standardized language is accepted and used, the value of the NMDS to describe nursing practice across sites and geographical locations can be realized.

A final issue for discussion is the alteration of elements within a minimum data set. There are two points that need to be considered. First, the NMDS was designed to be a *minimum* data set. Programs and agencies are free to add elements to the NMDS while maintaining the core of the data set. The Nursing Management Minimum Data Set (Huber, Delaney, Crossley, Mehmert, & Ellerbe, 1992) is an example of adding elements to achieve additional purposes. Nurse executives have identified additional data necessary to assist in administrative and system decision making. The NMMDS has built on the NMDS without altering the existing elements of the NMDS. Second, elements cannot be deleted from the NMDS without altering the comparability of data across sites and affecting the intended purposes of the NMDS.

Descriptions of nursing practice across health care delivery settings and geographical locations will enable the discipline of nursing to describe and compare nursing practice, and the requirements for patient care. Standardized data will enable nurses to discuss practice issues and allocation of resources across patient groups and clinical settings. Database descriptions will allow the practitioners to make informed choices about practice and documentation. Nurses currently are trying to evaluate the effectiveness of their practice through small samples of patient outcomes. Large databases including the elements of the NMDS will provide descriptions of outcomes.

DIRECTION FOR FUTURE RESEARCH ON THE NURSING MINIMUM DATA SET

Research efforts to test and use the NMDS have just begun. Additional research is needed to determine the availability and retrievability of the elements, linkage of the elements, electronic data retrieval, and estimates of reliability and validity. However, NMDS research is needed in two additional areas: specifically, research related to (a) testing of the NMDS and (b) the use of the NMDS. Testing the NMDS requires a commitment to the elements of the data set and the definition of these elements (Werley & Lang, 1988). The NMDS elements should not be altered to meet the needs of individuals or specialties before testing because altering the NMDS would destroy the standardization of the NMDS. The integrity of the NMDS should remain intact during testing. Revisions, if needed, should be based on replicated research findings.

TABLE 7.3 Directions for Research Using the Nursing Minimum Data Set

Purposes of the Nursing Minimum Data Set	Nursing Science		Outcomes		Systems	
	Nursing practice description	Nursing theory: prediction and control	Patient outcomes	Quality monitoring	Delivery systems	Organizations
Describe nursing care in a variety of settings						
Comparability of nursing data across clinical populations, settings, geographical areas, and time						
Project trends in nursing care and allocation of resources						
Research through links with other data bases						
Influence health policy decision making						

NMDS research can be used to describe and test nursing science, outcomes, and systems. Proposed directions for future research are identified in Table 7.3. Shaded boxes indicate where preliminary work has been done; however, this work needs to be replicated with different clinical populations, in different settings, and across geographical locations.

Research on the NMDS could be used to advance nursing science. Questions, such as: What are the common nursing diagnoses for patients with a specific clinical condition, and do these diagnoses differ across geographical locations?; or How have patient outcomes changed since the use of DRGs? could be answered. Outcome research using the NMDS could answer questions, such as: How do specific nursing interventions affect nurse-sensitive patient outcomes?; or How are nurse-sensitive patient outcomes affected by specific demographic characteristics of patients? System research using the NMDS could answer questions, such as: How are patient outcomes affected by the use of critical paths (or case management or changes in professional staff mix)?; or Do nursing diagnoses differ across organizational settings?

Clearly, the potential for research using the NMDS is great. Much research is necessary in which the NMDS is tested and used to describe and test nursing science and systems. This type of research will need support from all of nursing. Practicing nurses must realize the importance and value of consistent, complete documentation. Persons providing leadership in clinical arenas need to have a documentation system that contains elements of the NMDS, work toward the computerization of NIS, and request and use data from the NMDS to make decisions. Leadership is needed both in the United States and worldwide to continue to find solutions to issues, such as classification taxonomies and the development of comparable languages. Funding agencies need to support research using the NMDS. Issues, such as reliability and validity, are part of the NMDS research agenda, not issues that can be solved before NMDS research. The NMDS needs to be tested intact, and only after adequate testing should an evaluation of the effectiveness of the NMDS be made. And, finally, the NMDS needs to be represented at an international level as the work on nursing databases moves forth.

REFERENCES

American Nurses' Association. (1986). *Development of computerized nursing information systems in nursing science* (Resolution No. 24). Kansas City, MO: Author.

American Nurses' Association. (1991). *National data bases/sets to support clinical nursing practice* (Report to the Nursing Organization Liaison Forum, pp. 2–3). Unpublished manuscript.

Androwich, I. (1992, March). Data set initiatives: What has been done? In I. Androwich & K. Phillips (Eds.), *Report of the American Academy of Ambulatory Nursing Administration Pre-Conference Research Workshop: Strength in numbers: Positioning ambulatory nursing to maximize practice and reimbursement opportunities through research* (pp. 37–49). Pitman, NJ: American Academy of Ambulatory Nursing Administration.

Australian Council of Community Nursing Services. (1991). *Community Nursing Minimum Data Set—Australia*. Canberra, Australia: Department of Community Services and Health.

Canadian Nurses Association. (1993). *Papers from the Nursing Minimum Data Set Conference*. Edmonton, Alberta, Canada: Author.

Clark, J., & Lang, N. (1992). Nursing's next advance: An international classification for nursing practice. *International Nursing Review, 39*, 109–112, 128.

Coenen, A. (1993). *Case management at a community nursing center*. Unpublished doctoral dissertation, University of Wisconsin-Milwaukee.

Delaney, C. W., & Mehmert, P. (1990). Electronic transfer of clinical NMDS facilitates nursing diagnoses validation. In R. A. Miller (Ed.), *Fourteenth Annual Symposium on Computer Applications in Medical Care: Standards in Medical Informatics* (pp. 899–901). Los Alamitos, CA: IEEE Computer Society Press.

Delaney, C. W., & Mehmert, P. (1991). Utility of the Nursing Minimum Data Set in validation of computerized nursing diagnoses. In R. M. Carroll-Johnson (Ed.), *Classification of Nursing Diagnoses: Proceedings of the Ninth Conference* (pp. 175–179). Philadelphia: Lippincott.

Delaney, C., Mehmert, M., Prophet, C., & Crossley, J. (1994). Establishment of research utility of Nursing Minimum Data Set. In S. J. Grobe (Ed.), *Proceedings of the Fifth International Conference on Nursing Use of Computers and Information Science* (pp. 169–173). San Antonio, TX: International Medical Informatics Association.

Devine, E. C., & Werley, H. H. (1988). Test of the Nursing Minimum Data Set: Availability of data and reliability. *Research in Nursing & Health, 11*, 97–104.

Gliddon, T., & Weaver, C. (1994). The Community Nursing Minimum Data Set Australia—From definition to the real world. In S. J. Grobe (Ed.), *Proceedings of the Fifth International Conference on Nursing Use of Computers and Information Science* (pp. 163–168). San Antonio: International Medical Informatics Association.

Grier, J. B., Grier, M. I., Hickman, M. I., & Berry, R. D (1991). Linking components of the Nursing Minimum Data Set. In E. J. S. Hovenga, K. J. Hannah, F. A. McCormick, & J. S. Ronald (Eds.), *Proceedings of the Fourth International Conference on Nursing Use of Computers and Information Science* (pp. 87–90). Berlin: Springer-Verlag.

Grier, M. R., Grier, J. B., Greiner, P. A., & Stanhope, M. K. (1991). Savings form use of the Nursing Minimum Data Set. In E. J. S. Hovenga, K. J. Hannah, F. A. McCormick, & J. S. Ronald (Eds.), *Proceedings of the Fourth International Conference on Nursing Use of Computers and Information Science* (pp. 105–109). Berlin: Springer-Verlag.

Grobe, S. J. (1990). Nursing intervention lexicon and taxonomy study: Language and classification methods. *Advances in Nursing Science, 13*(2), 22–33.

Hays, B. J. (1992). Nursing care requirements and resource consumption in home health care. *Nursing Research, 41*, 138–143.

Health Information Policy Council. (1983). *Background paper: Uniform minimum health data sets*. Unpublished manuscript.

Helberg, J. L. (1993a). Factors influencing home care nursing problems and nursing care. *Research in Nursing & Health, 16*, 363–370.

Helberg, J. L. (1993b). Patients' status at home care discharge. *Image: Journal of Nursing Scholarship, 25*, 93–99.

Holzemer, W., & Henry, S. B. (1992). Computer-supported versus manually-generated nursing care plans: A comparison of patient problems, nursing interventions, and AIDS patient outcomes. *Computers in Nursing, 10*(1), 19–24.

Huber, D. G., Delaney, C., Crossley, J., Mehmert, M., & Ellerbe, S. (1992). A Nursing Management Minimum Data Set. *Journal of Nursing Administration, 22*(7/8), 35–40.

International Council of Nurses. (1993, October 8). *Nursing's next advance: An international classification for nursing practice (ICNP).* (working paper, pp. 105–106). Geneva: Author.

Kaplan, R., & Berry, C. (1990, May). Adjusting for confounding variables. Research methodology: Strengthening causal interpretations of non-experimental data. *AHCPR Conference Proceedings*, 105–114.

Karpiuk, K. L. (1995). *South Dakota Statewide Nursing Minimum Data Set Project*. South Dakota: Author.

Lundeen, S., Coenen, A., & Marek, K. (1993). *Clinical nursing data elements as predictors of primary care utilization in a community nursing center*. Unpublished manuscript.

Lutjens, L. R. J. (1991). Medical condition, nursing condition, nursing intensity, medical severity, and length of stay in hospitalized adults. *Nursing Administration Quarterly, 15*, 64–65.

Martin, K. S., Scheet, N. J., & Stegman, M. R. (1993). Home health clients: Characteristics, outcomes of care, and nursing interventions. *American Journal of Public Health, 83*, 1730–1734.

Marek, K. S. (1992). *Analysis of the relationships among nursing diagnoses and other selected patient factors, nursing interventions and other measures of utilization, and outcomes in home health care*. Unpublished doctoral dissertation, University of Wisconsin-Milwaukee.

McCloskey, J. C., & Bulechek, G. M. (Eds.). (1992). *Nursing Interventions Classification (NIC): Iowa Intervention Project*. St. Louis: Mosby.

McCloskey, J. C., Bulechek, G. M., Cohen, M. Z., Craft, M. J., Crossley, J. D., Delaney, J. A., Glick, O. J., Kruckeberg, T., Mass, M., Prophet, C. M., & Tripp-Reimer, T. (1990). Classification of nursing interventions. *Journal of Professional Nursing, 6*, 151–157.

McCormick, K. A., Lang, N., Zielstorff, R., Milholland, D. K., Saba, V., & Jacox, A. (1994). Toward standard classification schemes for nursing language: Recommendations of the American Nurses Association Steering Committee on databases to support clinical nursing practice. *Journal of the American Medical Informatics Association, 1*, 421–427.

Mehmert, P. A., & Delaney, C. W. (1991). Validating impaired physical mobility. *Nursing Diagnosis, 2*, 143–154.

Moorhead, S. A., McCloskey, J. C., & Bulechek, G. M. (1993). Nursing interventions classification: A comparison with the Omaha System and the Home Healthcare Classification. *Journal of Nursing Administration, 23*(10), 23–29.

Murnaghan, J. H. (Ed.). (1973). Ambulatory care data: Report of the conference on ambulatory medical records. *Medical Care, 11*(2, Suppl.), 1–205.

Murnaghan, J. H. (Ed.). (1976). Long-term care data: Report of the conference on long-term health care data. *Medical Care, 14*(5, Suppl.), 1–233.

Murnaghan, J. H., & White, K. L. (Eds.). (1970). Hospital discharge data: Report of conference on hospital discharge abstract system. *Medical Care, 8*(4, Suppl.), 1–215.

National Committee on Vital and Health Statistics. (1980a). *Long-term health care: Minimum data set* (DHHS Publication No. PHS 80-1158). Hyattsville, MD: U.S. Department of Health and Human Services, National Center for Health Statistics.

National Committee on Vital and Health Statistics. (1980b). *Uniform hospital discharge data: Minimum data set* (DHHS Publication No. PHS 80-1157). Hyattsville, MD: U.S. Department of Health and Human Services, National Center for Health Statistics.

National Committee on Vital and Health Statistics. (1981). *Uniform ambulatory medical care: Minimum data set* (DHHS Publication No. PHS 81-1161). Hyattsville, MD: U.S. Department of Health and Human Services, National Center for Health Statistics.

National Library of Medicine. (1992, August). *UMLS knowledge sources* (3rd experimental ed.). Bethesda, MD: U.S. Department of Health and Human Services, National Institutes of Health, National Library of Medicine.

Newcomb, J. B. (1981). Issues related to identifying and systemizing data—group discussions. In H. H. Werley & M. R. Grier (Eds.), *Nursing information systems* (pp. 278–296). New York: Springer Publishing.

Pascucci, M. A., Adams, M., Jacobson, S., Holtzen, V., & Knickerbocker, P. (1993). Nursing service data for research in patient care. *Journal of Professional Nursing, 9*, 284–289.

Rios, H., Delaney, C., Kruckeberg, T., Chung, Y., & Mehmert, P. A. (1991). Validation of defining characteristic of four nursing diagnoses using a computer data base. *Journal of Professional Nursing, 17*, 293–299.

Rubin, D., & Schenker, N. (1991). Multiple imputation in health-care data bases: An overview and some applications. *Statistics in Medicine, 10*, 585–598.

Ryan, P., Coenen, A., Devine, E. C., Werley, H. H., Sutton, J., & Kelber, S. (1994). Prevalence and relationships among elements of the Nursing Minimum Data Set. In S. J. Grobe (Ed.), *Proceedings of the Fifth International Conference on Nursing Use of Computers and Information Science* (pp. 174–178). San Antonio, TX: International Medical Informatics Association.

Saba, V. K. (1992, March). The classification of home health care nursing: Diagnoses and interventions. *Caring*, 50–57.

Saba, V. K., O'Hare, P. A., Zuckerman, A. E., Boondas, J., Levine, E., & Oatway, D. M. (1991). A nursing intervention taxonomy for home health care. *Nursing & Health Care, 12*, 296–299.

Saba, V. K., & Zuckerman, A. E. (1992, October). A new home health classification method. *Caring*, 27–34.

Sermeus, W. (1988). Nursing related groups: A research study. In K. J. Hannah

(Ed.), *Proceedings of Nursing and Computers: Third International Symposium on Nursing Use of Computers and Information Science* (pp. 177–182). St. Louis: Mosby.

Sheil, E. P., & Wierenga, M. E. (1994). The use of the Nursing Minimum Data Set in several clinical populations. In S. J. Grobe (Ed.), *Proceedings of the Fifth International Conference on Nursing Use of Computers and Information Science* (pp. 139–143). San Antonio: International Medical Informatics Association.

Tierney, W., & McDonald, C. (1991). Practice databases and their uses in clinical research. *Statistics in Medicine, 10*, 541–557.

Tillman, H. J. (1990). *Test of the Nursing Minimum Data Set in a nursing center*. Unpublished master's thesis, Marquette University, Milwaukee.

Visiting Nurses Association of Omaha. (1986). *Client management information system*. Washington, DC: U.S. Department of Health and Human Services, Health Resources & Services Administration, Division of Nursing.

Werley, H. H. (1986). National, invitational work conference to develop a Nursing Minimum Data Set. *Research Alert, 7*, 4, 8.

Werley, H. H. (1987). Nursing diagnosis and the Nursing Minimum Data Set. In A. M. McLane (Ed.), *Classification of Nursing Diagnoses: Proceedings of the Seventh National Conference* (pp. 21–36). St. Louis: Mosby.

Werley, H. H., & Devine, E. C. (1987). The Nursing Minimum Data Set: Status and implications. In K. J. Hannah, M. Reimer, W. C. Mills, & S. Letourneau (Eds.), *Clinical judgment and decision making: The future with nursing diagnosis* (pp. 540–551). New York: Wiley.

Werley, H. H., Devine, E. C., Westlake, S. K., & Maternach, C. A. (1986). Testing and refinement of the Nursing Minimum Data Set. In R. Salamon, B. Blum, & M. Jorgensen (Eds.), *Medinfo 86: Proceedings of the Fifth World Congress on Medical Informatics* (Pt. 2, pp. 816–817). Amsterdam, Holland: Elsevier Science.

Werley, H. H., Devine, E. C., & Zorn, C. R. (1988a). The Nursing Minimum Data Set: Effort to standardize collection of essential nursing data. In M. J. Ball, K. J. Hannah, U. Gerdin Jelger, & H. Peterson (Eds.), *Nursing informatics* (pp. 160–167). New York: Springer-Verlag.

Werley, H. H., Devine, E. C., & Zorn, C. R. (1988b). Nursing needs its own minimum data set. *American Journal of Nursing, 88*, 1651–1653.

Werley, H. H., Devine, E. C. & Zorn, C. R. (1989a). The Nursing Minimum Data Set: An abstraction tool for computerized nursing service data. In V. K. Saba, K. A. Rieder, & D. B. Pocklington (Eds.), *Nursing and computers: An anthology* (pp. 187–195). New York: Springer-Verlag.

Werley, H. H., Devine, E. C., & Zorn, C. R. (1989b). Status of the Nursing Minimum Data Set and its relationship to nursing diagnosis. In R. M. Carroll-Johnson (Ed.), *Classification of Nursing Diagnoses: Proceedings of the Eighth Conference* (pp. 89–97). Philadelphia: Lippincott.

Werley, H. H., Devine, E. C., & Zorn, C. R. (1990). The Nursing Minimum Data Set: Issues for the profession. In J. C. McCloskey & H. K. Grace (Eds.), *Current issues in nursing* (3rd ed., pp. 64–70). St. Louis: Mosby.

Werley, H. H., Devine, E. C., & Zorn, C. R. (1992). *The Nursing Minimum Data Set data collection manual*. Milwaukee: University of Wisconsin-Milwaukee School of Nursing. (Original work published 1988.)

Werley, H. H., Devine, E. C., Zorn, C. R,. Ryan, P., & Westra, B. L. (1991). The

Nursing Minimum Data Set: Abstraction tool for standardized, comparable, essential data. *American Journal of Public Health, 81*, 421–426. (Reprinted from J. H. van Bemmel & A. T. McCray (Eds.), *Year book '92 of medical informatics: Advances in an interdisciplinary science* [pp. 87–92]. The Netherlands: IMIA Publications).

Werley, H. H., & Grier, M. R. (Eds.). (1981). *Nursing information systems*. New York: Springer Publishing.

Werley, H. H., & Lang, N. M. (Eds.). (1988). *Identification of the Nursing Minimum Data Set*. New York: Springer Publishing.

Werley, H. H., Lang, N. M., & Westlake, S. K. (1986). The Nursing Minimum Data Set Conference: Executive summary. *Journal of Professional Nursing, 2*, 217–224.

Werley, H. H., Ryan, P., & Zorn, C. R. (in press). The Nursing Minimum Data Set: A framework for the organization of nursing data. In *An emerging framework for the profession: Data system advances for clinical practice*. Washington, DC: American Nurses Association.

Werley, H. H., Ryan, P., Zorn, C. R., & Devine, E. C. (1994). Why the Nursing Minimum Data Set? In J. C. McCloskey & H. K. Grace (Eds.), *Current issues in nursing* (4th ed, pp. 113–122). Hanover, MD: Mosby-Year Book.

Werley, H. H., & Zorn, C. R. (1989). The Nursing Minimum Data Set and its relationship to classifications for nursing practice. In *Classification systems for describing nursing practice* (pp. 50–54). Kansas City: American Nurses' Association.

Chapter 8

Pediatric Hospice Nursing

IDA M. MARTINSON
SCHOOL OF NURSING
UNIVERSITY OF CALIFORNIA, SAN FRANCISCO
AND
FRANCES PAYNE BOLTON SCHOOL OF NURSING
CASE WESTERN RESERVE UNIVERSITY

CONTENTS

This chapter includes a review of the research on pediatric hospice nursing. The principles of pediatric hospice nursing are defined, and the historical development is briefly described. A review of the major studies in which researchers addressed issues related to the care of the dying child and the bereavement experienced by parents and siblings following the death of a child in a home care or hospice program is included. Exclusion criteria included deaths of adult children, bereavement response of deaths of parents, and all suicide studies. The chapter concludes with suggestions concerning additional studies that may be fruitful for the field of pediatric hospice nursing.

The *Cumulative Index to Nursing and Allied Health Literature* (CINAHL) was reviewed for the last 10 years (1983–1993) using the term of *pediatric hospice*. This search identified only 5 articles; 2 met the criteria for inclusion and are included here. Using the term *child,* 55 articles were identified; 8 are included here. The Medical Literature Analysis and Retrieval System on Line (MEDLINE) review of 1966 to 1993 for the term *pediatric hospice* was identified in 4 articles; 2 are included here. Review for the term *dying child* was identified in 79 articles; 12 are included here. The references of all suitable articles were examined for additional potential articles. Thus, 21 references were located. In addition, references accumulated on children's death and home/hospice care from more than 20 years were checked, and 24 articles that met the criteria were located. The inclusion criteria were that the article was databased or essential for definition of this critical review.

PEDIATRIC HOSPICE PHILOSOPHY

The concept of hospice does not refer to a building, facility, or institution but rather to a philosophy of care. Hospice is a concept of care and can be given in hospitals, nursing homes, respite houses, or individual homes (Corr & Corr, 1992). Pediatric hospice philosophy is an approach focused on comfort care when cure is no longer a reasonable expectation. Pediatric hospice care addresses the physical, psychosocial, and spiritual needs of the dying child and provides support to family members during the illness and after the death of the child.

The philosophy of pediatric hospice care applies to children usually under the age of 18. Once infectious and communicable diseases are under control, childhood cancer is frequently the most common cause of disease and death of children in both developing and developed countries around the world. Children dying from acquired immunodeficiency syndrome (AIDS) is increasing worldwide and may surpass cancer as the leading cause of death for children in pediatric hospices in the near future. A key component of pediatric hospice care is that parents are involved, and the home is the setting. Parents are the primary caregivers; therefore, they require support and guidance in meeting the complex needs of the child and other family members.

Other environments than the home, hospital, or nursing home, in which hospice services are provided to dying children include "houses" located close to hospitals. The homes offer professional nursing services for a limited period that can be an excellent adjunct to hospice/home care. A home-like environment is made possible while remaining close to the acute care hospital. Terminally ill children who are unable to return home or where families need respite can be referred to these houses.

According to Children's Hospice International (1991) hospice care is currently defined as "both a concept for caring and a system of comprehensive interdisciplinary services" (p. 40). Children's Hospice International (CHI) published Standards of Hospice Care for Children. The standards speak to the principles and guidelines involved in access to care, the child and family as a unit of care, policies and procedures, interdisciplinary team services, continuity of care, pain and symptom management, bereavement program, and use review/quality improvement (CHI, 1993b). Children's Hospice International was founded in 1983 by Ann Armstrong-Dailey. Armstrong-Dailey, who had worked as a staff person in the National Hospice Organization, believed that a separate organization for children would be useful, and she invited health care professionals to join her in this endeavor. Over the years this organization, by cosponsoring conferences and having available materials regarding pediatric hospice/home care has raised the consciousness of both health care professionals and the public to the tragedy of the death of a child and to the resources that need to be available to the families (Dailey, 1985).

The International Work Group on Death, Dying and Bereavement (IWG) has recently published a statement pertaining to the principles of palliative care for children. Despite health care advances, children continue to die (IWG, 1993). The death of a child disrupts human development and is perceived as less acceptable than a death that occurs from being old. Children's needs are constantly changing because of the developmental process as well as the dying process, and effective care requires knowledge of childhood development. This statement may provide the guidelines in developing hospice services across cultures.

WHO will be publishing in 1995 guidelines on Cancer Pain Relief and Palliative Care for children with cancer that will be useful for the world governments. These guidelines will provide clearer criteria for expanding pediatric/hospice home care programs around the world especially in pain management issues.

There are three researchers, Waechter, Spinetta, and Bluebond-Langner who provided the research base for the greatly improved communication between the health care professionals, the family, and the dying child. The results of their research led to the openness in the United States that provided the environment for the development of pediatric hospice.

Waechter worked directly with dying children using projective techniques; she found that children with cancer were preoccupied with their future and told stories relating to death. It became apparent that the dilemma of clinicians as to whether they ought to tell a child that she or he has a potentially fatal illness was meaningless because the child was already concerned. Her research provided the major impetus for advocating a more open approach to children to express their concerns and have their questions answered honestly (Waechter, 1971, 1987a, 1987b, 1987c).

Spinetta's work supported Waechter's conclusions. His own studies as well as those of his collaborators, revealed that terminally ill children have a keen awareness of the hospital experience, its personnel, and procedures. In contrast to other chronically ill children, patients with leukemia expressed more hospital and nonhospital anxiety (Spinetta, 1974; Spinetta & Maloney, 1975; Spinetta, Rigler, & Karon, 1973, 1974).

Bluebond-Langner's anthropological work on the pediatric oncology ward revealed that children knew that they were dying. They acquired this knowledge through five consecutive stages regardless of age. Children in the first stage realized the seriousness of their illness. In the second stage, they learned from personal experience, through the side effects of treatment. In the third stage, they understood the purpose of the procedures and treatment. During the fourth stage, and as their condition deteriorated, children became aware of the cycles of relapses and remissions of their disease, but did not perceive yet that they were going to die. It is only when they learned or heard about the death of another child on the unit that they realized they would die too. Children accumulate information about their disease through experience and progressively come to an understanding of their disease and its prognosis (Bluebond-Langner, 1978). Her work did not acknowledge the influence of the child's perception of what was happening to their own physical bodies.

POTENTIAL NUMBERS FOR HOSPICE/HOME CARE

There are approximately 1.7 billion children in the world, and more than three fourths of these children live in developing countries. The death rates for children in most developing countries are high. There is a clear need for pediatric hospice services worldwide.

In the United States alone, more than 100,000 children die annually. However, most of these deaths are not amenable to pediatric hospice care. Deaths from accidents provide no opportunity for clinical services before the death occurs; this is also true for sudden infant death syndrome (SIDS), and factors related to pregnancy, childbirth, and complications following birth.

Pediatric cancers are the leading cause of disease-related death for children from the ages of 1 to 14. The death of children with pediatric cancers has decreased dramatically during recent years and accounts for less than 1,800 per year in the United States. When one includes birth defects, heart diseases, and death from AIDS, close to 15,000 children in the United States could use pediatric hospice clinical services.

Until the early part of the 20th century, children died at home in the United States. Hospitals were not common and the process of dying and the actual death of any family member, including a child, took place within the home. Between the 1930s and the 1960s, services for dying children became increasingly centered in the hospital. Dying children would increasingly be admitted to an acute, cure-oriented, technology-based system, the hospital, in part because of lack of home care services. This practice continued into the early 1970s when dying children were still being admitted to the hospital for care (Martinson, 1993).

PEDIATRIC HOSPICE/HOME CARE PROGRAMS

United States

In 1972, a home care program for dying children and their families was developed by Martinson in Minnesota. With funding from the National Cancer Institute in 1976, a nursing study was conducted (Martinson, 1976). About 80% of the children died at home with the family providing the primary care and most outside professional help facilitated by nurses. Physicians served as consultants primarily to the nurse. Both urban and rural families were part of the study. All children, regardless of the type of cancer, were included in the project. During a 2-year period, 58 families cared for the child under the home care project, and 46 of the children died at home. Only 11 families whose child was dying were not referred to the project because of one physician who was not willing to make the referral. These 11 families served as a convenient control group. Their costs were compared with the project group and found to be higher. The overall study served as a basis for pediatric hospice/home care. It was the first study to offer home care for the dying child systemically, regardless of where the family lived, the type of cancer the child had, the complexity of the symptoms, including difficult pain management problems, or the configuration of the family. There are numerous published reports from various aspects of his study (Martinson, 1976; Martinson et al., 1978, 1986; Martinson & Henry, 1980; Martinson, Nesbit, & Kersey, 1985; Moldow & Martinson, 1980).

Edwardson (1983, 1984, 1985) used this same study group. Edwardson examined the decision-making process of physicians and parents when they chose hospital or home care for the dying child from cancer. Looking at the total sample of 123 children who had died, the most significant variable that predicted the care option of home over hospital care was the physicians' experience with the option. When, however, the parents of the children who had died at home were interviewed to clarify what had influenced them to choose home care, a second determinant become important. Parents reported their child's and their own desires and beliefs about their ability to provide care influenced them with physicians having little impact over their decision. Edwardson pointed out that the choice of terminal care at home was in fact a "second" decision that was preceded by a critical first decision regarding the cessation of active treatment. Once the aggressive, curative approach was stopped, parents considered their own desires and abilities, and the child's desire to be of major importance.

The University of Virginia researchers, Fortunato and Komp (1979) retrospectively analyzed the medical records of 27 children who died from acute lymphoblastic leukemia during a 5-year period. Thirteen (44%) died at home and 14 (56%) died in the hospital. A comparison between the home and hospital group revealed no significant difference in age at death, distance from home to hospital, and the frequency of disease-related symptoms. A significant difference was found between the two groups for average length of survival from diagnosis to death. The home group mean was 32 months compared with 18 months for the hospital groups ($p < .02$). Possible reasons for the longer period in home care before dying could be the more supportive atmosphere of the home and the use of less toxic chemotherapy drugs. The authors concluded that with sufficient medical and psychosocial support, it is feasible for a child with acute lymphoblastic leukemia to die at home (Fortunato & Komp, 1979).

Since 1979, several studies have reported on home care for the dying child as an alternative to hospitalization. Adapted from the Minnesota project, the Midwest Children's Cancer Center at Milwaukee Children's Hospital developed a home care program to provide support for families who wished to care for their dying child at home. In the first 2 years of this program, 42 families received the home care option, and the children died at home. Only 6 families refused the option of home care (Lauer & Camitta, 1980; Lauer & Mulhern, 1984; Lauer, Mulhern, Bohne, & Camitta, 1985).

In the summer of 1979 an adult hospice, Hospice of Louisville Inc., cared for their first pediatric patient, and by August 1984, 79 children and their families had been served, with most of the children dying at home (Bertolone, Michal, & Morrell, 1982). In 1984, Nunneley reported that 100% of the 10 families who chose home care in her private practice were able to remain at home until the child's death (Nunneley, 1984).

Although the Martinson and Lauer studies examined care for children dying only of cancer in the mid-central part of the United States, more recent studies have included care for children with other terminal conditions as well as in other parts of the United States. In 1980 a formal home care program was started at Children's Hospital of Los Angeles, California. This hospital-based pediatric hospice program was designed to serve children with any terminal illness and was under the direction of Belinda Martin (Martin, 1986). The study team identified 167 patients who had received services from August 1980 to May 1985 and located 114 primary caretakers (68.3% of the sample population) to be part of the retrospective study. The prospective study included 46% or 78% of the 59 additional patients and families participating in the Home Care Program from mid-1985 to February 1988. Most of the children died from cancer (72.2%), whereas other diagnoses included neonatal deaths (14%), and AIDS (4.6%) (Martin, 1989). Families of diverse ethnic and cultural backgrounds were able to provide this home care with the assistance of nursing personnel.

Since 1980, all families whose infants died in the newborn intensive care unit (NICU) at the Children's Hospital in Denver, Colorado, have had available the hospice approach to care for the families. In a follow-up of 38 married mothers, 19 had participated in the hospice program. Mothers who had been in the hospice program were more positive about their experiences in the NICU. Among the hospice intervention mothers, 92% were contacted about autopsy results in comparison with only 60% of mothers before the hospice program began. This autopsy contact and explanation of the results had helped the mothers in their understanding of the reasons for their infant's death (Harmon, Glicken, & Siegel, 1984).

Lauer, Mulhern, Hoffman, and Camitta conducted a national survey of the use of hospice/home care in pediatric oncology in 1986. Data were received from 85 institutions in 47 states. Home care for the dying child was offered by 86% of the institutions, with 56% relying on community-based services and 44% provided their own programs of care. In the institutions that provided their own programs, home care was offered to more families, more of the families accepted the option of home care, and a smaller number of children returned to the hospital to die than in institutions that used community agencies. Their survey revealed that the community agencies' most frequent problems were with inexperience with pediatric issues, inadequate pain control, and the families' reluctance to work with new staff. Institutions that were hesitant to develop their own home care programs indicated that this was due to the anticipated problems with pain and other management of symptoms. Also, uncertainty as to the family competency to provide care and concerns over the effects of the child dying at home on the family were factors (Lauer et al., 1986).

In the United States, pediatric hospices are growing in numbers, and evaluation of the effectiveness of these programs is beginning in terms of clinical management of the child's symptoms, and the ability of the family members to be involved during the dying process and the death event. Generally, in the U.S. children are well aware of their prognosis, and usually no attempts are made to hide the reality of the impending death from the child.

Continued study needs to be done in this area because of changes in medical treatment that brings the child physically close to death but rescues the child with additional treatments. Cultural differences in communications with the family, the dying child, and the health care professionals need to be examined.

The study of home versus hospital care for the dying child continues to encourage the home care alternative (Dufour, 1989; Hutter, Farrel, & Meltzer, 1991). Wilson (1982) discussed the establishment of a pediatric hospice, and Corr and Corr (1992) revisited the concept of pediatric hospice care. However, no random clinical trial has been done. No multisystem comparison study has been conducted with the growing number of hospice programs in the United States that offer pediatric hospice services. Although the research question as to the feasibility of pediatric hospice has been answered, the more complex levels of research including identification of the significant variables have not been done.

Programs for pediatric hospice/home care have also been developed outside of the United States. Presentation of data from these international programs is discussed.

England

In England, home care for dying children developed later than hospice care for adults. In England, home care for the dying child is now more widely available. At Children's Hospital at Great Ormand Street in London, England, a team of three to four nurses provide home care for children with cancer throughout London from the time of diagnosis through the terminal stage of the illness including bereavement follow-up services (Goldman, Beardsmore, & Hunt, 1990).

Chambers, Oakhill, Cornish, and Curnick conducted a study in southwestern England of 12 children who died at home and one who was at home until the last 24 hours before death. The researchers concluded that most children who are terminally ill can be supported at home.

Kohler and Radford (1985) in Southampton, England, interviewed 18 families of children who had died of cancer during the previous 5 years. All of the families had chosen to take their child home when curative treatment was no longer effective. All but five of the children died at home. The main burden of care at home was psychological. The quality of the child's life was good up until the last few days.

In 1982 Helen House, a respite facility in Oxford, provided respite care primarily for families with long-term chronically ill children (Dominica, 1982, 1987). During a 5-year period (1983–1987), of the 30 children who died at Helen House, most deaths were due to degenerative disease and not to cancer (Hunt, 1990). In a follow-up study of the first 29 families who had been to Helen House, five of the children had died. The interviews of these five families were between 11 and 23 months after the child had died. Each child had spent between 3 days and up to 3 months in the year preceding the child's death in Helen House. The mean was 31 days. The families whose child had died at Helen House felt well supported at the time of the child's death. A variety of rituals surrounding the death, for example, bathing and laying out of the child after the death, provided the opportunity for the whole family to be with the child and to spend time with the body in an unhurried manner. Of the five bereaved families, two had marital problems. Two mothers and one father were rated as having psychological difficulties on the general health questionnaire. Three out of the five families recalled being worried about at least one symptom of the child (seizures, breathlessness, or pain most commonly mentioned). Several families reported difficulties with the surviving siblings (Stein, Forrest, Woolley, & Baum, 1989). The same team interviewed 24 out of 27 staff members at Helen House with a semistructured guide as well as the Goldberg's 60-item general health questionnaire. Four of the six high scores on the Goldberg scale had a death of a close relative or friend during the past year. Job satisfaction remained high despite experiencing stress in dealing with child and family. Although 80% of the staff reported difficulties in staff communication and that relationships were an important source of stress as well, the informal staff support was also the most important factor, which helped them to cope (Woolley, Stein, Forrest, & Baum, 1989).

In England both a respite house Helen House, and the home care hospice programs are providing pediatric hospice clinical services. All published reports are with a small number of children. A national study of all children who die in England, including where they die, would provide needed direction for the field. With the growing cultural diversity in England, comparison of family reactions during the crisis of the dying child and the death event would add basic needed knowledge to the field.

Canada

A home-based palliative care program for children was initiated in 1984 at the Hospital for Sick Children in Toronto, Canada, and provided care to 29 children. Most of these children (75.9%) had central nervous system tumors, and 17.2% had a myelomeningocele that led to complications resulting in death. All but 1 of the 29 children died at home (Duffy, Pollock, & Levy, 1990; Levy, Duffy, & Pollock, 1990).

A project is under way in Vancouver, British Columbia, in Canada to develop pediatric hospice services including a respite facility. Major fund raising is presently under way to construct the building, and plans are to begin providing services for terminally ill children in 1994. One of the major objectives will be to assist families to care for their dying child at home. This facility will be a respite center for the families as well as providing a consultative service to health care providers and families who are caring for their dying child at home.

In the preceding project in Vancouver, evaluation will be integral to the programs and should provide data that will clarify the issues in pediatric hospice care. More precise measurements of the changes that occur in both the child and family during the dying phase need to be done. Clinical trials in symptom management and psychosocial interventions need to be conducted.

Australia

In 1982, in Melbourne, Australia, a hospital's Hematology/Oncology Pediatric Unit suggested that the district nursing service expand its role to provide a 24-hour "on-call" service for the families of children dying from cancer. In a 15-month period, a total of 21 children—ages 2 to 18 years old—were included in the Pediatric Palliative Care Project. All but three died at home. Norman and Bennett (1986) concluded that in Australia, home is a viable alternative to hospitalization for the terminally ill child.

The deaths at Adelaide Children's Hospital were reviewed with identification of 80 deaths in a 1-year period, with 62 (82%) dying in the hospital. The four most common causes of death were cancer (27%), congenital abnormalities (19%), sudden infant death syndrome (16%), and trauma (11%). Besides the medical records review, 19 individuals were interviewed including parents and staff personnel. A series of recommendations were made including more referrals to hospices and home care services (Ashby, Kosky, Laver, & Sims, 1991).

The Australian programs have identified the feasibility of pediatric hospice for their country. Now more sophisticated research methodologies could be employed such as clinical trials.

Greece

In Greece, the Nursing School at the University of Athens, under the direction of Danai Papadatou and with partial funding from the European Economic Community, has developed a home-based palliative care program for children with cancer. During the first phase a feasibility study had been conducted. Based on the major findings the researchers suggested that home care is both feasible and desired by families, who despite the lack of home care services, tend to care for their child at home during the terminal phase of the disease (Papadatou, Yfantopoulos, Vassilatou-Kosmidis, & Maistros, 1992). The researchers identified a great need for families to care for their child at home during the terminal period, which was reinforced by the child's request, in 87% of the cases, to return home as he or she became aware that he or she was dying and expressed it directly, indirectly, or symbolically. Findings suggested that the experience at home was perceived as "very positive" by 4 families (40%) and "positive" by 6 (60%) of the 10 families who chose to care for the child at home.

Following the preceding report, funding was received to train health care professionals for pediatric hospice services. Plans are under way to begin pediatric hospice services with a strong evaluation component. Both the rural, mountain areas, and the urban large centers of population will be included in the service area and the results of their implementation of clinical services under diverse conditions will be useful to the field.

Sweden

Examination of the records for eight children who had died of cancer in Sweden showed that only one child died at home, one in the ambulance on the way back to the hospital, one soon after admission (within a matter of hours), four died after a few days in the hospital, and the last child died in the hospital 4 weeks after readmission to the hospital. The researchers reported that without a formal pediatric hospice program, most children would die in the hospital (Kreuger, Gyllenskold, Pehrsson, & Sjolin, 1983).

The Swedish experience would appear to be typical of well-developed health care systems that do not have a structured program. If a pediatric hospice program was now established, present data would provide a comparative base for the evaluation of the new program.

Asia

In Taiwan, nurses, with the support of the Childhood Cancer Foundation, have supported families as they have cared for their dying child at home (personal communication, 1983–1992). In June 1992, Dr. Susie Kim, a nurse and dean of the Ewha Womans' University in Seoul, Korea, established a pediatric hospice. Other adult-focused hospices in Korea also have established care for dying children at home (S. Kim, personal communication, 1992). Although there are established adult hospice programs, there is no known pediatric hospice program in Japan or Hong Kong. The Tianjin Hospice Program in China does include children and one of the nursing faculty of the School of Nursing where the hospice program is based has cared for a dying child at home (personal communication, 1991).

SELECTED STUDIES RELATED TO PEDIATRIC HOSPICE/HOME CARE

Cost of Pediatric Hospice/Home Care Programs

Regarding the costs of a pediatric hospice program, two studies and one newsletter report were located; each examined the issue of home care for the dying child. Moldow, Armstrong, Henry and Martinson (1982) documented that the costs of home care were from 22% to 207% less than hospital care. The variation in comparisons depended on whether home care was regarded as an alternative to inpatient hospitalization or a larger concept of care that included added services at a time when the child would not necessarily be hospitalized. More recently, data were provided from the Children's Hospital in Los Angeles on provider use and duration in a pediatric hospice program retrospectively on 177 children and prospectively from the families of 27 children enrolled in the pediatric hospice program. The mean total cost for the families was $4,808 per case assuming average direct costs. Incidental expenses were $446 with indirect costs of $1,478. Indirect costs included the foregone earnings of either the family, friends, or volunteers. These researchers concluded that children can be cared for at home whether or not they use hospital outpatient or intermittent inpatient care, and whether or not they continue with aggressive therapy. They also demonstrated that services can be made available to both single- and two-parent households with widely varying socioeconomic backgrounds (Schweitzer, Mitchell, Landsverk, & Laparan, 1993).

A 1993 newsletter of the Children's Hospice International (CHI) reported that in one member institution that treated 33 terminally ill children (AIDS, brain tumors, leukemia, spina bifida, osteopetrosis, and seizure disorders) the cost was $445,000. Without home care the cost would have been $860,000 in a skilled nursing facility, or more than $4 million in an acute care facility. "By caring for these children in their homes, there was an annual cost savings to the system of between $415,000 and $3.55 million, depending on the alternative treatment site" (CHI, 1993a). Although the site is not mentioned, the same newsletter reported on another CHI member organization that rendered 3,838 patient days of care to 17 terminally ill children in its palliative care unit at a cost of approximately $1.2 million. "In the absence of this unit, these children would have required hospitalization in an acute care setting at an estimated annual cost of at least $4 million ($800/patient/day). The annual savings totalled $1.8 million or $105,000 per patient" (CHI, 1993a). There has been no study reported that documents an increase in cost for pediatric hospice/home care. Clearly from the financial standpoint, there is no debate on the present cost effectiveness of pediatric hospice/home care. A randomized clinical trial would be useful to settle the financial concerns as well as psychological concerns.

Although all the studies had input into the analysis from health economists, the study done in Los Angeles included a health economist from the point of the initial design of the study to its completion and publication. As hospital costs continue to rise, the option of home care becomes a more viable alternative.

BEREAVEMENT FOLLOWING PEDIATRIC HOSPICE/HOME CARE

Parent

Little is known of the actual impact of the child's death on the surviving family, the length of time needed for resolution, or the variables that influence the particular outcomes achieved following the death of a child in pediatric hospice/home care. Much more research of the hospice health care system is needed.

In the one study where the families were involved in home care and actively participated in providing care for the dying child, no relationship was found between the length of the child's illness and the severity of the symptoms (Martinson, Davies, & McClowry, 1987; Moore, Gilliss, & Martinson, 1988). Similar results were found by Lauer and Mulhern (1984).

Research publications from Lauer and colleagues have been focused on family adjustment following a child's death at home. Lauer and associates interviewed 37 sets of parents between 3 and 28 months after the death of their child. When comparing 24 sets of parents who cared for their dying child at home to the 13 sets whose child died in the hospital, more favorable outcomes were achieved by the home care parents. Home care parents had comparatively less guilt, fewer regrets, and more positive views of themselves and their marriages than did the contrast group who had not participated in the home care option (Lauer, Mulhern, Wallskog, & Camitta, 1983). Mulhern, Lauer, and Hoffmann in 1983 reported that parents of children who died in the hospital were more anxious, depressed, defensive, and had greater tendencies toward somatic and interpersonal problems than the parents of children who died at home in the home care (hospice) program. Parents who had provided home care for their dying child reported significant reduction of guilt following the death of their child at both the 6- and 12-month periods. In contrast, parents who did not provide home care reported greater feelings of guilt, which were still unresolved 1 year after the child's death.

Six years later the same population was again contacted. Within the home care group, all parents who had been previously interviewed gave consent again to participate. Within the hospital care groups 92% of the previous sample also agreed. The early pattern of better adjustment of home care parents was a reliable predictor of long-term bereavement outcomes. Non–home care parents continued to exhibit more frequent indications of poor adjustment. Home care parents did not experience a delayed or otherwise complicated bereavement process (Lauer, Mulhern, Schell, & Camitta, 1989).

McClowry, Davies, May, Kulenkamp, and Martinson (1987) investigated families 7 to 9 years after the death of a child who had been involved in a home care for the dying child project and found that grieving to some degree may last that long. The families described their grief over an "empty space," and the researchers were able to identify three different grieving patterns used by parents: (a) getting over it by accepting the reality of the death and getting on with their life; (b) filling the emptiness by keeping busy and involved in various projects and activities; and (c) maintaining the connection, by integrating the "empty space" caused by the child's death into every day living and cherishing recollections of the child. It is evident from these studies however, that grief does not follow a set time table and seems to be an individual journey; therefore, clinically one needs to accept various patterns of grief expression among family members (McClowry et al., 1987). Other reports corroborated the finding that some grieving parents continue to experience intense symptoms 2 to 3 years after the death of their child (Miles, 1985; Moore et al., 1988; Spinetta, Swarner, & Sheposh, 1981).

In summary, the research indicates that bereavement is a long-term process for parents. Additional work needs to be done in identification and development of interventions that may lessen the difficulties for parents who have lost a child. Identification of high-risk parents is imperative.

Siblings' Responses

Few investigators have examined the immediate or long-term effects of the loss of a child through cancer in a pediatric hospice/home care program on the surviving, healthy siblings. In studies where pediatric hospice/home care was involved it was found that the self-concept of siblings was higher than normal (Martinson et al., 1987). The factors related to the positive responses and coping methods of siblings were good communication in the family, ability to share the death experience with others, expression of pleasure in the surviving siblings' company, and reliance on the family for economic support after death (Martinson & Campos, 1992). In the Martinson and Campos study, four out of five bereaved adolescents had no long-term negative effects.

The effect of a sibling dying at home as perceived by the surviving children was reported. Nineteen children whose sibling had participated in a home care program for dying children and 17 children whose sibling died in the hospital were interviewed 1 year after the death. Their data indicated that multiple factors influenced the positive adjustment of siblings who participated in home care. These children expressed their desire to be involved in the care of the dying child, and findings suggested increased family intimacy and communication in contrast to the children whose sibling had died in the hospital. These children described themselves as not being prepared for the death and had been isolated from the dying child and their parents and felt useless in terms of their own involvement (Lauer et al., 1985).

Concern for the vulnerability of the adolescent sibling (Adams & Deveau, 1987) and, most recently, studies on the response of the children to the dying and death of siblings have included the relationship of the parent and sibling communication and their coping with the death (Birenbaum, 1989). Sixty-one children ages 4 to 16 years were studied during the first year following the death of their sibling. Of interest are the variables related to behaviors indicative of depression, social withdrawal, anxiety, and somatic complaints. The behaviors were elevated at all points in their study for these children (Birenbaum, Robinson, Phillips, Stewart, & McCown, 1989). The question becomes is this recording the child's bereavement response and is this not normal? These children were involved in the home care project, but the data were not reported separately out if the child had died at home or in the hospital.

RECOMMENDATIONS FOR FURTHER RESEARCH

An evaluation of the effectiveness of services provided to children and families by various models of hospice care should be conducted. No random clinical trial has been done on pediatric hospice to date. Providing a control group would be useful to identify precisely the benefits and limitations of pediatric hospice care. More careful attention to the operational definitions of pediatric hospice care and to careful collection of data on process variables is needed.

There is a need to design instruments that measure quality of life in dying children because the essence of any hospice intervention is the enhancement of quality of life. Children, although verbal, may use indirect and symbolic ways to express their concerns and feelings. Thus, in designing instruments, researchers need to be sensitive to children's mode of communication and developmental concerns to assess their experience of "living until they die." Further research needs to also generate more knowledge on the quality of life of parents and siblings involved in caring for the dying child.

Careful attention needs to be given to the specifics of the desired outcomes for pediatric hospice care. Clinical trials in the area of pediatric symptom management including psychosocial interventions need to be conducted.

Another significant area that needs more exploration is parent and sibling bereavement after the child dies. Further longitudinal studies need to focus on how marital, parent-child, and family relationships evolve over time as a result of the loss of a child, and how their grief may be affected by their experiences throughout the illness and terminal care provided by hospice or home care.

REFERENCES

Adams, D. W., & Deveau, E. J. (1987). When a brother or sister is dying of cancer: The vulnerability of the adolescent sibling. *Death Studies, 11*, 279–295.

Ashby, M. A., Kosky, R. J., Laver, H. T., & Sims, E. B. (1991). An enquiry into death and dying at the Adelaide Children's Hospital: A useful model? *The Medical Journal of Australia, 154*, 165–170.

Bertolone, S. J., Michal, K., & Morrell, M. (1982). Development of a pediatric hospice program within an existing hospice program. *Psychosocial Aspects of Cancer*. (From American Society of Clinical Oncology Abstracts, C-199, Abstract No. 192)

Birenbaum, L. K. (1989). The relationship between parent-siblings' communication and siblings' coping with death experience. *Journal of Pediatric Oncology Nurses, 6*, 86–91.

Birenbaum, L. K., Robinson, M. A., Phillips, O. S., Stewart, B. J., & McCown, D. (1989). The response of children to the dying and death of a sibling. *Omega: Journal of Death and Dying, 20*, 213–228.

Bluebond-Langner, M. (1978). *The private worlds of dying children*. Princeton: Princeton University Press.

Chambers, E. J., Oakhill, A., Cornish, J. M., & Curnick, S. (1989). Terminal. *British Medical Journal, 298*, 937–940.

Children's Hospice International (1991). Board of Directors statement. In I. M. Martinson, B. B. Martin, M. E. Lauer, L. K. Birenbaum, & B. Eng (Eds.), *Children's hospice/home care: An implementation manual for nurses* (p. xv). Los Angeles: Children's Hospital of Los Angeles (original work published 1989)

Children's Hospice International (1993a, summer). The role of pediatric hospice care in health care reform. *CHI Newsletter*, 3.

Children's Hospice International. (1993b). Standards of hospice care for children. *Pediatric Nursing, 19*, 242–243.

Corr, C. A., & Corr, D. M. (1992). Children's hospice care. *Death Studies, 16*, 431–449.

Dailey, A. A. (1985). Hospice care and the role of Children's Hospice International. *Caring, 4*(5), 66–67.

Dominica, F. (1982). Helen House—a hospice for children. *Maternal Child Health Journal, 7*, 355–359.

Dominica, F. (1987). The role of the hospice for the dying child. *British Journal of Hospital Medicine, 38*, 334–343.

Duffy, C. M., Pollock, P., & Levy, M. (1990). Home-based palliative care for children: 2: The benefits of an established program. *Journal of Palliative Care, 6*(2), 8–14.

Dufour, D. F. (1989). Home or hospital care for the child with end-stage cancer:

Effects on the family. *Issues in Comprehensive Pediatric Nursing, 12*, 371–383.

Edwardson, S. R. (1983). The choice between hospital and home care for terminally ill children. *Nursing Research, 2*, 29–34.

Edwardson, S. R. (1984). Using research in practice: Factors associated with the adoption of a nursing innovation . . . home care as an alternative to hospital for children terminally ill. *Western Journal of Nursing Research, 6*, 141–143.

Edwardson, S. R. (1985). Physician acceptance of home care for terminally ill children. *Health Services Research, 20*, 83–101.

Fortunato, R., & Komp, D. (1979). Death at home for children with acute lymphoblastic leukemia. *Virginia Medical, 106*, 124–126.

Goldman, A., Beardsmore, S., & Hunt, J. (1990). Palliative care for children with cancer—home, hospital or hospice? *Archives of Diseases in Children, 65*, 641–643.

Harmon, R. J., Glicken, A. D., & Siegel, R. E. (1984). Neonatal loss in the intensive care nursery. *Journal of the American Academy of Child Psychiatry, 23*, 68–71.

Hunt, A. M. (1990). A survey of signs, symptoms and symptom control in 30 terminally ill children. *Development of Medical Child Neurology, 32*, 341–346.

Hutter, J. J., Farrel, F. Z., & Meltzer, P. S. (1991). Care of the child dying from cancer: Home vs. hospital. In D. Papadatou & C. Papadatos (Eds.), *Children and death* (pp. 197–208). Washington, DC: Hemisphere.

International Work Group on Death, Dying, and Bereavement. (1993). Position statement: Palliative care for children. *Death Studies, 17*, 277–280.

Kohler, J. A., & Radford, M. (1985). Terminal care for children dying of cancer: Quantity and quality of life. *British Medical Journal, 291*, 115–116.

Kreuger, A., Gyllenskold, K., Pehrsson, G., & Sjolin, S. (1983). Parent reactions to childhood malignant diseases: Experience in Sweden. *The American Journal of Pediatric Hematology/Oncology, 3*, 233–238.

Lauer, M. E., & Camitta, B. M. (1980). Home care for dying children: A nursing model. *Journal of Pediatrics, 97*, 1032–1035.

Lauer, M. E., & Mulhern, R. K. (1984). Parental self-selection versus psychosocial predictors of capability in home care referral: A case study. *American Journal of Hospice Care, 1*(1), 35–38.

Lauer, M. E., Mulhern, R. K., Bohne, J. M., & Camitta, B. M. (1985). Children's perceptions of their sibling's death at home or hospital: The precursors of differential adjustment. *Cancer Nursing, 8*, 21–27.

Lauer, M. E., Mulhern, R. K., Hoffman, R. G., & Camitta, B. M. (1986). Utilization of hospice/home care in pediatric oncology: A national survey. *Cancer Nursing, 9*, 102–107.

Lauer, M. E., Mulhern, R. K., Schell, M. J., & Camitta, B. M. (1987). Long term follow-up of parental adjustment following child's death at home or hospital. *Cancer, 63*, 988–994.

Lauer, M. E., Mulhern, R. K., Wallskog, J. M., & Camitta, B. M. (1983). A comparison study of parental adaptation following a child's death at home or in the hospital. *Pediatrics, 1*, 107–112.

Levy, M., Duffy, C. M., & Pollock, P. (1990). Home-based palliative care for children: 1: The institution of a program. *Journal of Palliative Care, 6*, 11–15.

Martin, B. B. (1986). Pediatric hospice care: An update. *Caring, 5*(12), 5–6.

Martin, B. B. (1989). *Implementation of a hospital-based pediatric hospice care program*. (Final Report to the Maternal and Child Health Program, Health and Human Services). Report #MCJ-063703-03-0. Los Angeles: Children's Hospital of Los Angeles.

Martinson, I. M. (1976). Why don't we let them die at home? *Registered Nurse, 39*, 57–65.

Martinson, I. M. (1993). Pediatric hospice: Past, present and future. *Journal of Pediatric Oncology Nursing, 10*, 93–98.

Martinson, I. M., Armstrong, G. D., Geis, D. P., Anglim, M. A., Gronseth, E., MacInnis, H., Kersey, J. H., & Nesbit, M. E. (1978). Home care for children dying of cancer. *Pediatrics, 62*, 106–113.

Martinson, I. M., & Campos, R. G. (1992). Adolescent bereavement: Long term responses to a sibling's death from cancer. *Journal of Adolescent Research, 6*, 54–69.

Martinson, I. M., Davies, E. B., & McClowry, S. G. (1987). The long-term effects of sibling death on self-concept. *Journal of Pediatric Nursing, 2*, 227–235.

Martinson, I. M., & Henry, W. F. (1980). Some possible societal consequences of changing the way in which we care for dying children. *Hastings Center Report, 10*(2), 5–8.

Martinson, I. M., Moldow, D. G., Armstrong, G. D., Henry, W. F., Nesbit, M. E., & Kersey, J. H. (1986). Home care for children dying of cancer. *Research in Nursing & Health, 9*, 11–16.

Martinson, I. M., Nesbit, M. E., & Kersey, J. H. (1985). Physician's role in home care for children with cancer. *Death Studies, 9*, 283–293.

McClowry, S. G., Davies, E. B., May, K. A., Kulenkamp, E. J., & Martinson, I. M. (1987). The empty space phenomenon: The process of grief in the bereaved family. *Death Studies, 11*, 361–363.

Miles, M. C. (1985). Emotional symptoms and physical health in bereaved parents. *Nursing Research, 34*, 76–81.

Moldow, D. G., Armstrong, G. D., Henry, W. F., & Martinson, I. M. (1982). The cost of home care for dying children. *Medical Care, 20*, 1114–1160.

Moldow, D. G., & Martinson, I. M. (1980). From research to reality. Home care for the dying child. *MCN: The American Journal of Maternal Child Nursing, 51*, 159–160, 162, 166.

Moore, I. M., Gilliss, C. L., & Martinson, I. M. (1988). Psychosomatic manifestations of bereavement in parents two years after the death of a child with cancer. *Nursing Research, 37*, 104–107.

Mulhern, R. K., Lauer, M. E., & Hoffman, R. G. (1983). Death of a child at home or in the hospital: Subsequent psychological adjustment of the family. *Pediatrics, 71*, 743–747.

Norman, R., & Bennett, M. (1986). Care of the dying child at home: A unique cooperative relationship. *Austrian Journal of Advanced Nursing, 3*(4), 3–16.

Nunneley, C. (1984). Home care of the child with cancer. *Journal of the Association of Pediatric Oncology Nurses, 1*, 11.

Papadatou, D., Yfantopoulos, J., Vassilatou-Kosmidis, E., & Maistros, Y.

(1992). *Feasibility study: A home based palliative care for children with cancer* (Final Report to Europe Against Cancer: European Economic Communities. Report B3-Y3OU. Athens: University of Athens.)

Schweitzwer, S., Mitchell, B., Landsverk, J., & Laparan, L. (1993). The costs of a pediatric hospice program. *Public Health Reports, 108*, 37–45.

Spinetta, J. J. (1974). The dying child's awareness of death. *Psychological Bulletin, 4*, 256–260.

Spinetta, J. J., & Maloney, L. J. (1975). Death anxiety in the outpatient leukemic child. *Pediatrics, 56*, 1034–1037.

Spinetta, J. J., Rigler, D., & Karon, M. (1973). Anxiety in the dying child. *Pediatrics, 52*, 127–131.

Spinetta, J. J., Rigler, D., & Karon, M. (1974). Personal space as a measure of a dying child's sense of isolation. *Journal of Counseling and Clinical Psychology, 42*, 751–756.

Spinetta, J. J., Swarner, J. A., & Sheposh, J. P. (1981). Effective parental coping following the death of a child from cancer. *Journal of Pediatric Psychology, 6*, 251–263.

Stein, A., Forrest, G., Woolley, H., & Baum, J. (1989). Life threatening illness and hospice care. *Archives of Disease in Childhood, 64*, 697–702.

Waechter, E. H. (1971). Children's awareness of fatal illness. *American Journal of Nursing, 71*, 1168–1172.

Waechter, E. H. (1987a). Children's reactions to fatal illness. In T. Krulik, B. Holaday, & I. M. Martinson (Eds.), *The child and family facing life-threatening illness* (pp. 108–119). Philadelphia: Lippincott.

Waechter, E. H. (1987b). Dying children: Patterns of coping. In T. Krulik, B. Holaday, & I. M. Martinson (Eds.), *The child and family facing life-threatening illness* (pp. 293–312). Philadelphia: Lippincott.

Waechter, E. H. (1987c). Working with parents of children with life-threatening illness. In T. Krulik, B. Holaday, & I. M. Martinson (Eds.), *The child and family facing life-threatening illness* (pp. 246–257). Philadelphia: Lippincott.

Wilson, D. C. (1982). The viability of pediatric hospices: A case study. *Death Education, 6*, 205–212.

Wooley, H., Stein, A., Forrest, G., & Baum, J. (1989). Staff stress and job satisfaction at a children's hospice. *Archives of Disease in Childhood, 64*, 114–118.

PART III

Research on Nursing Education

Chapter 9

Faculty Practice: Interest, Issues, and Impact

PATRICIA HINTON WALKER
SCHOOL OF NURSING
UNIVERSITY OF ROCHESTER

CONTENTS

Interest and issues related to faculty practice are moving to center stage in the educational literature, continuing education programs for nursing educators and administrators, and in determining new ways to generate revenue to support faculty salaries in higher education. Recent interest in more formally integrating faculty practice roles and responsibilities into traditional educational roles is occurring in all types of educational settings. This interest in faculty practice is not new. However, there is increased emphasis on the challenges created in defining faculty practice, designing faculty practice plans, and measuring the outcomes and impact of this important trend in nursing education and practice.

HISTORICAL OVERVIEW

The idea of faculty practice has early roots in nursing, because historically the practitioner served in the role of educator. During the diploma era, nursing education and nursing service were more closely intertwined, and the director of nursing service was commonly also the director of the School of Nursing. Later, although many of the theory classes were taught by "more educated nurses," most clinical expertise was still gained from nurses who worked in the hospitals and provided direct care to patients.

During World War II in the 1940s, nursing education clearly moved away from patient care settings and into educational institutions (Just, Adams, & DeYoung, 1989). Consequently, nurse educators became more involved with obtaining advanced education, and clinical practice took a back seat. Graduate education focused on curriculum development and acquisition of skills necessary for success in academia. This resulted in a shift away from advanced education for clinical practice and use of practicing faculty as educators—and the gap between "those who teach" and "those who practice" widened. Overall, the importance of faculty competence in the practice arena was not really seen as a problem and was not addressed until much later.

From the late 1970s to the early 1990s, nurse educators began moving closer to valuing practice to bridge the education/service gap. These efforts were supported and enhanced by a grant awarded to the American Nurses Foundation from The Robert Wood Johnson Foundation to conduct four symposia on faculty practice. Barger, Nugent, and Bridges (1992) credited these symposia with the important work of exploring the philosophical, theoretical, and practical issues related to faculty practice. Potash and Taylor (1993) wrote that the advent of nurse practitioner and clinical nurse specialist roles in the 1960s and 1970s provided stimulation to faculty practice. Advanced practice certification may also have played an important role in the need for clinically competent (practicing) faculty to teach advanced practice students. According to Millonig (1986), faculty recognize the need to "keep up" clinically to teach students. However, the nursing profession continues to struggle with the idea of faculty practice, how it should be structured, and what are the benefits.

Definitions of faculty practice vary in the literature. For some, faculty practice included activities related to patient care that are scholarly in nature (Millonig, 1986). Another definition included direct or indirect provision of care or service to the consumer, which must be scholarly and result in publication (Joel, 1983). Anderson and Pierson (1983) defined faculty practice as previously stated and beyond the expected teaching role accomplished through moonlighting or summer employment. Barger et al. (1992) in their operational definition included provision of direct service to clients with the goal of advancement of nursing practice and knowledge; practice occurring when faculty members were not teaching in the clinical setting; and practice contributing to individual growth of the faculty member rather than just maintaining clinical skills. More recently, Potash and Taylor (1993) provided a definition of faculty practice that includes all aspects of the delivery of nursing service through the roles of clinician, educator, researcher, consultant, and administrator.

Several different models have been used historically and continue to influence faculty practice today. Examples cited in the literature are unification, collaboration, the integrated model, and entrepreneurial model (Potash & Taylor, 1993). Other references to faculty practice models included joint appointments or dual appointments in education and practice, private practice, assuming patient care responsibilities while teaching students in the clinical settings, moonlighting, and development of practice organizations, such as nursing centers within a nursing education program. The unification model was usually described at the University of Rochester and Rush Presbyterian. In this model, administration of clinical agencies and the school of nursing are "unified," and faculty serve as both clinicians and educators. The collaborative model is usually described by joint or dual appointments. The most frequently cited early example of this model is Case Western Reserve University. The integrated model, in which faculty and graduate students share patient care responsibilities is evident at Pennsylvania State University and the University of Wisconsin Milwaukee (Stainton, 1989). In the entrepreneurial model, faculty design their own practices, which may also serve as a teaching or research site. Examples of this type of model are described at the University of Tennessee at Memphis (Potash & Taylor, 1993) and in the new community nursing center at the University of Rochester (Walker, 1991). Selected research findings related to nursing centers are highlighted in the section on support and barriers to faculty practice.

LITERATURE REVIEW

This review of faculty practice research reflects literature published from 1966 through 1993. The method of the search included *Cumulative Index of Nursing and Allied Health Literature* (CINAHL) and MEDLINE computer searches using faculty practice; faculty nursing; contracts;

practice. Also, a review of reference lists of the publications on faculty practice was conducted to identify additional sources. Because most academic nursing centers facilitate faculty practice, a review was also conducted related to nursing centers in academic settings to determine if there was research related to faculty practice in this body of literature. Of the 85 references reviewed, 17 were research articles.

Publications related to faculty practice clustered around several themes. Many articles simply described models and methods of instituting faculty practice in a variety of educational institutions. Faculty practice roles and responsibilities in a variety of settings with specific patient/client populations were highlighted. Joint practice arrangements, private practice, group practice, and development of nurse-managed centers within schools of nursing to facilitate faculty practice constituted another aspect of the literature. Benefits, outcomes, and issues of concern related to faculty practice began to dominate more recent publications. Development of faculty practice plans, administration of faculty practice, and issues related to revenue generation were the focus of the most recent publications.

SUMMARY OF RESEARCH METHODS

There is a dearth of research related to faculty practice. Just et al. (1989) reported that although much has been written about faculty practice, little research regarding frequency, outcomes, and implementation has been generated. It appears that in the developmental process, much of the research related to faculty practice was in the exploratory or descriptive stages. Most of these early studies would be classified as simple survey research, whereas more complex designs such as correlational studies, use of the Delphi technique, and semantic differential scale were used later. Use of survey instruments was the most common data collection technique. Sample sizes ranged from interviews of small numbers of faculty or student participants to significant numbers of faculty and administrators in schools of nursing in a region, or nationally, in the United States or Canada.

A general weakness in the design of much of the early research related to faculty practice is the lack of documentation or evidence of testing of the research instruments for validity and reliability. Also, many researchers tried to survey the population (in many cases, all faculty or administrators in schools of nursing); however, when this was not possible, they selected a convenience sample that may or may not have reflected accurate findings and conclusions. In later research on factors contributing to practice, support for practice, and benefits and outcomes of practice, researchers more frequently used instruments tested for validity and reliability.

Sound conceptual frameworks were not evident in early studies; however, conceptual or theoretical approaches were used as a basis for research related to faculty practice in later studies. These included role theory, including role perception, role strain, and role conflict and ambiguity; status-risk theory of receptivity; social support; and professional craftsmanship. The statistical analysis most frequently used was simple descriptive statistics, especially in those studies that were exploratory in design. Other researchers used correlational statistical analyses, factor analysis, *t*-tests, multiple regression, and analysis of variance.

FACULTY PRACTICE RESEARCH

For the purpose of this research review, themes most commonly occurring in the research publications about faculty practice are grouped into the following subtopics: (a) occurrence and characteristics of faculty practice; (b) attitudes, views, and perceptions of practicing faculty; (c) support and barriers to practice in schools of nursing; and (d) benefits and outcomes for faculty and students. Within these groupings, research reports were assessed for the following: purpose of study, conceptual framework, study design, data collection procedures, instrumentation, and reported findings.

Faculty Practice Characteristics and Descriptions

This section of the research literature answers such questions as: What is faculty practice?; What are the definitions of faculty practice?; What are the characteristics of faculty who practice?; and How many faculty are involved in faculty practice? Most of this research was exploratory, and administrators and faculty of schools of nursing were surveyed with questions related to faculty practice.

Rosswurm (1981) conducted one of the earliest studies. This author chose practitioner programs to survey on the assumption that faculty in these programs would be involved in some type of clinical practice. The purpose of the survey was to determine characteristics of group nursing practices, the nurses in practice, and the clients. Respondents were also asked to identify major benefits and problems experienced. Of the 114 questionnaires sent to practitioner programs listed in *A Directory of Expanded Role Programs for Registered Nurses* (1979), the response rate was 70%.

Questionnaires were sent to deans with a request to forward to faculty members involved in practice or to indicate that no group faculty practice existed. Results of the survey indicated that 23 contained descriptions of group faculty practices. The remaining 57 responses verified by the deans that no faculty were engaged in group practices, but were involved in independent, joint, or multidisciplinary group practices. Most of the practices were within nonprofit health agencies, health maintenance organizations (HMOs), or ambulatory care units of hospitals with clients paying fees for service to the agency. Characteristics of the client served were evenly distributed across the age span primarily from middle and lower socioeconomic classes. Services offered included health assessments, counseling, and health education. The most important benefits were independence, enjoyment, and excitement of practicing nursing in a group practice. Major problems, consistent with the results of other studies centered around lack of time for both education and practice, workload, and lack of third-party reimbursement.

In a second descriptive survey, Anderson and Pierson (1983) surveyed 986 baccalaureate nursing faculty to determine how many faculty were involved in faculty practice. This study was designed to explore facilitating and inhibiting factors for faculty practice, where practice was implemented, and whether or not the school had policies related to faculty practice. Results indicated that more than 50% of the faculty were practicing approximately 8 hours per week, and 48% of these were moonlighting. Practice in inpatient settings for personal reasons was identified by most practicing faculty. Reimbursement and policy related to reward systems in most schools of nursing were nonexistent. Faculty workload was considered to be the major barrier to faculty practice while administrative support facilitated practice.

In another nationwide study, Just et al. (1989) surveyed a random sample of 909 associate degree and baccalaureate degree educators. The purposes of the study were to (a) determine how faculty conceptualize faculty practice, (b) determine the extent of implementation of faculty practice, and (c) identify differences/similarities between associate degree and baccalaureate educators on the preceding variables. Researchers randomly selected 136 baccalaureate- and 136 associate-degree schools of nursing to obtain a representative sample. From these, 71 baccalaureate- and 67 associate-degree programs agreed to participate. Sixty-nine percent of the faculty in the programs participated, with 529 baccalaureate- and 372 associate-degree respondents.

Based on their own definitions, 60% of faculty surveyed said they were involved in practice, and 63% reported part-time work. Eighty to ninety percent of the faculty identified consultation, clinical research, volunteering professional services, and committee work in a health care agency as faculty practice. Approximately 70% listed part-time staffing in agencies or private duty and conducting staff development programs as faculty practice. Most of the faculty (79%) believed that teachers should not be required to care for patients while teaching but 69% listed teaching students in the clinical area as practice. Other results of this research indicated that 94% of faculty practice to maintain clinical skills. Personal satisfaction and earning extra money were additional reasons for practicing.

Potash and Taylor (1993) surveyed National Organization of Nurse Practitioner Faculties members with 36 respondents representing 26 college and university schools of nursing. Of these, 66% reported faculty practice in their schools. Ninety-seven percent described practice as providing direct care, whereas 38% and 33%, respectively, listed consultation and education as description of practice. Faculty (ranging from 38% to 47%) identified consulting, volunteering services, clinical research, and working part-time as staff as faculty practice. Only 2% to 3% reported that faculty practice was highly recommended or encouraged by administration, whereas lack of time, lack of support from administrators, and too few academic rewards were listed as reasons for lack of faculty practice. Also, 41% listed additional income or benefits when asked how faculty practice was compensated.

Attitudes, Views, and Perceptions of Practicing Faculty

Most studies in this area relate to some aspect of role development, analysis of role strain, role conflict, or role ambiguity. Role theory and related concepts including status-risk theory of receptivity were used as a theoretical base.

The first empirical work in this area was conducted by Yarcheski and Mahon (1985). This study analyzed faculty receptivity to proposed introduction of the unification model to nurse educators. This research focused on three status groups: deans, tenured faculty, and nontenured faculty. Data were collected from a random sample of accredited baccalaureate schools in the United States excluding seven schools identified in the literature as having unification or collaborative practice models. From each of 88 schools responding, 1 faculty name from tenured and nontenure lists was randomly selected per 10 faculty—resulting in 210 faculty and 88 administrators surveyed. A description of a unification model was composed based on the literature and was sent to participants in the study.

Yarcheski and Mahon (1985) used a semantic differential scale to measure receptivity and perceived risk according to the following hypotheses: (a) that differences in receptivity would exist between the three status groups; (b) differences in level of risk would also exist between three status groups; (c) that the greater the perceived risk, the lower the degree of receptivity; and (d) that nontenured faculty would demonstrate highest level of perceived risk, deans would exhibit lowest level of risk, and tenured faculty would demonstrate less risk than nontenured faculty.

Factor analysis was used to analyze responses from 222 educators. Results did not support any of the previously listed hypotheses. There was no significant difference in degree of perceived risk or receptivity among status groups. However, means indicated moderately positive receptivity to unification and that all three groups perceived moderately high benefits accruing to status with unification; a high correlation was found between receptivity to unification and level of direct risk/benefit perceived by all groups.

A second study was published by Steele (1991), which explored attitudes about faculty practice, role, and role strain. The population surveyed was a random sample of faculty from 53 schools who agreed to participate based on letters sent to 100 deans or administrators of National League for Nursing (NLN)-approved programs from four geographical areas. A questionnaire, the Deans Demographic Questionnaire, was designed by the researcher to determine deans' perceptions of the importance of various faculty roles and was subsequently sent to 550 individual faculty members with a response rate of 55%. Of these, 292 were usable and included in data analysis.

Demographics of respondents indicated that 55% of the faculty were tenured, with the remaining 37.2% on the tenure track. Of the 302 responding, 40% or 122 indicated that they were involved in practice. Comparisons of the differences in perceptions of the two groups (practicing and nonpracticing faculty) were measured. Perception of practice was measured by the Faculty Perception of Practice Questionnaire.

Steele's (1991) results indicated that deans and nonpracticing faculty rank ordered perception of importance of role functions in the following way: (a) teaching, (b) research, (c) practice, and (d) service. Practicing faculty ranked practice second. When ranking reward structures related to each role function in terms of personal satisfaction, financial reward, and academic advancement, the two groups differed significantly on rewards related to practice. Nonpracticing faculty ranked personal satisfaction from teaching, service, research, and practice in that order, and rank-ordered research, teaching, service, and practice as relevant for academic advancement. However, practicing faculty ranked personal satisfaction in order of teaching, practice, service, and research. Practicing faculty (52%) felt more clinically competent than nonpracticing faculty (24.7%).

Practicing faculty also reported being perceived as student role models, and they experienced enhanced credibility with students significantly more than nonpracticing faculty. Faculty who practiced perceived that emphasis on practice should increase and enhance scholarly productivity and improve patient care. These beliefs were not as strongly held by nonpracticing faculty.

When measuring perceptions about role strain, there was no significant difference between the groups of practicing and nonpracticing faculty; however, nonpracticing faculty indicated a higher level of strain. The greatest amount of role strain was perceived by assistant professors (61%), whereas associate professors and instructors perceived less strain (56% and 50% respectively). Role strain definitely increased with number of years teaching experience (from 40% for 1 year to 92.5% for up to 7 years). Although this study had limitations, the researcher demonstrated the need for clarification of reward systems, incentives, and organizational commitment to faculty practice.

More recent research addressing role strain was conducted and reported by Lambert and Lambert (1993). The purpose of this study was to measure role stress and psychological hardiness in educators involved in practice. A demographic questionnaires and instruments measuring role stress and hardiness were returned by 871 faculty from 34 randomly selected NLN-accredited schools of nursing. The instruments used in the study were the Role Conflict and Role Ambiguity Scale developed by Rizzo, House, and Lirtzman (1970) and the Personal Views Survey (Kobasa, 1985). Results of the study indicated significant negative correlations between role stress, and the components of psychological hardiness for educators involved in practice and educators not involved in practice. The authors concluded that psychological hardiness is not a determinant of participation in faculty practice and that role stress was related to lack of a sense of control for nurse educators, regardless of their involvement in faculty practice.

A fourth study was conducted by Acorn (1991) with a sample of 113 nursing faculty from five Canadian universities. Hypotheses of the study were designed to determine whether joint appointment faculty would experience (a) higher role conflict and ambiguity than traditional faculty appointment faculty; (b) higher scholarly productivity; (c) greater role conflict than role ambiguity; and (d) higher job satisfaction. In addition, the research hypothesized that there would be an inverse relationship between role conflict and ambiguity and perceived social support and job satisfaction; and that there would be a positive relationship between role conflict and ambiguity and the propensity to leave a joint appointment position.

The sample was drawn from 5 of 10 schools in Canada reporting use of joint appointment faculties. Of these 162 faculty responded to the study with 69.8% (113 questionnaires) usable. Instruments used to measure role conflict and ambiguity was a 14-item index developed by Rizzo et al. (1970). Social support was assessed with a questionnaire developed by Dickens (1983). Job satisfaction and propensity to leave were measured each with single items with a Likert response scale. Scholarly productivity for the previous 3 years was measured by numbers of articles and chapters in books published (research and nonresearch), conference papers and posters presented, and funding of external research grants. Data were analyzed using descriptive statistics, *t*-tests, and correlations.

Twenty-nine percent of the faculty surveyed were in joint appointments, and 80% held traditional appointments. Most (62.5%) held a master's degree, and 59% were tenured. The researcher reported no significant differences in role conflict, role ambiguity, scholarly productivity, and job satisfaction between joint appointment faculty and traditional faculty as predicted. However, two of the hypotheses were supported in Acorn's (1991) study. Results indicated that role conflict was significantly higher than role ambiguity for joint appointees, which may suggest incongruity or incompatibility of role expectations for this group. Role conflict and ambiguity significantly correlated with a decrease in job satisfaction, with a significant inverse relationship between role conflict and social support. There also was a significant relationship between role conflict and ambiguity with a desire to leave a joint appointment. The results of this study reinforce the need for clarification of role expectations and the need for both administrative and peer support for practicing faculty.

Support and Barriers to Faculty Practice

This section of the research describes studies related to support and barriers to faculty practice. According to Diers (1980), mechanisms of institutional support are important to the merging of teaching, scholarship, and practice, in addition to the perseverance and coherent efforts of the individual faculty member. For institutions to support faculty practice, Chicadonz, Bush, Korthus, and Utz (1981) identified four areas in which change must occur in higher education settings: (a) communication and clarification of role expectations and responsibilities; (b) support for role transitions and changes; (c) provision of some type of structure supporting practice; and (d) development of incentive or rewards in performance systems. This section includes research directed toward organizational or administrative responses to faculty practice in schools of nursing.

The earliest exploratory research identified in the literature was designed to identify institutional support for faculty practice. This study was conducted and published by Dickens (1983) in which she surveyed 113 baccalaureate- and higher-degree programs of the Southern Council on Collegiate Education for Nursing. The purposes of the study were to (a) review models for faculty practice, (b) determine evidence of social support for faculty who practice, and (c) report findings of survey conducted to discover mechanisms of social support put into place by administrators to support faculty practice.

Using four broad categories of social support identified by House (1981) information, emotional, instrumental, and appraisal support, Dickens (1983) operationalized these categories for purposes of her research on faculty practice. A clear statement of definition, expectations, and determinations related to time for faculty practice for faculty interested in practice was considered evidence of informational support. Evidence of emotional support was operationalized as a willingness of administration to support practice activities and networking among faculty who were practicing. Instrumental support included compensation for practicing faculty, including such specifics as granting release time or varied types of faculty leaves, altering schedules for practice, and providing financial remuneration of some type for practice. Lastly, mechanisms for comparative evaluation of practicing faculty with other faculty and providing institutional recognition were considered evidence of appraisal support for the purposes of this research study.

Dickens (1983) reported a 65.8% response rate from the 113 administrators targeted in the survey. These administrators reported that 32% of their full-time faculty (671 of 2116) and 42% of part-time faculty (118 of 285) were involved in some form of clinical practice. There were 145 answers related to instrumental support that included 2%, release time; 23%, altered schedules; 9%, sabbaticals; 17%, leaves of absence without pay; and 5%, other financial remuneration. Regarding a policy on compensation, 14% identified a policy in their school with some type of formal structure for collaborative practice with a service institution.

Thirty-two percent of 72 respondents reported existence of written definitions and expectations as informational support, and 68% said none existed. Additionally, 93% reported no specified time for expectations of clinical practice, and 94% identified no definition of what constituted clinical practice. These data also indicated that 100% of the administrators believed in faculty practice and encouraged it (emotional support); 68% did not require practice. Thirty-one percent of those responding reported networking activities, and 78.5% reported mutual trust or caring among other faculty members (emotional support).

Lastly, Dickens (1983) reported that 85% of respondents indicated no mechanism for evaluation of clinical practice, whereas 15% reported evidence of appraisal support. Mechanisms for recognition were reported as follows: 23%, in promotion policies; 47%, as part of the annual evaluation process; and 22%, in the tenure policy. The researcher concluded there was little evidence of instrumental, informational, or appraisal support. Emotional support requires further study.

Bellinger and Sanders (1985) conducted another study to examine institutional faculty practice policies. Their survey of 287 NLN baccalaureate-accredited programs resulted in responses from 118 of the schools. Of these, only 30% ($n = 35$) reported that some type of policy was in place, whereas clearly 70% ($n = 82$) had no policy and no plan to develop one. Of the schools reporting existing policies, there were a variety of responses including faculty obtaining approval from administration for clinical practice; regulating work outside the institution, which included clinical practice; limiting practice to a number of hours or percentage of salary; policies prohibiting faculty from engaging in practice during the contract period. Consequently, most of these policies would not be categorized as supportive. For the 82 administrators reporting no formal policy related to faculty practice, there was little evidence of support for faculty practice. Eighteen reported occurrence of faculty practice but did not provide explanations. The researchers concluded that most educators either do not practice or practice without a policy or institutional support.

Faculty Practice in Community Nursing Centers

An emerging body of literature and research influencing faculty practice is related to development of nursing centers. Three research reports that have implications related to faculty practice and directions for the future. Higgs (1988) conducted a descriptive study related to nursing centers, which have implications for faculty practice, with semistructured telephone interviews. She surveyed 65 schools that currently or previously had nursing centers and 12 schools planning a nursing center. Faculty interviewed indicated concerns about the time and energy commitments that nurse-managed centers take and questioned the negative impact on efforts needed for promotion, tenure, and personal/family well-being. Faculty indicated that nursing-managed centers provided opportunities for clinical research but were only incorporated into a few centers. Support was needed for computerization of client data and program data to develop research.

A more in-depth study of institutional facilitators and inhibitors for faculty practice in nursing centers was conducted and published by Barger and Bridges (1987). In this study, the researchers explored the relationship between specific organizational barriers and personal factors of individual faculty members to faculty practice. From 427 NLN schools responding to an initial survey regarding nursing centers, 41 were selected to participate in the second phase of the study. A faculty questionnaire was constructed and pretested by practicing and nonpracticing faculty, then a total of 1507 questionnaires were sent out with a response rate of 68.7% from 1036 faculty. Of these participants, 462 or 44.6% had engaged in practice during the past year. Of these, 27.8% were tenured, whereas 39.6% of those who did not practice were tenured. The percentage of faculty members engaged in research was almost equal between practicing and nonpracticing faculty (51% and 56%, respectively). The largest areas of difference between practicing and nonpracticing faculty was in educational preparation; only 22.4% of the practicing faculty had doctorates, whereas 38.9% of nonpracticing faculty reported doctoral preparation.

There was no significant difference in the number of faculty practice hours generated in a year among schools with nursing centers and those schools without nursing centers as sites for practice. Also, there was no significant difference in the extent of faculty practice between those schools reporting administrative policies and those reporting none. Further, schools that required practice had a mean of only 97.17 practice hours, whereas those schools not requiring practice reported a mean of 132.33 hours. However, for schools that considered practice a promotion criterion, faculty reported an average of 150.39 hours compared with 79.11 hours when practice did not count for promotion. There was however, no significant difference in this relationship between practice and promotion credit.

Other institutional variables studied by Barger and Bridges (1987) included the size of the faculty; private or public status of the school of nursing; presence of health science center within university or college; and the type of academic programs offered. Findings indicated two significant differences: There were significantly more practice hours in public versus private schools, and faculty members in schools with doctoral programs practiced more hours than in schools without doctoral programs (168.5 hours to only 61 hours, respectively). Neither the size of faculty, presence of a master's program, nor presence of health science center related significantly to the extent of faculty practice.

When reporting the personal factors of the faculty, such as age, marital status, earned doctorate, and area of clinical expertise, Barger and Bridges (1987) reported that all factors but one (clinical practice area) were significant. Age had an inverse effect on practice with practicing faculty having a younger mean age (40.7 years) than nonpracticing faculty (43.9 years). The doctorate significantly affected the extent of practice adversely. There were 164.7 practice hours reported for those without doctorate, whereas doctorally prepared faculty practiced only 64.8 hours. Results of this study indicated that there was a significant difference in marital status with divorced faculty having practiced significantly more than other groups: married, widowed, or single.

Lastly, reporting on differences in productivity related to research and publication, there was not significant difference between practicing and nonpracticing faculty. Berger and Bridges (1987) suggest that faculty perceive that administrative support is the greatest facilitator of faculty practice and express concern regarding role overload and role strain. They also question whether it is realistic to expect role integration of clinical research with faculty practice, because faculty are not generating research from their practice. Based on their findings, these researchers identify relevant challenges for the future. Because schools that have doctoral programs seem to stimulate more faculty practice, how will the profession prevent faculty practice from declining if doctorally prepared faculty are less likely to practice? A second challenge relates to the need for integration of practice and research roles of faculty. Here, the authors suggest development of clinical practice sites where faculty can collect research data while practicing for the profession to realize the benefit of practice-based research from faculty practice.

In 1992, Barger et al. conducted a follow-up study on faculty practice, focusing on organizational factors facilitating or inhibiting faculty practice. Of the 462 survey questionnaires sent to NLN-accredited schools, data from 354 respondents were reported in the findings. Of these, only 63.3% reported faculty who were practicing, but only 8.8%, or 20 schools, required faculty practice. In response to questions regarding formal or informal faculty practice plans, only 23 schools reported a written plan, with 53 schools reporting an informal plan and 149 schools (66.2%) listing no plan. Several formalized practice arrangements were reported, including those within hospitals, clinics, and health departments, and nursing centers. Sixteen percent reported faculty-generated income; however in 53.8% of the schools, the income was kept by the schools, whereas 12 schools reported that a percentage of revenue was kept by faculty.

Several organizational factors influencing faculty practice were reported by Barger et al. (1992). These included the presence of master's and doctoral programs, those with the master's program were more significant; size of school, with larger schools reporting more practice faculty; having a practice plan and generating revenue; and requiring practice for promotion and tenure. In this area, only 15% required practice for promotion and tenure. Results of the study indicated strong relationships between requiring practice, and rewarding practice through promotion and tenure. On the contrary, existence of a formalized practice plan, generating revenue, and having a nursing center were not significant.

Another study reported by Barger, Nugent, and Bridges (1993) focused on faculty practice policies within the context of schools of nursing and nursing centers. Barger found that policies related to faculty practice had not changed significantly in 5 years. Also, faculty practice was still not a criterion for promotion or tenure in most schools. The relationship between schools with nursing centers and use of faculty practice as a criterion for promotion was significant, but as criterion for tenure was not. Additionally, most schools reported no formalized faculty practice plan, and there was no significant difference between schools with nursing centers and other schools reporting practice plans. In the area of revenue generation, Barger et al. (1993) reported an inverse relationship between amount of revenue generated for practice and schools with nursing centers. This area of concern that schools with nursing centers seemed to generate less revenue than schools that have other faculty practice arrangements was also confirmed by Higgs (1988) in a previous study. Barger et al. (1993) concluded that nursing centers facilitate faculty practice, which provides obvious benefits in student education and potential benefits of clinical research. However, there is a critical need for institutional commitments to develop policies that support integration of practice, education, and research roles of faculty; reward structures for promotion and tenure; and formalized practice plans.

Nugent, Barger, and Bridges (1993) reported results of a study related to facilitators and inhibitors of faculty practice using a Delphi procedure. For this study, faculty from NLN-accredited baccalaureate programs that had participated in earlier faculty practice studies were contacted. Of the 470 faculty participating in round 1 of the survey, 299 participants representing 170 schools completed all three rounds. Of these, most (58%) respondents were nontenured, with 39% holding a doctoral degree. The top five reasons reported for faculty practice were remaining current in knowledge and skills, personal satisfaction, credibility, improvement in clinical teaching, and contact with patients. Results related to personal attributes facilitating practice included competence, commitment to practice and the profession, caring, and organizational skills. As expected, opposite personal attributes were identified as inhibiting practice. Multiple roles and role conflict was ranked first, with lack of personal value of practice, lack of time, confidence, and commitment also ranked, respectively.

Organizational factors facilitating practice were in order ranked as follows: flexible workload in the school, flexible scheduling by the agency, practice being valued, support from administration, and having practice addressed in tenure and promotion criteria. Again, as anticipated, opposing perspectives dominated organizational inhibitors. At the top of the list was faculty workload, followed by lack of release time, recognition, administrative support, and tenure requirements focusing on other dimensions of the faculty role. The findings of this research are consistent with other reports of facilitators and inhibitors to faculty practice in the literature.

Benefits and Outcomes for Faculty and Students

What are the expected benefits and outcomes of faculty practice? Several authors have described these in the literature; however, limited research has been done in this area. In numerous articles included in the review of the literature, many of the benefits of faculty practice were identified. Ryan and Barger-Lux (1985) reported increase in faculty research and publications/presentations of 32% and 36%, respectively, among their faculty. Frazer (1980) described benefits of private practice with peer, interdisciplinary, and student recognition as clinical role models. In addition, she emphasized the value of personal satisfaction and contributions in both education and service settings. Jezek (1980) suggested potential economic benefit of increasing faculty size without increasing cost, with more clinical specialties and decreased costs related to clinically expert teachers in the classroom. This theme is beginning to dominate much of the current literature with emphasis on opportunities for the direct and indirect economic benefits of faculty practice both to the individual faculty members and to institutions through revenue generation and potential research dollars. Additionally, some of the data from previously reported research in this chapter have implications relevant to benefits of faculty practice.

Only two studies could be identified that specifically were focused on benefits and outcomes of faculty practice. The first study was conducted as an evaluative component of the Robert Wood Johnson Teaching Nursing Home Project (TNHP). One of the purposes of this project was to involve nurse faculty/clinicians expert in clinical care and research in nursing home care. Mezey, Lynaugh, and Cartier (1988) published results of a three-stage Delphi study of 116 faculty and 11 deans to achieve group consensus about the teaching nursing home project's impact on participating schools of nursing and faculties. Of those surveyed, 107 subjects (87%) completed one round, and 70 or (55%) responded to two or more rounds of the Delphi study. There were 40 items related to profession and career, specifically to faculty practice. Of these, the top six (15%) emphasized the importance of clinical practice to faculty members participating. Overall, the two greatest outcomes or benefits were (a) the undergraduate and graduate student education was strengthened, and (b) the creation of clinical positions for faculty was effective in encouraging students to seek clinical rotations in nursing homes. Another significant impact of the TNHP was the opportunity for clinical research. From 1984 to 1986, TNHP faculty increased research funding from $382,000 to approximately $2 million. Deans of participating schools also believed that the TNHP increased schools' prestige and opportunity to impact health policy through research. Overall conclusions of the researchers were that the TNHP provided insights into the importance of faculty practice and that faculty practice was both rewarding and workable.

Kramer, Polifroni, and Organek (1986) conducted the most significant research related to benefits and outcomes of faculty practice. The purpose of this study was to explore the relationship between faculty practice and student acquisition of values, beliefs, and attributes associated with professional craftsmanship. Faculty practice was viewed in two ways in this study: first, as a treatment variable for faculty who were engaged in practice while clinically teaching students; and, second, as a continuous variable referring to the amount of exposure students had to faculty engaged in practice. A number of instruments were administered to 137 senior baccalaureate nursing students to measure the dependent variable "professional craftsmanship." Of these students, 59 students were taught by faculty involved in practice and 74 students did not have practicing faculty.

Several subvariables were identified as indicators of professional craftsmanship. Instruments used to measure these included: Levinson's (1973) Perception of Events to measure locus of control; a researcher-developed and tested 60-item "nurse self-concept instrument" measured concept of self in the role of nurse and self-esteem; another researcher designed instrument, "the role behavior scale," measured ability to professional and bicultural behavior; autonomy was measured with the Pankratz and Pankratz (1974) 69-item attitude scale; and a seven-item, self-report rating scale was devised from characteristics of professionalism found in the literature. It was hypothesized that students taught by faculty engaged in practice will score higher on previously mentioned indicators of professional craftsmanship than students taught by faculty not engaged in practice. Results confirmed the hypothesis that the treatment group scored significantly higher than the nontreatment group on the self-rating scale of professional characteristics, self-concept and self-esteem, locus of control, and professional and bicultural behavior scale, and the autonomy tool. Researchers concluded that there is a definite effect of faculty practice on the development of professional characteristics in students. Three specific areas highlighted were integration of theory into practice, realistic perception of the work environment, and use of nursing research. Additionally, comments of students supported the theory of modeling as a process by which students learn professional craftsmanship.

SUMMARY AND DIRECTIONS FOR THE FUTURE

In summary, major issues influencing current research related to faculty practice are in many cases further study of the areas already identified in this review of nursing research. However, emphasis in the future will clearly shift from descriptive research related to type and models of practice to more studies on the benefits and outcomes of these practices. Further studies of the barriers to integration of practice and research roles and problems with the reward systems are critical for continuation of faculty practice in many institutions. More cost studies that analyze the economic impact and contributions of faculty practice in educational institutions must also be done. Also, opportunities for studies demonstrating comparisons of quality and cost-effective care among practicing nursing and medical faculty must also be high on the agenda in the context of health care reform. The potential of the new health care agenda to increase nursing's involvement in managed care, primary care, and community-based care will require the profession to measure the outcomes of these practices. Consumer involvement and outcomes of preventive and health promotion services provided by nursing faculty in various practice arrangements must be evaluated. As more schools of nursing become involved in nurse-managed practices, through nursing centers and other faculty practice arrangements, health services and clinical research must accompany these efforts. The development of computerized databases to track and analyze client data, cost of care, and effectiveness of outcomes will be the next challenge for the nursing profession, and, specifically, nurse educators. It is this author's belief that the integration of faculty practice and research roles and the degree of institutional commitment to support through policies and dollars for data systems will determine the future of faculty practice.

REFERENCES

Acorn, S. (1991). Relationship of role conflict and role ambiguity to selected job dimensions among joint appointees. *Journal of Professional Nursing, 7*, 221-227.

Anderson, E., & Pierson, P. (1983). An exploratory study of faculty practice: Views of those faculty engaged in practice who teach in an NLN-accredited baccalaureate program. *Western Journal Nursing Research, 5*, 129-140.

Barger, S. E., & Bridges, W.C. (1987). Nursing faculty practice: Institutional and individual facilitators and inhibitors. *Journal of Professional Nursing, 3*, 338-346.

Barger, S. E., Nugent, K. E., & Bridges, W. C. (1992). Nursing faculty practice: An organizational perspective. *Journal of Professional Nursing, 8*, 263-270.

Barger, S. E., Nugent, K. E., & Bridges, W. C. (1993). Schools with nursing centers: A 5-year follow-up study. *Journal of Professional Nursing, 9*, 7-13.

Bellinger, K., & Sanders, D. H. (1985). Faculty practice policy. *Journal of Nursing Education, 24*, 214-216.

Bennett, S. J. (1990). Blending the entrepreneurial and faculty roles. *Nurse Educator, 15*(4), 34-37.

Chicadonz, G. H., Bush, E. E., Korthus, K., & Utz, S. W. (1981). Mobilizing faculty toward integration of practice into faculty roles. *Nursing & Health Care, 2*, 548-553.

Dickens, M. R. (1983). Faculty practice and social support. *Nursing Leadership, 6*, 121-128.

Diers, D. (1980). Faculty practice: Models, methods and madness. In*Cognitive dissonance: Interpreting and implementing faculty practice roles in nursing education* (Report No. 15, pp. 7-15). New York: National League for Nursing.

Frazer, J. (1980). Future perspectives for faculty practice: Credibility, visibility, accountability. In *Cognitive dissonance: Interpreting and implementing faculty practice roles in nursing education* (Report No. 15-1831, pp. 43-48). New York: National League for Nursing.

Government Printing Office (1979). *A directory of expanded role programs for registered nurses* (Department of Higher Education Publication No. HRA 79-10). Washington, DC: Author.

Higgs, Z. R. (1988). The academic nurse-managed center movement: A survey report. *Journal of Professional Nursing, 4*, 422-429.

House, J. S. (1981). *Work stress and social support*. Reading, MA: Addison-Wesley.

Jezek, J. (1980). Economic realities of faculty practice. In *Cognitive dissonance: Interpreting and implementing faculty practice roles in nursing education* (Report No. 15-1831, pp. 37–41). New York: National League for Nursing.

Joel, L. A. (1983). Stepchildren in the family: Aiming toward synergy between nursing education and service—from the faculty perspective. In D. E. Barnard & G. R. Smith (Eds.), *Structure to outcome: Making it work* (pp. 23–57). Kansas City, MO: American Academy of Nursing.

Just, G., Adams, E., & DeYoung, S. (1989). Faculty practice: Nurse educators' views and proposed models. *Journal of Nursing Education, 28*, 161–168.

Kobasa, S. (1985). *The Personal Views Survey*. Chicago: The Hardiness Institute.

Kramer, M., Polifroni, E. C., & Organek, N. (1986). Effects of faculty practice on student learning outcomes. *Journal of Professional Nursing, 2*, 289–301.

Lambert, C., & Lambert, V. A. (1993). Relationships among faculty practice involvement: Perception of role stress, and psychological hardiness of nurse educators. *Journal of Nursing Education, 32*, 171–179.

Levinson, M. (1973). Multidimensional locus of control in psychiatric patients. *Journal of Consulting and Clinical Psychology, 41*, 397–404.

Mezey, M. D., Lynaugh, J. E., & Cartier, M. M. (1988). The teaching nursing home program, 1982–87: A report card. *Nursing Outlook, 36*, 285–288.

Millonig, V. L. (1986). Faculty practice: A view of its development, current benefits, and barriers. *Journal of Professional Nursing, 2*, 166–172.

Nugent, K. E., Barger, S. E., & Bridges, W. E. (1993). Facilitators and inhibitors of practice: A faculty perspective. *Journal of Nursing Education, 32*, 293–300.

Pankratz, L., & Pankratz, D. (1974). Nursing autonomy and patient's rights: Development of a nursing attitude scale. *Journal of Health and Social Behavior, 15*, 211–216.

Potash, M., & Taylor, D. (1993). *Nursing faculty practice: Models and methods*. Washington, DC: National Organization of Nurse Practitioner Faculties.

Rosswurm, M. A. (1981). Characteristics of 23 faculty group nurse practices. *Nursing & Health Care, 2*, 327–330.

Rizzo, J., House, R., & Lirtzman, S. (1970). Role conflict and ambiguity in complex organizations. *Administrative Science Quarterly, 15*, 150–163.

Ryan, S., & Barger-Lux, M. (1985). Faculty expertise in practice: A school succeeding. *Nursing Outlook, 28*, 75–78.

Stainton, M. C. (1989). The development of a practicing nursing faculty. *Journal of Advanced Nursing, 14*, 20–26.

Steele, R. L. (1991). Attitudes about faculty practice, perceptions of role, and role strain. *Journal of Nursing Education, 30*, 15–22.

Walker, P. H. (1991, fall). The community nursing center: For nurse practitioners, an opportunity to develop entrepreneurial skills. *Rochester Nursing*, 18–19.

Yarcheski, A., & Mahon, N. E. (1985). The unification model in nursing: A study of receptivity among nurse educators in the United States. *Nursing Research, 34*, 120–125.

PART IV

Research on the Profession of Nursing

Chapter 10

Professionalization of Nurse Practitioners

Bonnie Bullough
Department of Nursing
University of Southern California

CONTENTS

The research describing nurse practitioners is reviewed here in its historical context. The primary goal was to critically review the research literature, but in this process the history of the nurse practitioner movement also has been analyzed. A broad search was done, including material from nursing and non-nursing sources, and a review of all of the standard nursing and medical computerized databases was carried out. The search yielded too many items to include in this brief review. Studies were selected on the basis of the quality of the research and the topic of the study; those articles without a primary database were excluded. Although nurse midwives have similar roles and legal coverage in many state nurse practice acts, they were excluded from this review for two reasons: The literature about nurse midwives and nurse practitioners is generally separate and the midwifery literature was reviewed in an earlier volume of this series. A theoretical framework drawn from the sociological study of the professions is proposed to put the literature into perspective.

CURRENT DEFINITION

Nurse practitioners are nurses in advanced practice with education beyond the basic level of the registered nurse, which enables them to take on an expanded scope of function in the diagnosis and treatment of patients. Originally, their role was limited to primary ambulatory care settings and definitions tended to exclude roles in other settings (American Academy of Nursing, 1976; American Nurses' Association [ANA], 1981), but a growing minority of nurse practitioners are now filling positions in acute care hospitals, long-term–care institutions, and home care so any definition of the role that included only primary care would be outdated (Rogers, Sweeting, Davis, 1989; Towers, 1989).

The comprehensive literature review done by Shamansky in 1984 indicated that there was a controversy over whether the nurse practitioner should be thought of as an extension of or a replacement for physicians (Shamansky, 1984). Although this issue still is being discussed, most definitions of the role, particularly those that appear in the state nurse practice acts indicate a significant and growing overlap with medicine. In fact, nurse practitioners are able to replace physicians in a variety of settings (Bullough, 1980; Pearson, 1993; Pearson, 1994). This overlap with medicine's role differentiates nurse practitioners from most clinical nurse specialists who have carved out a set of roles distinct from medicine and are focused on traditional nursing skills with an augmented role in patient support, administration, and the teaching of personnel (Fenton & Brykczynski, 1993). Thus, the growing advanced practice movement in nursing includes two separate models of care, the clinical nurse specialist, in contrast to practitioners whose roles overlap with medicine. These latter include nurse practitioners, nurse anesthetists, nurse midwives, and some psychiatric nurses (Bullough, 1992). However, even with this framework, nurse practitioners retain the basic characteristics of nurses in their interactional styles; they manage to carry out the technical procedures yet still retain a focus on the psychosocial issues (Campbell, Mauksch, Neikirk, & Hosokawa, 1990). Using data from a qualitative study of nurse practitioners, Brykczynski characterized their practice as "holistic personalized assessment, participatory care, health maintenance and promotion, along with illness treatment and detection, and teaching, counseling, and supportive interventions" (1989).

DESCRIPTION OF THE LITERATURE

The literature about nurse practitioners is voluminous, particularly the work published during the first 10 to 15 years after the development of the role. The goal of the studies and the quality of the research varied widely. A variety of research designs were used, including case studies about a single-practice, descriptive studies and behavioral science approaches-testing hypotheses with statistical analysis. In the last decade, there have been fewer studies comparing nurses with physicians, more descriptive studies, a few qualitative studies, and some historical studies. There have also been two recent excellent literature reviews, one done by the Office of Technology Assessment (1986) and the other by Mezey and McGivern and the authors who contributed to the 1993 edition of *Nurses: Nurse Practitioners* (1993). Although theory seldom guided the recent studies of nurse practitioners, the methodologies were usually congruent with the goals of the studies, so research of the last 10 to 15 years is for the most part both valid and reliable.

Early History of Nurse Practitioners

Recognition of a nurse practitioner role is dated from 1965 with the beginning of the Colorado Pediatric Nurse Practitioner and Associate Program. Although there were nurses whose roles overlapped with those of physicians throughout the 20th century, including early settlement nurses (Wald, 1915), public health nurses (Buhler-Wilkerson, 1993; Siegel & Bryson, 1963), and clinic nurses (Noonan, 1972), their expanded role was not publicized. This means, however, that the expansion of the nursing role was not as sudden as it seems when the Colorado program is studied in isolation.

A major impetus for the development of the nurse practitioner role was a shortage of physicians, particularly those in primary care (Fein, 1967). This was due to a reform movement in medicine that had started at the turn of the century, raising the standards of medical education and limiting the number of physicians. At the same time the growing complexity of medicine had led to specialization and subspecialization so physicians were drawn away from general practice and into the specialties. By 1970, specialist physicians outnumbered generalists by three to one (U.S. National Center for Health Statistics, 1973). In addition, improvements in nursing education fostered the development of an advanced level of nursing (Bullough, 1976).

Education of Nurse Practitioners

The Colorado program was initiated by a physician, Henry Silver, and a nursing professor, Loretta Ford (Ford, 1982; Ford & Silver, 1967; Silver, Ford, & Day, 1968). Registered nurses were prepared as nurse associates (later called nurse practitioners) in a 4-month intensive program that was followed by a preceptorship with a physician. They were taught to do health histories, physical examinations, handle minor illnesses, and gather data that would facilitate physician interactions with children who had more serious illnesses (American Academy of Pediatrics & ANA, 1971). Using the model of this program, which was a continuing education offering, the early nurse practitioner programs were placed outside the mainstream of nursing education in departments of continuing education, medical schools, or hospitals (Andrus & Fenley, 1976). Changes in the educational system were traced by Harry Sultz and his colleagues in a series of comprehensive and carefully executed longitudinal studies of cohorts or nurse practitioner students who started in 1973, 1977, and 1980 (Sultz, Henry, Kinyon, Buck, & Bullough, 1983a, 1983b; Sultz, Zielezny, Gentry, & Kinyon, 1978; Sultz, Zielezny, & Kinyon, 1976). Although the first programs almost all awarded certificates, by 1973 there were 45 master's-degree programs and 86 certificate programs. By 1980, the 112 master's-degree programs outnumbered the 77 certificate programs. The trend to replace certificates with master's-degree programs and institutionalize them in the schools of nursing has continued in all majors except family planning that remains primarily a certificate program (Sultz et al., 1983b).

When the movement started in the 1960s, more than one half of the programs were in pediatrics. By 1980, other specialties had expanded such that family nurse practitioners and adult nurse practitioners were the most numerous. The major nurse practitioner specialties in the 1990s are adult, family, women's health, family planning, pediatrics, and geriatrics (Garrard et al., 1990; Kane, Garrard, & Skay, 1989). As master's education became the norm in all but family planning, the programs were lengthened (Sultz et al., 1983b; Towers 1989, 1990).

Early Evaluative Studies

A primary agenda of the early researchers was to evaluate the level of competence of nurse practitioners and to compare the outcomes of care with those of physicians. In 1971, Andrews and Yankauer reviewed 14 outcome studies and reported uniformly positive findings in all of them. However, as they pointed out many of these studies were done by the early promoters of the new role, and most were describing a single-practice setting (Andrews & Yankauer, 1971). This was also true of the review done by Sox (1979) of studies comparing physician care with nurse practitioner care. Many of the authors of these studies were the physician originators of the projects to prepare or use nurse practitioners. Notwithstanding the apparent conflict of interest, the research was of high quality and Sox indicated that there were no systematic differences between the process or outcomes of care given by nurse practitioners and physicians (Sox, 1979).

The most comprehensive early review of the literature was done by Edmunds in 1978, which covered 471 books and articles. Although she criticized the methodologies of many of the studies because of their inadequate sample sizes, or improper methodological or statistical treatment of the data, she was nevertheless able to find enough good studies to conclude that nurse practitioners were competent in the delivery of quality care. In addition, she found that they had been accepted fully by patients as a source of care.

Patient acceptance was also evaluated in a Missouri study of 492 patients from a multispecialty clinic who were randomly placed with either nurse practitioners or physicians for an examination. Questionnaires were used to assess the patients' response, which was significantly more favorable if they saw a nurse practitioner (Brown, Brown, & Jones, 1979). Other studies documenting patient satisfaction included early studies by Lewis and Resnick (1967), and Linn (1976). In the Lewis and Resnick study (1967), patients with negative opinions about nurses performing tasks, such as explaining results of tests, explaining the medical diagnosis, examining the throat, and instructing about medications, reversed the opinions after 1 year of care by a nurse practitioner. The randomly assigned control group made no changes.

The acceptance by physicians during this period became mixed. A survey of 4,000 pediatricians found only 13% had an unsuccessful experience with a nurse practitioner; most were pleased and reported that working with a nurse practitioner gave them more free time or time to care for seriously ill patients (Yankauer, Tripp, Andrews, & Connelly, 1972). A survey by Heiman and Dempsey (1976) reported that physicians were pleased with the performance of nurse practitioners when they carried out the simpler tasks, suggesting that they believed the more complex procedures required a physician. This implies that the enthusiasm of physicians, even in this early era was limited to certain settings or certain patient populations, including not just less complex procedures, but tending also to focus on underserved rural and inner-city practice settings (Master et al., 1980; Miller & Goldstein, 1972; Morgan & Sullivan, 1980).

Among the early outcome studies that stand out because of their solid methodologies were some of those in which researchers compared nurse practitioners with physicians. Levin et al. (1976) used a follow-up survey of providers and patients in a prepaid group practice to compare the resolution of acute problems in patients seen by nurse practitioners and physicians. The study was carefully planned and executed. The researchers found that the patients seen by nurse practitioners reported feeling less anxious and were more free of pain than those seen by physicians. Perrin and Goodman (1978) reported that pediatric nurse practitioners did better telephone management, were more effective in interpersonal interactions, and that patients learned more about their conditions than if they were seen by a physician. Hastings et al. (1980) used a chart review over a 3-year period to demonstrate that the quality of care provided by nurse practitioners was equal to that of subspecialty fellows and that their addition to the health service allowed doubling of the patient capacity while the average cost per visit was reduced by one third.

Runyon (1975) set up a nurse practitioner clinic for patients with diabetes, hypertension, or cardiac disease, and did vigorous study comparing the outcomes of care for the nurse practitioner patients and patients seen in the outpatient clinics of the city of Memphis hospital. A sample of 1,500 patients was followed for 2 years. The rate of hospitalization among the patients seen by the nurse practitioners fell dramatically (Runyon, 1975). However, this study and those like it that used the existing standards of care were criticized by later critics who argued that the usual standard of care in city hospitals is resident care, and nurse practitioners should be held to the standard of attending physicians.

Probably the best comparison study of this period was conducted in Burlington, Ontario. The investigators used random sampling that was a rarity in the early comparison studies. The standard of care used for comparisons was physician care. A group of 1,598 families who were receiving clinical services from two family physicians in a middle-class suburb were randomly assigned to either continue with their conventional care or reassigned to a nurse practitioner group. The nurse practitioners managed the care, although when needed, they requested consultation from the associated physician(s). Only seven families refused assignment to a nurse practitioner. Measurement of mortality rates, and physical, social, and emotional functioning after 1 year supported the conclusion that the patients in the nurse practitioner group were cared for as effectively as those in the physician group (Sackett, Spitzer, Gent, & Roberts, 1974). The study also showed nurse practitioners to be cost-effective from the viewpoint of society, but the rigid state reimbursement mechanisms that did now allow nurse practitioners to be reimbursed forced the physicians in the study to pay the nurse practitioners out of their salaries (Spitzer et al., 1974). Thus, the most carefully controlled study from the standpoint of research methodology was a failure in the political arena. The fact that the physicians in the study were forced to pay the salaries of the nurse practitioners out of their own pockets was widely publicized among Canadian physicians, and this was a significant factor in delaying the further development of nurse practitioners in Canada for more than 20 years (Bullough, 1994).

There also have been several more recent comprehensive literature reviews that evaluated the quality of this research as well as the quality of nurse practitioner care. In 1985 the Institute of Medicine (1985) reviewed the literature about low-birthweight infants and drew up a report with recommendations for its prevention. The document is carefully documented and well written. It recommended that more reliance be placed on nurse midwives and nurse practitioners to provide prenatal care to more high-risk mothers. The implication here seemed to be on nurse practitioners in underserved urban and rural areas.

An information synthesis study sponsored by the Veterans Administration was done by Feldman, Ventura, and Crosby (1987). After starting with a comprehensive review of the literature about nurse practitioners, the researchers analyzed the methodological characteristics of the articles and reports. They reviewed the sample sizes, the use of comparison groups, the appropriate use of statistics, and other methodological characteristics of the corpus of studies. In their final report to the Veterans Administration, they gave each item a deficit score for its methodological flaws. However, they (1987) also published an article in the nursing literature synthesizing only those articles published between 1973 and 1987 that had low deficit scores. They then summarized the findings of this body of literature reporting positive findings related to the use of nurse practitioners, their productivity, and consumer satisfaction.

The most widely distributed critical review and evaluation of the quality of care provided by nurse practitioners, nurse midwives, and physicians assistants was done by the Office of Technology Assessment

(1986) in response to a request from the Senate Appropriations Committee. In general the review criticized the large body of literature for its use of small samples, focusing on short-term outcomes, and use of nonrandom samples, applying single evaluation criteria, using incomplete and unstandardized medical records, and choosing nonrepresentative sample sites. They also noted that too often comparisons were made with house staff instead of attending physicians. However, despite these criticisms, they noted that many investigators had used sound methodology, and their findings appeared to be valid and reliable. Two of the studies mentioned for their sound methodology and vigor were the Canadian randomized trials (Sackett et al., 1974; Spitzer et al., 1974), which have already been discussed and a study of "new health practitioners" (nurse practitioners and physicians assistants) done in a prepaid group practice in Maryland (Levine, Morlock, Mushlin, Shapiro, & Malitz, 1976). A variety of outcomes were studied including patient satisfaction, changes in patient status, pain, and anxiety. All of the outcome measures were positive. In terms of practice, the most important finding was the fact that the new health professionals could carry 75% of the well-person care, and 56% of the problem-oriented care. Hence, patient access to care was greatly increased without additional physician staff.

The Office of Technology Assessment (1986) reviewed these many studies and concluded that within their area of competence, nurse practitioners, nurse midwives, and physicians' assistants provided care that was equivalent to that provided by physicians. It was noted however, that restrictive third-party reimbursement mechanisms were preventing full use of these workers. The Office of Technology Assessment recommended extending third-party reimbursement for their services, arguing that this could increase their use and result in cost savings to consumers (Office of Technology Assessment, 1986).

Changing State Nurse Practice Acts

One reason the role expansion of the early nurse practitioners was so modest was that many of the state nurse practice acts prohibited diagnosis and treatment by nurses. Changes in the state nurse practice acts were needed before significant expansion of the role could occur. Accomplishing these changes involved prolonged political activity at the state level by nurse practitioners. By 1975, there were 21 states that had revised their practice acts to allow nurse practitioners to diagnose and treat in some type of collaborative arrangements with physicians. By 1980, 41 states had revised their practice acts (Bullough, 1980). At the present time all of the states except Ohio and Illinois have authorized or recognized nurse practitioners in laws or regulations, or significantly expanded the scope of function of all nurses (Pearson, 1994). Although the ANA (1981) opposed a second licensure for nurses in advanced practice, the National Council of State Boards of Nursing (1986) favored it. Surveys and histories of the changing nurse practice acts indicate that as the laws changed over time, the states have gradually developed either a separate license or certification for nurse practitioners and other advanced nursing specialties (Bullough, 1984a; Megel, 1994; Safriet, 1992).

Changes in the Literature

Beginning in about 1980, the volume of literature about nurse practitioners started to gradually diminish. Most of the case studies of one practice disappeared, and studies comparing nurse practitioners to physicians appeared somewhat less frequently. For example, the *New England Journal of Medicine, The Annals of Internal Medicine, Pediatrics,* and *The Journal of the American Medical Association* had each published several articles each year about nurse practitioners in the 1960s and 1970s, but by 1985 these articles had dwindled to only an occasional offering. The Public health journals. *American Journal of Public Health* and *Medical Care*, continued to publish articles but not as frequently as in the earlier era. Instead, most of the articles about nurse practitioners appeared in the nursing journals, including *Nursing Research* and those aimed at nurse practitioner audiences: *Nurse Practitioner, Journal of the Academy of Nurse Practitioners*, and the *Journal of Pediatric Health Care*. Some of this decline in volume can be attributed to the fact that the concept was no longer news, and the body of research documenting patient satisfaction and the comparability of nurse practitioners to physicians was already large. However, the loss of interest in the medical journals could have been due to a changing climate of medical opinion regarding nurse practitioners. This occurred, even as nurse practitioners became more competent, more autonomous, and more accepted through the state nurse practice acts.

PHYSICIAN CONCERNS

The increasing supply of physicians was apparently a key element in this change of opinion. The growing number of physicians was documented in the "Graduate Medical National Advisory Committee (GMENAC) Report" published in 1980. The authors recommended that in light of an anticipated oversupply of physicians by 1990 it would be wise to curtail further expansion of programs to prepare nurse practitioners, physicians' assistants, and nurse midwives. The report also called for more control of these workers by physicians, including a recommendation that third-party reimbursement be made to the employer (the physician) rather than directly to the worker (GMENAC, 1980; Whitney, 1983).

The medical associations were supportive of nurse practitioners in the 1960s and 1970s. The American Academy of Pediatrics, in 1971, issued a set of joint guidelines with the ANA for the training of pediatric nurse practitioners. The American Medical Association's (AMA's) Committee on Nursing (1970) issued a position statement in 1970 that favored the nurse practitioner role. However, the threatened oversupply of physicians changed the climate, and boards of medicine and medical societies initiated a variety of activities aimed at controlling or eliminating nurse practitioners. Bullough followed the history of these backlash activities and reported them at an ANA conference and in published articles (Bullough, 1984a, 1984b). The physician backlash was first noticed in 1978 when the New Jersey Board of Medicine charged two nurse practitioners and four physicians with the illegal practice of medicine because their employer, the Rutgers Community Health Plan, allowed nurse practitioners to do medical diagnoses and prescribe medications. The case was settled 2 years later when the HMO agreed to prevent nurse practitioners from doing histories and physical examinations or using presigned prescription pads (Administrative action, State of New Jersey, 1980).

In 1980 the Missouri Board of Registration for the Healing Arts charged five physicians with aiding and abetting the illegal practice of medicine. At that time, the Missouri law did not specifically allow nurse practitioner practice, although it described nursing in broader terms than it had in the prenurse practitioner era. The five physicians were serving as consultants to two nurse practitioners who used protocols to guide their practice in family planning clinics in rural Missouri. In 1982 the County Circuit Court ruled against the five physicians and the two nurse practitioners. When the case was reviewed by the State Supreme court, it attracted nationwide attention, and 36 nursing and health care organizations wrote amicus curiae briefs. The Missouri supreme court decided in favor of the two nurses (Greenlow, 1984; Sermchief v. Gonzales, 1982, 1983).

In 1980, the Arkansas State Medical Board passed a regulation prohibiting any physician or group of physicians from employing or collaborating with more than two nurse practitioners (Bullough, 1985). The regulations not only called for a review of nurse practitioner credentials by the board of medicine, but indicated any violation of these rules would constitute malpractice and subject the physicians involved to penalties. The Arkansas State Nurses Association filed suit against the medical board charging them with restraint of trade. The medical board lost the suit at the circuit court level but won in the state supreme court (Arkansas Supreme Court, 1984; Bullough, 1985). The regulation was then rewritten by the Medical Board and titled Regulation 15. Again they were challenged by the Arkansas Nurses Association and the circuit court ruled in favor of the nurses in late 1984 (State News, Arkansas, 1984).

In 1981, the Kansas medical society brought a suit against the board of nursing charging that the nurse practitioner regulations were unconstitutional. The court agreed, and the board of nursing was not allowed to write the regulations for nurse practitioners until 1983 when the language of the state nurse practice act was changed. In 1981 the Louisiana Medical Society brought a suit against the board of nursing for writing regulations for nurse practitioners. The medical society lost that case and again in 1983 brought a petition to add the words "under the supervision of a physician" to the regulations. They were unsuccessful in this action as well (Louisiana State Board of Nursing: Judgement, 1983). In 1982, the Ohio medical board brought a suit against an HMO that used nurse practitioners. The medical board won the case because Ohio had not changed its law to allow nurse practitioner practice (Bullough, 1984b).

These various activities suggested a perception of threat on the part of organized medicine about the developing nurse practitioner specialty (Bullough, 1984b). Culminating these state actions, the Board of Trustees of the AMA in 1990 recommended that the AMA monitor state and federal legislation to oppose independent practice or the direct reimbursement of nurses (AMA, 1990; Safriet, 1992).

CURRENT FOCUS OF THE RESEARCH LITERATURE

Most of the research literature is now written by nurse practitioners, other nurses, and social scientists. There are still physician members of research teams, but they are usually not the first author. There are a few articles comparing physicians and nurse practitioners, but there are also a wide variety of other topics covered including the following: third-party reimbursement for nurse practitioners, the laws covering nurse practitioner practice including continued research on prescription writing privileges, economic issues, the incomes and distribution of nurse practitioners, the issue of merger of the roles of nurse practitioners with clinical specialists, communication patterns between nurse practitioners and their clients, and new areas of nurse practitioner specialization.

THIRD-PARTY REIMBURSEMENT

As the practice of nurse practitioners expanded, third-party reimbursement emerged as an important mechanism for survival. Hence, descriptive studies surveying these practices are a feature of the more recent literature (LeBar, 1986; Knox, 1988; Sullivan; 1992, Mittelstadt, 1993). The first recognition of nurse practitioner reimbursement was in the Social Security Act of 1972 ([PL] 92603, 86 Stat 1329), and it was a negative notice. A government official realized that some doctors had billed for services performed by nurse practitioners; the 1972 law restricted this billing and indicated that the services were covered only if they were performed under the direct supervision of the physician. Expansion of federal reimbursement to cover nurse practitioners first occurred in the Rural Health Clinic Services Act of 1977 (PL 95 210, 91 Stat 1485); it waived the on-site supervision by physicians for nurse practitioners and physicians assistants. In 1979 CHAMPUS, a federal program for members of the armed services and their dependents, covered certified nurse midwives and initiated an experimental program (PL 95-457, 1979) reimbursing nurse practitioners for primary health services and showed a 31% decrease in costs when services were performed by nurse practitioners. As a result of the successful pilot project, nurse practitioner services for CHAMPUS patients were authorized (PL 97-114, 1982). A similar experimental use of nurse practitioners by the Federal Employees Health Benefits Program was carried out from 1980 to 1984 with successful outcomes in terms of cost and satisfaction with services. Eventually a law was passed (PL 101-509, 1990) requiring reimbursement of nurse practitioners for their services; this law was passed in response to nonreimbursement policies under President Reagan. Reimbursement was put into effect again after he left office (Hardy, Havens, & Hestvick, 1991; Knox, 1988).

Nurse practitioners were not covered by Medicaid until 1990 when the services of pediatric and family nurse practitioners were authorized. The additional progress made through 1993 included payment for work in nursing homes, rural health clinics, health maintenance organizations, federally qualified health centers, and certain other ambulatory care settings. The nursing home and rural area provisions were, however, the only ones providing direct reimbursement (Mittelstadt, 1993).

Legislation has also been passed in 26 states requiring private companies including Blue Cross/Blue Shield, to reimburse nurse practitioners for functions that would be reimbursed if performed by physicians. Such legislation was not always immediately effective, however, as shown by a survey of the plans offered by research universities in 1990. This study indicated that 70% of the plans surveyed did not reimburse nurse practitioners; only traditional nursing was covered (Scott & Harrison, 1990). This lack of insurance coverage is emphasized by the statistics from the national surveys. The National Association of Pediatric Nurse Associates and Practitioners (NAPNAP) survey (Dunn, 1993) indicated that only 8% of the respondents reported they could bill in their own names, although 53% are able to bill through the physician or agency where they work.

CURRENT STATE POLITICAL ACTIVITY: PRESCRIPTIVE AUTHORITY

As soon as basic authorization of nurse practitioner practice was achieved in most of the states, the next political goal of nurse practitioners was recognition of their right to write prescriptions. The first laws authorizing nurse practitioners to order drugs were written in 1973 in Arizona and Washington. By 1983, 14 states had authorized nurse practitioners or other nurses in advanced practice to prescribe, but the early laws tended to give only limited privileges (Bullough, 1983). The 1994 survey done by *Nurse Practitioner* reported that 45 states (including the District of Columbia) gave nurse practitioners some sort of prescriptive authority (Pearson, 1994). The 1992 NAPNAP survey of 800 pediatric nurse practitioners reported 60% of the respondents had full prescriptive privileges, whereas 14% were in some sort of transitional phase with the law changing or new regulations pending, and 26% did not have prescriptive authority (Dunn, 1993).

It is clear that prescription privileges vary widely even in the states with statutory coverage. Safriet (1992) published a comprehensive historical study of the laws, regulations, and other barriers that impede full and usual practice for advanced practice nurses. She found that the degree of autonomy or professional decision making varied widely from state to state. States, such as Oregon, Washington, and Alaska, allow nurse practitioners full prescriptive privileges, whereas other states employ various devices to limit nurse practitioners including mandating the use of protocols, formularies, or prohibiting the prescription of all or certain controlled substances. Safriet (1992) noted that organized medicine has played a central role in shaping the provisions of prescriptive authority for nurses by consistently lobbying against prescriptive authority. In 1992, the AMA published state model legislation that defines prescribing as a medical function that nurses should carry out only under protocols and only for institutionalized or medically underserved patients (AMA, 1991).

When nurse practitioners actually are empowered to prescribe, their practices are similar to those of physicians. Batey and Holland studied log recordings by 89 nurse practitioners from five western states in 1981 and compared the findings with those from the National Ambulatory Medical Care Report. They found that the nurse practitioners used the same range of drugs as the physicians who were surveyed but prescribed drugs in only 49% of all visits, whereas physicians prescribed in 63% of their visits. Nurse practitioners sought physician consultation or referral 13% of the time (Batey & Holland, 1985).

ECONOMIC VIABILITY OF NURSE PRACTITIONERS

In 1993 there were approximately 27,000 nurse practitioners (Morgan, 1993). The number has grown slowly since 1980 when Sultz and his associates estimated that there were approximately 20,000 (Sultz et al., 1983a). A salary study of 382 certified nurse practitioners done in North Carolina in 1989 reported that two thirds of the sample received less than $30,000 a year in compensation (Rogers et al., 1989). A 1990 survey of 597 New York state nurse practitioners reported a median of $35,000 with $39,000 in New York City and $30,000 in rural areas (Abt & Bullough, 1990). Although many nurse practitioners buy malpractice insurance the rates are modest in comparison with those for physicians. The American Academy of Nursing 1989 survey found that less than 1% of the 5,964 respondents had been named as primary defendants in a malpractice suit (Towers, 1989).

The modest salaries and the lack of malpractice suits makes the employment of practitioners a bargain for health care institutions. Two studies of private companies that used occupational health nurse practitioners to provide primary care to employees documented significant savings when costs were compared with what it would have cost to use physicians to provide the same services (Dellinger, Zentner, McDowell, & Annas, 1986; Scharon, Tsai, & Bernacki, 1987).

An HMO study published in 1982 found a 20% cost saving for pediatric patients and a 52% saving for women patients (Salkever, Skinner, Steinwachs, & Katz, 1982). The HMOs seem well aware of the possible savings, and the job market within HMOs has increased steadily (Coslow, 1992) with approximately 8% of the nurse practitioners now employed by HMOs (Towers, 1989, 1990).

In a study of a geriatric nurse practitioners working in nursing homes, cost savings were realized because fewer hospitalizations were needed (Garrard et al. 1990). A county hospital diabetes clinic saved admissions (and money) by adding a nurse practitioner telephone consultation service and a nurse practitioner or resident preadmission screening service (Miller & Goldstein, 1972).

It is important to note, however, that the studies that showed cost savings were done in sites where third-party reimbursement is available in nursing homes, or it is not an issue, as is the case with HMOs, governmental agencies, or the private companies that employed nurse practitioners directly instead of going through an insurance carrier. Reimbursement of nurse practitioners in all work sites would be needed to bring the cost savings to the total market. Nichols (1992) estimated an annual cost saving between $6.4 billion and $8.75 billion to the United States if all of the reimbursement and legal barriers were removed and nurse practitioners were used at their full potential.

INTEGRATION OF NURSE PRACTITIONERS AND CLINICAL SPECIALISTS

The second edition of the book *Nurses: Nurse Practitioners* (Mezey & McGivern, 1993) included a comprehensive historical review of the literature about nurse practitioners and the other nursing specialties. The editors argued that the roles of nurse practitioners, clinical nurse specialists, nurse midwives, and nurse anesthetists should be conceptualized as an advanced practice role and that the role of the nurse practitioner and clinical specialist should be integrated. This issue was brought to public attention in 1986 when the American Nurses Association merged its Councils of Clinical Specialists and Primary Health Care Nurse Practitioners and suggested that merger of the two positions should be seriously considered (Sparacino and Durand, 1986). Representatives of the National Organization of Nurse Practitioner Faculty were more cautious in their recommendations (Hanson & Martin, 1990). The American Association of Colleges of Nursing (AACN) appears to be in favor of advanced-practice nurses who combine to some degree the skills of nurse practitioners and clinical nurse specialists (AACN, 1994).

One of the research questions suggested by this proposed policy is how similar are the two roles? A survey of nurse practitioner and clinical nurse specialist (CNS) programs sponsored by the ANA was published in 1990 (Forbes, Rafson, Spross, & Kozlowski, 1990a, 1990b). Sixty nurse practitioner programs and 195 CNS programs were analyzed to assess the similarities in content. Although the nurse practitioner programs reported more emphasis on pharmacology, primary care, physical assessment, health promotion, nutrition, and history taking, most of the content in the two types of programs was the same.

The national survey of nurse practitioners done by the American Academy of Nursing sheds additional light on this issue (Towers, 1989). The survey was sent to 12,000 nurse practitioners, and 5,964 responses were received. The findings suggested significant variations in practice site by nurse practitioner specialty. Family nurse practitioners most often were employed in free-standing clinics or private medical practices; pediatric nurse practitioners were in hospital outpatient clinics, public clinics, or physicians' offices; womens' health care nurse practitioners were in free-standing and public clinics (including specialized family planning clinics); gerontological nurse practitioners were in extended care facilities; school and college nurse practitioners were in schools; and adult nurse practitioners were employed in various sites, including HMOs and home health care agencies. The specialties that were most likely to work in hospital inpatient units were the psychiatric mental health nurse practitioners (13.8%), adult nurse practitioners (6.1%), and geriatric nurse practitioners (6.1%). The geriatric nurse practitioners are the most likely to be institution-based, with extended care facilities accounting for 35.3% of their practices (Towers, 1989).

Elder and Bullough (1990) followed the nurse practitioners and clinical nurse specialists who graduated from a single master's program over a 10-year period. The job market for the two groups differed in that about one half of the clinical specialists were in administrative or teaching roles, whereas most of the nurse practitioners were in clinical roles. When the hands-on patient care roles were surveyed it was found that the two types of specialists were similar in many ways, however. There were no significant differences between the two groups in 17 of 25 work activities, including psychosocial assessments, teaching patients and their families, counseling, giving physical care, doing research, and publishing manuscripts. The two groups differed significantly on 8 tasks. Nurse practitioners were more likely to do physical examinations, order laboratory tests, prescribe medications, prescribe treatments, and make referrals. The clinical specialists were more likely to establish support groups, teach staff, and do psychotherapy. The authors recognized there were political differences between the two groups so they did not see an immediate merger, but predicted that a gradual merger would take place over the next 20 years.

Another comparison of the two positions compared the results of a study of clinical specialists done by Fenton (1985) and of nurse practitioners done by Brykczynski (1989). The purpose of both studies was to identify expert domains of nursing practice for the CNS and the nurse practitioner, using the approach Benner (1984) had used to identify expert practice domains for nurses. Fenton and Brykczynski (1993) then compared the results and conclusions of their two studies.

Data for Fenton's study included 105 situation-based interviews and 53 participant observations. Data for Brykczynski's study consisted of 62 hours of situation-based interviews and 80 hours of participant observations. The two methodologies were similar, and the comparisons of the two data sets seem reasonable.

Both of the investigators identified the seven domains used by Benner to describe expert nurses: (a) the diagnostic and patient monitoring function, (b) administering and monitoring therapeutic interventions and regimes, (c) monitoring and ensuring the quality of health care practices, (d) organization and work role competencies, (e) the helping role of the nurse, (f) the teaching/coaching function, and (g) effective management of rapidly changing situations (Benner, 1984). The fact that these domains were present in both roles documents that a significant component of advanced nursing practice exists in both roles.

There were, however, significant differences. The first domain identified by Benner (1984), "diagnostic and patient monitoring function," was demonstrated differently in the two roles with diagnosis being an important component of nurse practitioner expertise and monitoring a function of the clinical specialists. Fenton identified an additional domain of CNS practice, that of consulting. The nurse practitioners were more health oriented, while clinical specialists focused more on illness. Clinical specialists were responsible for promoting the overall functions of the organization, whereas the nurse practitioners focused on the patient. The authors' curriculum recommendation was to merge the common elements in the two specialty curriculums but separate them for the specialized elements.

INTERACTIONS WITH PATIENTS

There is a significant body of research literature looking at the relationships between nurse practitioners and their clients, often comparing them with physicians. The study by Campbell et al. (1990) was mentioned in the section on definition because a difference in styles of interaction seems to be one way nurse practitioners differentiate themselves from physicians, even when the technical roles overlap significantly. The difference tends to be consistent across studies but there are not extreme differences. Campbell et al. (1990) analyzed 412 patient visits (including

276 with physicians and 136 with nurse practitioners). Although there was little overall difference in the interaction styles of the two providers, the nurse practitioners focused more on psychosocial issues.

In a study of pediatric nurse practitioners, 70 audiotapes of well-child visits completed by 35 nurse practitioners were analyzed to describe the interpersonal process. Results suggested that nurse practitioners conducted a comprehensive and thorough assessment, but during that process they dominated the interaction by asking questions, giving opinions, and giving commands. Only rarely was the mother encouraged to ask questions or share her knowledge or problem solve. Because these are behaviors nurses sometimes accuse physicians of using, this study was sobering (Webster-Stratton, Glascock, & McCarthy, 1986).

A not too dissimilar picture of the interactional styles of nurse practitioners and physicians was reported by Taylor, Pickens, and Geden (1989) who studied the videotaped interactions of 85 physicians and 42 nurse practitioners to see what approaches each group used to influence their patients. These researchers wanted to separate the influence of the job role from that of gender in determining different interactional styles. Each of the professions included subsamples of males and females. However, only 3 of the nurse practitioners were male, and only 5 of the physicians were female, so this aspect of the study was problematic. Incidents of interactions were coded using one of three approaches: commands, fear-provoking consequences, or concordance. All groups used more command and consequence statements than concordance statements. However, males and physicians used more command statements and fewer consequence statements than females and nurse practitioners, so both gender and occupational role influenced the interaction patterns (Taylor, Pickens, & Genden, 1989).

PROFESSIONALIZATION OF NURSE PRACTITIONERS

Although most of the research literature about nurse practitioners is not conceptually oriented nor does it often invoke theory, the data that have been amassed over the last 3 decades are voluminous and multifaceted in their coverage. They can be used as primary data to trace the history and the process of professionalization as it relates to nurse practitioners.

Clearly, nurse practitioners have become more autonomous during the last three decades. Their level of knowledge and expertise is beyond that of the undergraduate trained nurses, and it has increased over time. Nurse practitioners have shown their worth to the public, and they have gained power through a separate level of licensure. Consequently they have become more professional. However, the process has also been marked by conflict. Supporting this generalization is the body of research literature that has ben collected at the University of Missouri-Columbia related to joint practice issues. It was assembled between 1981 and 1987 (Koch, Pazaki, & Campbell, 1992). The study group identified five dominant themes in the literature: nurse practitioner roles, education, health care crisis, evaluation, and legal issues, but the relative emphasis among these issues changed over time. The authors concluded that two interrelated factors influenced the nurse practitioner movement: labor market competition and professionalization. Shortages, or perceived shortages of primary care physicians supported the early development of the role. Physicians believed they could control nurse practitioners and that their use would increase profits and provide health care for less desirable markets. However, as the perception of shortage gave way to fear of an oversupply, anti–nurse practitioner sentiments were more often voiced. The physician dominated health care system was for a time able to halt expansion of funds to nurse practitioner education, but they were not able to get rid of nurse practitioners. The researchers now see evidence of an increasingly competitive health market as nurse practitioners seek autonomous practice, unfettered economic reimbursement, hospital privileges, and prescriptive authority.

Professionalization as a theoretical framework explaining the current situation is an aspect of the research literature that merits further exploration. The pioneer sociological work on theory related to professions was done by Carr-Sauners and Wilson in 1933. They compared law and medicine with other occupations and concluded that the key attribute of a profession was its possession of specialized techniques for giving service to clients. These techniques were acquired through a substantial program of academic study. In addition, members of professions tend to band together in some type of organization or occupational community to enforce standards and control access to the occupation. Often this process of control is carried out in cooperation with the state by the use of licensure laws. These authors differentiated the professional workers from business by the fact that business made a profit, whereas professionals were salaried or received fees for services. They considered nursing a borderline profession because in 1933 nurses were focused on the techniques of care rather than focusing on the knowledge basic to those techniques (Carr-Saunders & Wilson, 1933). Other sociologists writing on the subject of the professions drew up similar lists of attributes and began to define the professions as special elite occupations which were given special privileges because of their prestige and special contributions to the society. The approach was congruent with the structural functional theoretical approach that described the social relationships from a static point of view and assumed that the structures and relationships developed the way they did because of their positive functions.

Conversely, sociological theorists who focus on conflict and change have a less laudatory view of the professions, and they see occupations in more dynamic relationships. Probably the leading figure in this group is Eliot Freidson who argued that the crucial attribute of a highly professionalized occupation is its power to control the terms, conditions, and content of its work, and to protect its boundaries from interlopers who would lessen its power (Freidson, 1970, 1977). Freidson has been particularly interested in medicine and has analyzed its domination over the other health professions. (Freidson, 1971). Following Freidson's lead, Stewart and Cantor (1982) focused on autonomy as the key attribute of a profession, explaining that the other elements often included in the definitions are either means for achieving autonomy or benefits that flow from having power. The level of autonomy changes over time as occupations gain knowledge or their knowledge becomes obsolete, as their services become more or less valuable to society, and as they gain or lose power through licensure and other governmental actions.

Nurse practitioners have in fact furnished a challenge to the total domination of medicine. Freidson's thesis would predict the rift that surfaced in 1980 with the GMENAC Report. As the nurse practitioners became more knowledgeable and less willing to be dominated by their physician sponsors, as the programs moved out of the medical schools, hospitals, and agencies and into the nursing schools, and nurse practitioners sought laws that would give them more autonomy in the patient care decision-making process, they became a threat to physicians. Although at first the laws were limited by provisions requiring supervision or collaborative relationships with physicians, nurse practitioners can now replace physicians in some areas and that constitutes a threat to physicians' pocketbooks. Obviously the process of professionalization is not a smooth course. As the supply of physicians increased, the early facilitative stance of physicians changed to one that is more protective of their turf. Moreover, as other advanced specialties developed: nurse anesthetists, nurse midwives, and psychiatric nurses, these workers also sought to fulfill a significant component of the physicians' role at salaries that were much lower than physicians' salaries. The negative position papers and lobbying of medicine is not surprising under these conditions.

SUMMARY AND CONCLUSIONS

The research literature about nurse practitioners from 1965 through 1993 was reviewed. The literature of the early years was voluminous, it covered a variety of topics that emphasized the evaluation of the quality of care given by nurse practitioners and compared them to physicians. The current emphasis is broader. It emphasizes descriptive and historical studies, although some evaluative studies still are being conducted, including those that focus on the interactive styles of nurse practitioners. Increasingly research is focused on issues of concern to nurse practitioners, including third-party reimbursement, prescriptive authority, the economic viability of nurse practitioners, patient interactions, and consideration of a possible merger with clinical nurse specialists.

The review ends with a proposed theoretical framework for the events of the last 30 years, arguing that nurse practitioners are in the process of professionalization, and that process is sometimes painful because it involves an invasion of the turf of the medical profession and members of that profession are naturally protective of their turf. As health care reform continues and the possibility emerges for nurse practitioners to fill a more significant role in health care in the future then they have in the past, the struggle between physicians and nurse practitioners may continue to escalate.

REFERENCES

Abt, K., & Bullough, B. (1990, July). Survey of New York nurse practitioners. *The Coalition Communique*, pp. 1–4.

Administrative Action, Final Order, State of New Jersey. (1980). Department of Board of Medical Examiners, Dockett H-78-5022.

American Academy of Nursing. (1976). *Primary care by nurses: Sphere of responsibility and accountability*. Kansas City: The American Nurses' Association.

American Academy of Pediatrics and the American Nurses' Association. (1971). Guidelines on short-term continuing education programs for pediatric nurse associates. *American Journal of Nursing, 71*, 509–512.

American Medical Association, Board of Trustees. (1990). *Proceedings of the House of Delegates, 139th annual meeting*. Washington, DC: Author.

American Medical Association, Committee on Nursing. (1970). Medicine and nursing in the 1970s: A position paper. *Journal of the American Medical Association, 213*, 1881–1883.

American Medical Association, State Legislation, Legislative Activities. (1991, Feb). *An act to grant prescription writing authority to nurse practitioners and to regulate such prescription practices*. Washington, DC: Author.

American Nurses' Association. (1981). *The nursing practice act: Suggested state legislation*. Kansas City, MO: Author.

American Nurses' Association. (1987). *Standards of practice for primary health care nurse practitioners*. Kansas City, MO: Author.

Andrews, P. M., & Yankauer, A. (1971). The pediatric practitioner: 1. Growth of the concept. *American Journal of Nursing, 71*, 504–506.

Andrus, L. H., & Fenley, (1976). Evolution of a family nurse practitioner program to improve primary care distribution. *Journal of Medical Education, 51* (4), 317-324.

Arkansas Supreme Court. (1984, October 16). Rule struck down. *Arkansas Gazette*, p. 3.

Batey, M. J., & Holland, J. M. (1985). Prescribing practices among nurse practitioners in adult and family health. *American Journal of Public Health, 75*, 258-262.

Benner, P. (1984). *From novice to expert: Excellence and power in clinical nursing practice (p. 307)*. Reading, MA: Addison-Wesley.

Brown, J. D., Brown, M. I., & Jones F. (1979). Evaluation of a nurse practitioner-staffed preventive medicine program in a fee-for-service multispecialty clinic. *Preventive Medicine, 8*, 53-64.

Brykczynski, K. A. (1989). An interpretive study describing the clinical judgement of nurse practitioners. *Scholarly Inquiry for Nursing Practice: An International Journal, 3* (2), 75-104.

Buhler-Wilkerson, K. (1993). Bringing care to the people: Lillian Wald's legacy to public health nursing. *American Journal of Public Health, 83*, 1778-1786.

Bullough, B. (1976). Influences on role expansion. *American Journal of Nursing, 76*, 1476-1481.

Bullough, B. (1980). *The law and the expanding nursing role*. New York: Appleton-Century Crofts. (2nd ed).

Bullough, B. (1983). Prescribing authority for nurses. *Nursing Economics, 1*, 122-125.

Bullough, B. (1984a). The current phase in the development of nurse practice acts. *Saint Louis University Law Journal, 28*, 365-395.

Bullough, B. (1984b). Legal restrictions as a barrier to nurse practitioner role development. *Pediatric Nursing, 9*, 228.

Bullough, B. (1985). Legislative update: State supreme court rules in favor of Arkansas nurse practitioners. *Pediatric Nursing, 11*, 229.

Bullough, B. (1992). Alternative models for specialty nursing practice. *Nursing & Health Care, 13*, 254-259.

Bullough, V. (1994). The uses of history—a Canadian case study. *Journal of Professional Nursing*.

Campbell, J. D., Mauksch, H. O., Neikirk, H. J., & Hosokawa, M. C. (1990). Collaborative practice and provider styles of delivering health care. *Social Science and Medicine, 30*, 1359-1365.

Carr-Saunders, A. M., & Wilson, P. A. (1933). *The professions*. Oxford: Clarendon Press.

Coslow, F. (1992). The nurse practitioner in the HMO. *HMO Practice, 6*, 25-28.

Dellinger, C. J., Zentner, J. P., McDowell, P. H., & Annas, A. W. (1986). The family nurse practitioner in industry. *American Association of Occupational Health Nursing Journal, 34*, 323-325.

Dunn, A. M. (1993). 1992 NAPNAP membership survey: 2. Practice characteristics of pediatric nurse practitioners indicate greater autonomy for PNPs. *Journal of Pediatric Health Care, 7*, 296-302.

Edmunds, M. W. (1978). Evaluation of nurse practitioner effectiveness: An overview of the literature. *Evaluation of the Health Professions, 1*, 69-82.

Elder, R., & Bullough, B. (1990). Nurse practitioners and clinical specialists: Are the roles merging? *Clinical Nurse Specialist, 4*, 78–84.
Fein, R (1967). *The doctor shortage: An economic diagnosis*. Washington, DC: The Brookings Institute.
Feldman, M. J., Ventura, M. R., & Crosby, F. (1987). Studies of nurse practitioner effectiveness. *Nursing Research, 36*, 303–308.
Fenton, M. V (1985). Identifying competencies of clinical nurse specialists. *Journal of Nursing Administration, 15*, 31–37.
Fenton, M. V., & Brykczynski, K. A (1993). Qualitative distinctions and similarities in the practice of clinical nurse specialists and nurse practitioners. *Journal of Professional Nursing, 9*, 313–326.
Forbes, K. E., Rafson, J., Spross, J. A., & Kozlowski, D. (1990a). Clinical nurse specialist and nurse practitioner: Core curriculum survey results. *Nurse Practitioner, 15*, 45–48.
Forbes, K., Rafson, J., Spross, J., & Kozlowski, D. (1990b). The clinical nurse specialist and nurse practitioner: Core curriculum survey results. *Clinical Nurse Specialist, 4*, 63–66.
Ford, L. C. (1982). Nurse practitioners: History of a new idea and predictions for the future. In L. H. Aiken & S. R. Gortner (Eds.), *Nursing in the 1980's: Crises, opportunities, challenges* (pp. 231–247). Philadelphia: Lippincott.
Ford, L. C., & Silver, H. E. (1967). Expanded role of the nurse in health care. *Nursing Outlook, 15*, 43–45.
Freidson, E. (1970). *Professional dominance: The social structure of medical care*. New York: Atherton Press.
Freidson, E. (1971). *The professions and their prospects*. Beverly Hills: Sage.
Freidson, E. (1977). The future of professionalization. In M. Stacey (Ed.), *Health and the division of labor*. New York: Prodist.
Garrard, J., Kane, R. L., Radosevich, D. M., Skay, C. L., Arnold, S., Kepferle, L., McDermott, S., & Buchanan, J. L. (1990). Impact of geriatric nurse practitioners on nursing-home residents' functional status, satisfaction, and discharge outcomes. *Medical Care, 28*, 271–283.
Graduate Medical National Advisory Committee. (1980). *Report summary* (Vols. 1-7, HRA Publication No. 81-651-657). Washington, DC: U.S. Public Health Service.
Greenlaw, J. (1984). Commentary: Sermchief v. Gonzales and the debate over advanced nursing practice legislation. *Law, Medicine, and Health Care, 12*, 930–931.
Gunderson, L., & Kenner, C. (1992). Case management in the neonatal intensive care unit. *AACN Clinical Issues Critical Care Nurse, 3*, 769–776.
Hanson, C., & Martin, L. I. (1990). The nurse practitioner and the clinical specialist: Should the roles be merged? *Journal of the American Academy of Nurse Practitioners, 2*, 2–9.
Hardy Havens, D., & Hestvik, L. (1991). Federal reimbursement for nurse practitioners. *Journal of Pediatric Health Care, 5*, 47–49.
Hastings, G. E., Vick, L., Lee, G., Sasmor, L., Natiello, T. A., & Sanders, J. H. (1980). Nurse practitioners in a jailhouse clinic. *Medical Care, 18*, 731–744.
Heiman, E. M., & Dempsey, M. K. (1976). Independent behavior of nurse prac-

titioners: A survey of physician and nurse attitudes. *American Journal of Public Health 66* (6), 587–589.

Hobbie, W. L., & Hollen, P. J. (1993). Pediatric nurse practitioners specializing with survivors of childhood cancer. *Journal of Pediatric Health Care, 7,* 24–30.

Institute of Medicine. (1985). *Preventing low birthweight.* Washington, DC: National Academy Press.

Kane, R. L., Garrard, J., & Skay, C. L. (1989). Effect of a geriatric nurse practitioner program on the process and outcomes of nursing home care. *American Journal of Public Health, 79,* 1271–1277.

Knox, J. T. (1988). Direct reimbursement to nurse practitioners: The importance of the federal employees freedom of choice act (House of Representatives 382). *Nurse Practitioner, 13,* 52–53.

Koch, L. W., Pazaki, S. H., & Campbell, J. D. (1992). The first 20 years of nurse practitioner literature: An evolution of joint practice issues. *Nurse Practitioner, 17,* 62, 64, 65–66, 68.

LeBar, C. (1986). Third party reimbursement for services of nurses. In M. D. Mezey & D. O. McGivern (Eds.), *Nurses: Nurse Practitioners* (pp. 450–470). Boston: Little, Brown.

Levine, D. M., Morlock, L. L., Mushlin, A. I., Shapiro, S., & Malitz, F. E. (1976). The role of new health practitioners in prepaid group practice: Provider differences in process and outcomes of medical care. *Medical Care, 14* (4), 326–347.

Lewis, C. E., & Resnick, B. A. (1967). Nurse clinics and progressive ambulatory patient-care. *New England Journal of Medicine, 277,* 1236–1241.

Linn, L. S. (1976). Patient acceptance of the family nurse practitioner. *Medical Care, 14,* 357–364.

Louisiana State Board of Nursing: Judgement. (1983, November 4). The Matter of the Louisiana State Medical Society Requesting Review of R. N. 3.041.

Master, R. J., Feltin, M., Jainchill, J., Mark, R., Kavesh, W., Rabkin, M. T., Turner, B., Bachrach, S., & Lennox, S. (1980). A continuum of care for the inner city. *New England Journal of Medicine, 302,* 1434–1440.

Megel, M., & Nursing Licensure and Regulation. (1994). In B. Bullough & V. Bullough (Eds.), *Nursing issues for the nineties and beyond* (pp. 32–43). New York: Springer Publishing Co.

Melillo, K. D. (1993). Utilizing nurse practitioners to provide health care for elderly patients in Massachusetts nursing homes. *Journal of the Academy of Nurse Practitioners, 5,* 27–33.

Mezey, M. D., & McGivern, D. O. (Eds.). 1993). *Nurses, nurse practitioners: Evolution to advanced practice.* New York: Springer Publishing Co.

Miller, L. V., & Goldstein, J. (1972). More efficient care of diabetic patients in a country-hospital setting. *New England Journal of Medicine, 286,* 1388–1391.

Mittelstadt, P. J. (1993). Third-party reimbursement for services of nurses in advanced practice; Obtaining payment for your services. In M. D. Mezey & D. O. McGivern (Eds.), *Nurses: Nurse practitioners: Evolution to advanced practice* (pp. 322–341) New York: Springer Publishing Co.

Morgan, W. A. (1993). Using state board data to estimate the number of nurse practitioners in United States. *Nurse Practitioner, 18,* 65–66, 69–70, 73–74.

Morgan, W. A., & Sullivan, N. D. (1980). Nurse practitioner and physicians' assistant clinics in rural California: 1. Issues. *Western Journal of Medicine, 132*, 171–178.

National Council of State Boards of Nursing. (1986). *Position paper on the licensure of advanced nursing practice*. Chicago: Author.

Nichols, L. M. (1992). Estimating the cost of underusing advanced practice nurses. *Nursing Economics, 10*, 343–351.

Noonan, B. R. (1972). Eight years in a medical nurse clinic. *American Journal of Nursing, 72*, 1128–1130.

Office of Technology Assessment. (1986). *Nurse practitioners, physicians assistants, and certified nurse-midwives: A policy analysis* (Health Technology Case Study 3, OTA-HCS-37). Washington, DC: U.S. Government Printing Office.

Pearson, L. J. (1993). 1992-93 Update: How each state stands on legislative issues affecting advanced nursing practice. *The Nurse Practitioner, 18*, 23–28, 30–33, 35–36, 38.

Pearson, L. J. (1994). Annual update of how each state stands on legislative issues affecting advanced nursing practice. *The Nurse Practitioner, 19*, 11–13, 17–18, 21–22, 24–27, 31–34, 39–40, 42–44.

Perrin, E. C., & Goodman, H. C. (1978). Telephone management of acute pediatric illness. *New England Journal of Medicine, 298*, 130–135.

Rogers, B., Sweeting, S., & Davis, B. (1989). Employment and salary characteristics of nurse practitioners. *Nurse Practitioner, 14*, 56, 58, 60, 62–63.

Runyon, J. W. (1975). The Memphis chronic disease program: Comparisons in outcome and the nurse's extended roles. *Journal of the American Medical Association, 231*, 264–270.

Sackett, D. L., Spitzer, W. O., Gent, M., & Roberts, R. S. (1974). The Burlington randomized trial of the nurse practitioner: Health outcomes of patients. *Annals of Internal Medicine, 80*, 142–173.

Safriet, B. J. (1992). Health care dollars and regulatory sense: The role of advanced practice nursing. *Yale Journal on Regulation, 9*, 472–488.

Salkever, D., Skinner, E., Steinwachs, D., & Katz, K. (1982). Episode-based efficiency comparisons for physicians and nurse practitioners. *Medical Care, 20*, 143–153.

Scharon, G. M., Tsai, S., & Bernacki, E. (1987). Nurse practitioners in an occupational setting: Utilizing patterns for the delivery of primary care. *American Association of Occupational Health Nurses Journal, 35*, 280–284.

Scott, C. L., & Harrison, A. O. (1990). Direct reimbursement of nurse practitioners in health insurance plans of research universities. *Journal of Professional Nursing, 6*, 21–32.

Sermchief v. Gonzales. (1982, November 15). 4544455 (Cir. Ct. St. Louis County Division, 19).

Sermchief v. Gonzales. (1983, November 22). 660S.W.2d 683.

Shamansky, S. L. (1984). Nurse practitioners and primary care research: Promises and pitfalls. *Annual Review of Nursing Research* (Vol. 3), (pp. 107–125). New York: Springer Publishing.

Siegel, E., & Bryson, S. C. (1963). Redefinition of the role of the public health nurse in child health supervision. *American Journal of Public Health, 53*, 1015–1024.

Silver, H. K., Ford, L. C., & Day, L R. (1968). The pediatric nurse-practitioner program. *The Journal of the American Medical Association, 204*, 298–302.

Sparacino, P., & Durand, B. (1986). Specialization in advanced nursing practice. *Council of Primary Care Health Care Nurse Practitioners/Council of Nurse Specialists Newsletter, 4*, 3.

Spitzer, W. O., Kergin, D. J., Yoshida, M. A., Russel, W. A. M., Hackett, H. C., & Goldsmith, C. H. (1974). Nurse practitioners in primary care—the Southern Ontario randomized trial. *Canadian Medical Association Journal, 108*, 1005–1016.

State news, Arkansas. (1984) *NP News, 2*, 13.

Stewart, P. L., & Cantor, M. G. (1982). *Varieties of work* (pp. 13–37). Beverly Hills: Sage.

Sox, H. C., Jr. (1979). Quality of patient care by nurse practitioners and physician's assistants: A ten year perspective. *Annals of Internal Medicine, 91*, 459–468.

Sullivan, E. M. (1992). Nurse practitioners and reimbursement, *Nursing & Health Care, 13*, 236–241.

Sultz, H. A., Henry, O. M., Kinyon, L. J., Buck, G. M., & Bullough, B. (1983a). A decade of change for nurse practitioners: 1. *Nursing Outlook, 31*, 138–141, 188.

Sultz, H. A., Henry, O. M., Kinyon, L. J., Buck, G. M., & Bullough, B. (1983b). Nurse practitioners: A decade of change: 2. *Nursing Outlook, 31*, 216–219.

Sultz, H. A., Zielezny, M., & Kinyon, L. J. (1976). *Longitudinal study of nurse practitioners: Phase I* (Department of Health, Education and Welfare Publication No. HRA 76-43). Bethesda, MD: U.S. Department of Health, Education and Welfare.

Sultz, H. A., Zielezny, M., Gentry, J. M., & Kinyon, L. J. (1978). *Longitudinal study of nurse practitioners: Phase II* (Department of Health, Education and Welfare Publication No. 78-92). Hyattsville, MD: U.S. Department of Health, Education and Welfare.

Taylor, S. G., Pickens, J. M., & Geden, E. A. (1989). Regarding patient decision making. *Nursing Research, 38*, 50–55.

Towers, J. (1989). Report of the American Academy of nurse practitioners' national nurse practitioner survey: 1. *Journal of the Academy of Nurse Practitioners, 1*, 91–94.

Towers, J. (1990). Report of the national survey of the American Academy of Nurse Practitioners: 3. Comparison of nurse practitioner characteristics according to education. *Journal of the Academy of Nurse Practitioners, 2*, 121–124.

United States National Center for Health Statistics. (1973). *Health Resource Statistics: Health Manpower and Health Facilities* (U.S. Public Health Services Publication No. HAM 73-1509). Washington, DC: U.S. Government Printing Office.

Wald, L. (1915). *The house on Henry Street*. New York: Henry Holt.

Webster-Stratton, C., Glascock, J., & McCarthy, A. M. (1986). Nurse practitioner-patient interactional analysis during well child visits. *Nursing Research, 35*, 247–249.

Whitney, F. (1983). The GMENAC report: An opportunity for nursing. In B.

Bullough, V. Bullough, & M. C. Soucup (Eds.), *Nursing issues and nursing strategies for the eighties* (pp. 138–155). New York: Springer Publishing.

Yankauer, A., Tripp, S., Andrews, P., & Connelly, J. P. (1972). The outcomes and service impact of a pediatric nurse practitioner training program—nurse practitioner training outcomes. *American Journal of Public Health, 62*, 347–353.

Chapter 11

Feminism and Nursing

Peggy L. Chinn
School of Nursing
University of Colorado Health Sciences Center

CONTENTS

Feminism is increasingly recognized as a valuable perspective for nursing practice, education, and scholarship. The nursing literature on feminism has developed from a relatively defensive posture favoring the value of a broad feminist perspective to a more substantive application of feminist tenets and methods. This review focuses on research and scholarly writings that relate feminism and nursing practice, nursing as a profession, and the development of nursing knowledge. Literature that addressed feminist nursing education, which was reviewed but not reported here, reflected analogous themes found in the literature selected for this report.

The works reviewed span the 22-year period from 1971 through 1993. Articles and books were selected based on the following criteria: (a) citations, when they were given, included major feminist works identified by this reviewer; (b) explicit reference to feminism or feminist ideas appeared in the text; and (c) identifiable content was discerned that reflected a feminist perspective. The works reviewed were identified by computer search of nursing periodical and general literature on feminism and nursing, and by direct perusal of major nursing journals.

Using the criteria listed previously limited this review in one important aspect. Increasingly, works appear in the nursing literature that are derived from a feminist perspective, but the author does not state this perspective explicitly and does not cite feminist literature. These works, which were not included in this review, reflect the fact that feminism consists not only of explicit theoretical and philosophic constructions, but also that feminism is a point of view, or a consciousness, not unlike viewpoints that are not feminist in nature, not stated explicitly, and, therefore, must be identified by the critical reader as implicit assumptions. An example of this type of literature is the book *Lesbian Health: What are the Issues*? (Stern, 1993). The substantive content of this publication addresses the needs of a largely invisible group of women, treats the issues and concerns of women as valid and important, and challenges existing stereotypes and assumptions and treatment of women by the dominant culture and medical establishment. These perspectives place the work clearly in the realm of feminism, yet the authors limited their citations to works related to their own substantive focus (i.e., lesbian health) and their feminist perspectives remain implicit rather than explicit.

The author acknowledges the influence of her own perspective favoring feminism, particularly in the selection of materials identified by direct perusal of the major nursing journals, in the selection of those works that are reported here, and in the interpretations made concerning the works reviewed. The criteria used for selection of relevant literature assisted in maintaining consistency in the selection process and in identifying literature as feminist when it was not indexed as such.

OVERVIEW OF FEMINIST PERSPECTIVES IN NURSING SCHOLARSHIP

In feminist scholarship, the viewpoint assumed by the author is of central importance, in that the viewpoint, or perspective, is recognized as forming the nature of knowledge, as well as the type of action or practice that emerges from what is assumed to be known. Feminist scholars typically state their own viewpoints explicitly so as to inform the reader of the foundation for the work reported. Critical analyses of other points of view form the basis for much of the philosophical and theoretical discourse found in feminist literature. Feminist nursing literature draws on many of the feminist perspectives identified by feminist scholars (Donovan, 1985; Tong, 1989); the most common views found are liberal feminism, cultural feminism, and critical social feminism.

Liberal feminism predominated the early nursing literature, in part due to the historical context of the time. The third president of the National Organization for Women (NOW), Wilma Scott Heide, was a nurse and political activist (Haney, 1985). Heide's article appearing in the *American Journal of Nursing* in 1973, published during her NOW presidency, reflected both the liberal feminist political activism of the decade and recognition that nurses and women were not receiving a fair shake in legal social and political arenas (Ashley, 1975; Heide, 1973; Miller & Mothner, 1978).

By the early 1980s the feminist nursing literature had grown to reflect diverse feminist views. Cultural feminism, which can also embrace ideas shared with radical, poststructural, and social feminism, celebrates rather than denigrates that which has been associated with being female in patriarchal cultures, and offers visions of transformation rooted in a concern for the social and psychological liberation of women that will ultimately benefit all (Donovan, 1985; Hoffman, 1991; Rutnam, 1991). The shift away from liberal feminism reflected growing realization that while legal and political equity for women is important, equity alone fails to adequately address the experiences of women, including women who are nurses. Theories of cultural oppression struck a powerful chord of recognition for nurse scholars during the 1980s (Ashley, 1980; Roberts, 1983). The transformations envisioned by cultural feminist writers reflected values and traditions that had long been part of nursing's ideology but were not treated with due respect in the mainstream cultural mores of the systems in which nurses lived and worked (Ashley, 1980; Cohen, 1993; Wheeler & Chinn, 1991).

Critical social feminism addresses fundamental social change and explanations of prevailing social forces, particularly class and gender, that sustain oppression (Allen, 1987; Bent, 1993; Campbell & Bunting, 1991; DeMarco, 1993), but shifts away from broad theoretical assumptions of women's universal experience. For example, the value of caring as theoretically good for all is challenged. The burden of caring, its social relegation to women's sphere, and the potential oppressive nature of caring for the one providing care are issues raised by a critical social feminist perspective (Allen, Allman, & Powers, 1991; Sherwin, 1989). Further, critical social feminism emphasizes grass-roots actions or strategies, usually empowerment strategies, that are required to bring about desired transformations (Bunting & Campbell, 1990; Carryer, 1992; Stevens, 1989).

Two other important perspectives, less emphasized but emerging in the nursing literature, are eco-feminism and poststructuralist feminism. Eco-feminism places the environment at the center of the analysis, recognizing that women and nature are abused by patriarchal dominance in parallel ways. Eco-feminism emphasizes strategies for change at the macro, political and global levels in contrast to the micro and individual levels stressed in other approaches to feminist action (Kleffel, 1991).

Poststructural feminism forms its critique around the limits of any attempt to structure human experience in intellectual theories, including theories constructed within feminism itself. From this perspective, the existence of oppressive social and political systems is sustained by unequal power relationships structured into theories of human behavior. Deconstructing embedded power relationships in existing theories and revealing avenues for resisting that which sustains the status quo is a key to moving toward liberation (Anderson, 1991a; Dickson, 1990; Doering, 1992).

APPROACHES TO KNOWLEDGE DEVELOPMENT

Just as perspective influences the nature of knowledge and the approaches used to develop knowledge, what is accepted as the knowledge of the discipline influences the practice of the discipline. Chinn's (1989) analysis of the fundamental tenets of nursing and feminism illustrates a typical feminist approach to bring together knowing and doing, thinking, and practice. Starting with an imaginary dream of a "healing house," Chinn developed an explanation of how the feminist tenet "the personal is political" and the nursing tenet "health is wholeness" merge to create the foundation for new directions in practice and research. As this review shows, feminist literature that addressed the development of nursing knowledge has been explicit in drawing links between how nursing knowledge is developed, the nature of that knowledge, and how nursing is practiced. The literature reviewed focused on two major concerns: (a) challenges to prevailing methods of science, and (b) the development of feminist approaches to nursing scholarship.

Challenges to Prevailing Methods of Science

The first works to challenge prevailing methods of nursing science from a feminist perspective appeared in 1985. Chinn's (1985a) critical analysis of myths that have surrounded the ideals of science revealed how prevailing ideals emerge from a male worldview and provided specific recommendations for nursing scholarship that are grounded in values derived from women's and nursing's perspectives. Duffy's (1985) analysis more specifically focused on the male bias that persists in research on women since 1970. Three areas of concern emerged from her analysis: the impact of male bias on the development of research on women, the politics of research in general, and feminist directives for research. Duffy's directives included a political commitment to conduct research leading to positive change for women, theoretical grounding in women's experience and in the assumption that multiple realities exist, and methods that consider context.

Meleis (1987) challenged directions in nursing knowledge development and called for a shift in nursing theory away from broad macrolevel theory, toward substantive midrange theory that is also gender and culture sensitive. Chinn (1987), in response to Meleis' article, affirmed Meleis's position but also presented an analysis that moved the idea of gender sensitivity in knowledge development to an explicit awareness of women's knowledge and experience and in developing nursing knowledge. Hagell (1989), using a sociological perspective, also based her argument concerning method on the premise that women's knowledge must be incorporated into nursing's approaches to knowledge development. In Hagell's analysis, knowledge development methods that incorporate women's knowledge account for context, subjectivity, and caring.

Three critical analyses of existing research in specific substantive areas not only exposed specific ways in which androcentric bias operates to influence the nature of knowledge development, but also substantiate the earlier, more general claim of Chinn (1985a), Duffy (1985), Meleis (1987), and Hagell (1989). Allen et al. (1991) using poststructuralist methods of deconstruction, revealed ways in which the assumption of sex and gender dichotomies in research actually reproduce damaging social relations based on gender. Their analysis showed how deconstructing the dichotomy of gender can lead to inclusion of diverse contemporary and historical forms of gendered existence, and complex cultural and political aspects of human experience.

Pohl and Boyd (1993) analyzed the nursing and feminist literature vis-à-vis aging women, finding that both bodies of literature, with few exceptions, essentially ignored aging and defined the central issues for women from the perspective of women of child-bearing age. Although Pohl and Boyd advocated in favor of each discipline taking steps to remedy distortions based on ageism, they also noted the unique position of nurse scholars to pursue issues of aging women and to contribute to the discourse on aging and women in the feminist literature, by virtue of nursing's direct involvement with aging women, experience with their lack of parity in the health care system, and the ability to conduct research on the important interface of aging and health.

The idea of noncompliance formed the basis for Wuest's (1993) critical analysis of research literature, exposing ethnocentric and androcentric biases in the literature. Wuest concluded that feminist interpretations of human behavior in research would create relationships of reciprocity and partnership, and would incorporate the values and personal, social and political factors that determine what the person views as possible and desirable.

Emergence of Feminist Approaches

Explanations of how research methods can be designed to reflect feminist values and perspectives build on the widely cited work of MacPherson (1983). MacPherson did not claim to present a "feminist method" for research but did specify values of advocacy for women that influence the choices that a researcher makes in selecting the research problem, implementation of the research methods, and interpretation of findings. Parker and McFarlane (1991) reported on their development of a feminist consortium model for nursing research that reflected the values and principles of feminist research previously outlined in the nursing literature by MacPherson (1983) and Duffy (1985). Likewise, Webb (1993) drew on MacPherson's (1983) work, exploring contrasting opinions and methods that attempt to reduce power inequalities, report women's experience in their own terms, offer a structural analysis of conditions of women's lives, and that include the role and influence of the researcher. Hall and Stevens (1991) addressed the issue of rigor in feminist research. They proposed the criteria of reflexivity, credibility, consensus, relevance, honesty and mutuality, naming, and relationality to discern rigor.

Thompson's (1991) report of her study of gender and culture with Khmer refugee women included her commentary on the development and implementation of a participatory feminist research method that reflected many of the aspects of method that Hall and Stevens (1991) proposed as criteria for rigor. An explicit contribution of Thompson's work is her commentary on the method, showing how it provided a form of scholarly work in which daily experience, practice, and research came together, thereby accounting for and incorporating complexity, context, knowing, and doing.

The issue of researcher-participant relationship figures prominently in all of the literature on feminist research methods, but two authors specifically addressed this relationship as a central concern. Connors (1988) reported a critical philosophical analysis of the nature of researcher-participant relationship in three contrasting published nursing studies, ranging from a distanced and objectified relationship to a relationship that moves toward equal parity that is consistent with feminist values. Moccia (1988) began with a critical analysis of the methods debate in nursing, developing the premise that choices of method in research are fundamentally choices through which researchers make and remake themselves as human beings in relationship with what or whom they study. Using a framework grounded in feminist philosophy, Moccia questioned the extent to which nurse researchers can adopt methods, or even debate methods that undermine human relationship and human dignity.

There is a strong influence of critical social theory in the development of feminist methods for both empirical and analytic or philosophic approaches to scholarship (Anderson, 1991b; Campbell & Bunting, 1991; Carryer, 1992; Stevens, 1989; Thompson, 1987). Approaches to both empirical databased research and analyses from a critical social tradition emphasize context in its broadest sense—physical environment, politics, social structures, cultures, values, power relationships at all levels, and social dynamics of oppression, liberation, and empowerment. In addition, feminist critical social theory brings to method an explicit political dimension of creating change in favor of women's well-being.

PROFESSIONAL ISSUES AND NURSING HISTORY

The scholarly literature on professional issues and nursing history is important for nursing practice in that it addressed nurses' ability to control practice, the knowledge needed for practice, and the values and trends that influence the conditions under which nurses practice. The scholarly methods used in this body of literature were predominantly feminist historiography and feminist critical analysis grounded in critical social feminist theory and philosophic methods of discourse, debate, and dialogue. Feminist methods of historiography and critical social analysis deliberately set about to expose gender inequities, social structures that maintain dominance, and to reveal that which is hidden from view by systematic and institutionalized structures that maintain the status quo.

Two important books addressing professional issues were published in the early 1980s. The widely cited book *Socialization, Sexism, and Stereotyping* (Muff, 1982) served as a catalyst for other feminist writings of the later 1980s and 1990s. In this edited volume the authors addressed issues of female development, career choice and nursing stereotypes, social and political issues, psychological issues, and specific examples of approaches used to move "out from under." Although most, but not all, of the contributors to this volume wrote explicitly from a feminist perspective, the book was conceived out of the editor's recognition of the frustration of being a woman in the male-dominated health care system and the prevalent paternalism of that system. Consistent with trends seen in the journal literature, a liberal feminist perspective predominated, although some authors reflected the emerging trend toward cultural feminism. Wilma Scott Heide, a contributor to the Muff book, also authored a book not widely distributed, titled *Feminism for the Health of It* (Heide, 1985). Based on her doctoral dissertation and her years of experience as a leading feminist activist throughout the 1970s, her research reflected her sharp-witted humor, her creative style in confronting inequities and injustices, and provides a model of activism and "future search" that spans individual and global concerns.

The literature related to professional issues from a feminist perspective addressed two main concerns: critical analysis of the existing health care system and approaches to empowerment for change and transformation. Nursing history viewed from a feminist perspective also reflected these two themes, but focused on historical data and scholarly analysis that revealed both inadequacies and strengths in the evolution of nursing.

Critical Analyses of the Existing Health Care System

Feminist critical analyses of the health care system focused on the central theme of patriarchal or masculinist values, actions, and world views that structure not only the system as a system, but also ways in which individuals experience the existing system. These analyses identified deep cultural and social values and structures that underlie the structure and function of the health care system.

Writing in the early 1980s, Ashley (1980), Connors (1980), and Lovell (1980, 1981) presented critical analyses of the health care system that drew on existentialist and radical feminist methods of critical discourse. The major theme of these writings is a critique of a patriarchally defined medical system that systematically exploits women as patients, wives, and nurses. Each of these authors acknowledged the root of patriarchal dominance and exploitation in the broader cultural contexts of philosophy, religion and scientific theories, and on historical evidence that illustrates long-standing and persistent practices of exploitation. These analyses identified the remedy as residing not in massive changes in medicine or health care but rather in nurses shifting loyalties to their own values of nursing. Lovell (1981) also stressed the importance of breaking the traditional silence of nurses in the face of exploitation and abuse, but in her work Lovell approached an analysis that included implications for social and political change.

Ten years later in the early 1990s, critical feminist analyses of the health care system assumed a broader social stance that was inclusive of structures of patriarchal systems in general, and the social structures that sustain distance between nursing and feminism. Watson (1990) focused her analysis on the moral failure of patriarchy and advocated social revolution grounded in valuing of women and women's work, specifically emphasizing caring associated with women and women's work. Valentine (1992), Keddy (1993), and Reverby (1993) addressed specific factors that sustain distance between nursing and feminism. They critiqued ways in which women in each group assume as true stereotypes reflected in public discourse about the other, and called for each group to take steps to understand the perspectives of the other.

Approaches to Empowerment and Liberation

The most prevalent theme found in feminist scholarship on nursing as a profession is that of overcoming the oppressive conditions of patriarchal structures, and in so doing identifying specific and reachable goals and approaches for righting the wrongs of oppression. Widely cited for its analysis of nursing as an oppressed group, Roberts (1983) presented a model to identify elements in patterns of oppression and behaviors that arise from that oppression. Roberts argued that once nurses recognized dynamics of oppression, liberating actions were possible, including grass-roots leadership, reclaiming nursing's culture and heritage, and engaging in dialogue with other nurses to develop consensus on values and priorities in nursing practice.

Greenleaf (1980), in her critical social analysis of nursing's sex-segregated occupational status, called for health policy change. Rather than advocating the superficial remedy of more men in nursing, Greenleaf's analysis showed the potential for broad social policy change that values work typically relegated to women. More recently Rutnam (1991) challenged the adequacy of equity as a principle for developing health policy and argued that policy needs to be developed from broad feminist criteria that bridge ethical, political, and scientific concerns for the benefit of women.

The image of the nurse in both the general public and in the women's movement was analyzed by Hughes (1980), Baer (1991), Gordon (1991), and Reverby (1993). Although these analyses offered broad suggestions for change in health policy and social relationships, other than the ideas of public and self-education, they fell short of offering specific avenues whereby nurses can bring about broad social and policy change, and they do not cite feminist literature that might guide action. The book *Peace and Power: A Handbook of Feminist Process* (Wheeler & Chinn, 1991) focused on actions that flow from feminist values. This analysis emerged from critical discourse and experience with women working in activist groups, research teams, and classrooms. The actions that flow from feminist values are viewed by the authors as fundamental to creating broader and more far-reaching social transformation.

Several authors reported philosophic and critical social analyses that identified fundamental links in the ideologies of nursing and feminism, despite a persistent shroud of resistance to feminist ideas in nursing. These authors proposed specific ways in which nursing practice and nursing knowledge could be transformed by embracing feminist tenets more fully (Bunting & Campbell 1990; Chinn, 1989; Chinn & Wheeler, 1985; Keddy, 1993; Mason, Backer, & Georges, 1991; Sohier, 1992; Valentine, 1992). Lovell (1980, 1981) traced the historical relationships between medicine and nursing, concluding that nurses need to question the nature of their ties with physicians, acknowledge exploitation and sexism in these ties, and move to what she called the most political act of seeing through deceptions and becoming free to think and act on behalf of ourselves and clients. Doering (1992) used a feminist poststructuralist analysis to reach similar conclusions concerning the power relations between medicine and nursing.

Allen (1987) using critical social analysis, and Hughes (1990) using historiography, reached similar conclusions concerning the efforts of nurses to achieve professional status. In each analysis, the ideal of professionalism is shown as failing to address and incorporate values and concerns that are central to the practice of nursing. Glazer (1991) analyzed job segmentation within nursing based on class and race and advocated emancipation as an alternative to equity to support working class women and women of color. In an extensive empirical study using interviews of unionized hospital workers, Sexton (1981) also addressed issues of job segmentation and advocated networking to overcome class divisiveness in nursing.

Relationships between nurses were addressed by Chinn and colleagues (Chinn, Wheeler, Roy, & Wheeler, 1987; Chinn, Wheeler, Roy, Berrey, & Madsen, 1988) using a survey of nurses' experiences of friendship developed from Raymond's (1986) philosophy of female friendship.

The results of the survey suggested that positive factors of friendship were related to personal and political empowerment. In a critical feminist examination of existing nursing research on mentoring, DeMarco (1993) addressed mentoring relationships among nurses. Her analysis revealed how existing research fails to incorporate women's experience, and race, class, or age diversity. Using a feminist framework of reciprocity, empowerment, and solidarity, DeMarco concluded that emancipative interests need to be incorporated into research on mentoring in order to move toward a model of mentoring that is in the interest of nurses and women.

Philosophic discourse and critical analyses of the concept of caring has generated several approaches to empowerment for nurses and nursing. The development of moral and ethical theory that incorporates caring is viewed by some authors as prerequisite to establishing the right and responsibility to determine how care is delivered (Huggins & Scalzi, 1988; Laing, 1993; Liaschenko, 1993; Reverby, 1987a; Sherwin, 1989). Watson (1990) made an explicit connection between her views on caring and feminism in a critical analysis of the moral failure of the patriarchy to value women and caring. Bevis (1993) and Moccia (1993), in critical philosophic analyses of the problems of giving care to the elderly, focused on nurses working proactively to create a different future for elder care. Bevis (1993) identified barriers to care as bureaucracy and profit, and power; moved to a proposal of empowerment that requires refusing to take the given as destiny; promoted empowerment and sharing, health, and healing as life projects; and embraced the power of friendship.

Feminist Perspectives on Nursing History

Three landmark books based on historical research examined the history of nursing from the mid-1800s through the mid-1990s (Ashley, 1976; Melosh, 1982; Reverby, 1987b). As Hughes (1990) noted, each of these important historical works offered contrasting explanations of the dilemma posed by the conflicting ideological assumptions of domesticity and of professionalism. Ashley (1976), drawing largely on evidence of the lives of nurse leaders and professional organizations and their conflicts with hospitals and medical organizations, identified gender as the issue underlying conflicts between nurses and the dominant cultures. Melosh (1982), drawing on evidence of the lives and records of working nurses, identified class as the underlying issue that disempowered nurses in forming a shared vision for nursing. Reverby (1987b) identified both gender and class as underlying issues, forming her arguments primarily around the mandate to care that is culturally assigned to both women and lower-class working people.

Less widely recognized but equally important historical works are focused on the experiences of Black women in nursing by Carnegie (1986) and Hine (1989). Drawing on extensive evidence typically overlooked from a white historian's perspective or from a male historian's perspective, each of these authors drew insightful pictures of the remarkable contributions of Black nurses in their work lives, despite the social conditions of their time. These authors presented compelling evidence of the need to account for race and class, as well as gender, if future research and practice is to reflect inclusiveness and diversity.

Several feminist studies of individual nurses in history provided strong counterevidence to damaging myths concerning nursing's history. The earliest feminist perspective on the life and work of Nightingale appeared in 1981 (Smith, 1981). In this interpretive work, the author identified four prevailing features of Nightingale's work that imply feminist motives: her resistance to the prescribed role for women of her class, her commitment to education for women and women entering the work force, her belief that women could make significant contributions to society, and her concept of social classlessness. Wheeler (1984), in response to the republication of Woodham-Smith's biography of Nightingale, cited evidence from the biography that contradicts demeaning Nightingale myths found in nursing and other literature and highlighted biographical evidence affirming the feminist nature of many of Nightingale's motives and beliefs.

Sarnecky (1993), based on her historical study of the life of Julia Catherine Stimson, offered a counterpoint to the fallacious judgment that nurses have made few and insignificant contributions to feminist causes. Sarnecky described the oppressive and paternalistic contexts in which Stimson lived and worked that were similar to those in which Nightingale worked—the upper-class Victorian home, the hospital, and the military. This study revealed significant ways in which Stimson resisted the oppressive conditions of these contexts and worked to create feminist alternatives. The life of early 20-century feminist Lavinia Dock was examined by Chinn (1985b) and Poslusny (1989). Chinn focused on Dock's feminist political activism as reflected in her writings in the *American Journal of Nursing*. Poslusny focused on the friendships among Dock and her contemporaries Robb and Nutting. In each analysis, the authors presented evidence of political and social action that resulted in remarkable contributions to social and individual health and well-being.

Accounts of feminist historical research focused on professional socialization and social conflict also contradict prevailing myths about nursings' heritage. Wheeler (1985) reported an analysis of the editorial position and content of the *American Journal of Nursing* during its first 20 years, 1900 to 1920. Contrary to popular belief that early nurse leaders were subservient and unknowledgeable, Wheeler presented evidence reflecting courageous and independent actions on behalf of nursing against incredible odds from a broad base of solidarity with the broader community of activist women of the time. Baer (1992) presented an interpretation that differs from that of Wheeler. In Baer's work, the focus shifts from evidence of the political activism of nurse leaders to the conflicts internal to nursing between nurse leaders and working class nurses that detracted from forming a unified vision and purpose.

Baer's (1992) work illustrates the difficult challenge of simultaneously incorporating the diverse experiences of women, accounting faithfully for the contexts and situations in which women live and work, and remaining an advocate for women. Baer accounted for a broad scope of social and contextual factors that influenced the work of nurse leaders and ordinary nurses and commended the efforts of both groups in working toward disparate goals and ideals. There remains, however, a recurring theme in Baer's work of victim blaming, in that despite her recognition of the social and economic pressures underlying divisiveness among nurses, Baer attributed nurses' lack of ability to overcome divisiveness to specific acts or omissions of nurse leaders who failed to articulate to staff nurses how difficult their positions were.

Dickson's (1993) historical analysis of nurse leaders' actions to establish nursing as a profession is an example of scholarly balance that avoids both victim blaming and idealization. Dickson focused on the social, economic, and political factors that influenced and motivated the choices that nurse leaders made over time. Dickson incorporated evidence that professionhood for nursing based on a male ideology does not gain the hoped-for consequences of greater social respect and standing for nurses and instead has the unintended consequence of divisiveness within nursing. Both the enabling and the constraining sides of the professional ideology advocated by nurse leaders are acknowledged, and the moral and practical basis for nursing's authority is recognized as deriving from its work culture.

In a study of both working nurses and nurse leaders who participated in World War I, Beeber (1990) acknowledged the beliefs held by nurse leaders that participating in war would benefit nurses and nursing and lead to greater economic and social status. Despite this hope, participation in war did not bring about lasting benefits for nurses and nursing, nor did it enhance the image of the nurse. From the accounts of the nurses who did participate, the benefits of nurses' participation in war grew out of their confrontation with contradictions between war and healing, confrontation with differentness, and from actions by nursing on its own behalf. Beeber concluded that processes of change come from nurses' own actions to challenge constricting structures and create a process of self-definition and differentiation.

The feminist nursing literature on professional issues and nursing history has developed predominantly using methods of historiography and critical discourse. These methods, explicitly developed from and applied with a feminist commitment to emancipatory interest, systematically challenge prevailing patriarchal assumptions about women, nurses, and the practice of nursing. The applications of the methods are generally sound and thorough, resulting in a body of literature that contains significant conclusions concerning empowerment and liberation in nursing.

NURSING PRACTICE AND FEMINISM

The literature that focused specifically on the implications of feminism for nursing practice was found in scholarly journals, not journals intended to reach practicing nurses. Therefore, the actual influence of feminist ideas on nursing practice remains obscure. Of the 26 articles identified and reviewed here, 19 presented critical analyses of concepts, theories, and other scholarly literature related to nursing practice; 7 reported completed research related to practice that were conducted using feminist perspectives and methods. This literature reflected three main themes: challenges to prevailing paradigms in practice, nurse-client defined health issues, and emancipatory actions.

Challenges to Prevailing Paradigms in Practice

A reprint of previous work by Jean Baker Miller and Ira Mothner (1978), published in *Nursing Digest*, was the earliest work published in the nursing literature related to practice. This critical review of prevailing mental health practice called for behavioral scientists and practitioners to redefine what is normal behavior and good mental health in light of experiences of inequality and subordination, particularly for women. Although not explicitly citing the Miller and Mothner work, Connors (1985) and White (1991) addressed concepts related to defining what is normal, sick, or abnormal behavior for women. Connors (1985) analyzed theories of the sick role, challenging the notion that sickness yields secondary gains for women and exposing the primary losses for women who have been socialized to view one another as enemies rather than friends, to internalize blame, and to be passive rather than politically involved. White (1991) focused her critical analysis on biomedical and psychiatric approaches to eating disorders. She concluded that these approaches are damaging to women and fail to account for the cultural, political, and social factors that influence disordered eating behavior. A feminist perspective, she argued, would stress a contextual approach, affirm a positive view of women and their bodies, use a broad spectrum of research methods, and apply the findings for social change.

Williams (1989) and Kleffel (1991) reported critical feminist analyses of health promotion and directions for change in health promotion concepts and practices. Williams (1989) examined assumptions grounding individualistic self-care theory and classical liberal political theory, concluding that health promotion may have more to do with the preconditions for self-care than with self-care itself. Williams demonstrated that a feminist perspective on health promotion requires connecting the social structure to individual health promotion behaviors and would reorient health promotion thinking and action. Based on her critical feminist analysis of existing concepts of the environment in nursing theories, Kleffel (1991) advocated a shift in nursing's consciousness that would place the environment at the center of health promotion activities and move the profession to social, political, economic, and global arenas as the focus for health promotion.

MacPherson's (1981, 1985, 1990) and Dickson's (1990) extensive critical analyses of menopause challenged the medicalization of menopause as a means of social control and proposed reconstructions of menopause grounded in women's experience. MacPherson's (1981, 1985) critical social analyses and clinical research emphasized the need for nurses to form alliances with the women's health movement, to form women's self-help groups to empower women to assume the role of menopausal experts, and to educate women about developmental processes of menopause and dangers of medical intervention. Dickson (1990) conducted a study comparing knowledge reflected in scientific/medical discourse about menopause and knowledge in everyday discourse of midlife women about menopause. In women's discourse she found different images of menopause, resistance to the manipulation of women's bodies, displacement of women's knowledge by scientific/medical knowledge, a cloak of silence surrounding women's discussion of menopause with other women, and recognition of deviation from the male norm (Dickson, 1990).

Sandelowski (1988), Shattuck and Schwarz (1991), and Hagell

(1993) addressed the medicalization of reproduction and reproductive technologies. In the most extensive of these analyses, Sandelowski (1988) reported her critical analysis of the paradigm conflict between nursing and reproductive technology and of nurses' uncritical acceptance of medical technology while maintaining hope of humanizing increasingly machine-oriented health care. She identified vision as the paradigmatic sensory modality and distance as the paradigmatic relation between caregiver and client in technological care. In contrast, in the nursing tradition, touch is the paradigmatic sensory modality and connection the paradigmatic relation. Sandelowski concluded that technology, therefore, challenges the foundation of nursing and requires critical examination as a modality for nursing practice.

Nurse–Client-Defined Health Issues

A broad scope of health issues is presented in the literature that reflect redefinitions and practices from a feminist perspective, particularly the feminist move to view women and their health beyond the narrow scope of women's reproduction. The health issues addressed include mothering (Lovell & Fiorino, 1979), women's inner strength (Rose, 1990), concepts of health (Campbell, 1980; Travis, Gresskey, & Crumpler, 1991), violence (Campbell, 1981; Noel & Yam, 1992), sexual harassment (Lucas, 1991), help seeking (Anderson, 1985), menstrual self-care (Patterson & Hale, 1985), obesity and weight control (Allan, 1988; White & Schroeder, 1986), compliance (Wuest 1993) and choice (Sandelowski, 1981). Although this literature challenged prevailing views and practices, the primary purpose of these writings was to present research findings or analytical models that have implications for nursing practice. A predominant variable in this literature is nurse-client interactions that foster mutual understanding of the health issue from the client's perspective. The analytical models that emerge from this literature are grounded in client perception and informed by knowledge of the client's social, cultural, and political context. Although women are not the only people affected by contexts, these authors were primarily concerned with women's experience in the health care system.

Sandelowski's (1981) text focused on nursing practice and knowledge from a feminist perspective. Far ahead of its time, in most respects this important book remains pertinent to nursing practiced in the 1990s. Written from the conviction of women's right to health and right to choose, Sandelowski presented a comprehensive critical review of menstruation, menopause, maternity, women's choices in achieving health, relationships among women, the women's health movement, women in nursing, major health issues for women, including the use of estrogens, violence against women, drug abuse, and nursing assessment of women.

The research literature focusing on nurse-client health defined issues is particularly notable for the consistency of findings that coincide with the analytical literature that challenges prevailing paradigms. In particular, research findings consistently documented the contradictions that exist between women's experience and perceptions, and that represented in the scientific/medical paradigm and prevailing cultural stereotypes (Allan, 1988; Anderson, 1985; Lovell & Fiorino, 1979; Patterson & Hale, 1985; Rose, 1990; White & Schroeder, 1986). Silence surrounding women's experience is either implied or explicit in each of these studies. The contexts that influence women's experience are clearly reflected by virtue of the use of research methods that are inclusive of contextual factors.

Emancipatory Actions

Emancipation is central to feminist perspectives, and is reflected in nursing literature as actions that lead to emancipation for nurses in practice, or for clients (Kendall, 1992; Malloy & Berkery, 1993; Sampselle, 1990; Thompson, 1991; Wiens, 1993). Sampselle (1990) and Thompson (1991) provided examples of practice grounded in feminist philosophy that is designed to challenge traditional attitudes and values, enables nurses to provide care to women that positively affects self-concept and sense of self-ownership, and enables women to become full partners in sexual, social and economic relationships. Kendall (1992) and Wiens (1993) presented models of emancipatory nursing actions that include critical awareness, unity and social activism, meaning and negotiation, and patient autonomy. Malloy and Berkery (1993) analyzed theories that pathologize relationship needs and offer an alternative "growth in connection" view in which relationship needs are seen as a strength and also dysfunction in relationships is recognized.

SUMMARY AND RECOMMENDATIONS

Taken as a whole, the scholarly literature on feminism and nursing is diverse in scope, and approach or method. In this diversity, there emerges a consistent pattern of themes that can be in part attributed to consistent feminist premises. The limited but growing research evidence that is reported suggests, however, that the consistency of themes is not solely attributable to the use of feminist perspectives, but to the validity of these perspectives in the felt and lived experiences of women.

Although this literature spans more than 30 years, the frequency of publications that reflect feminist perspectives has grown steadily from a scattered number of articles found in the 1970s, to frequent appearances of feminist writings in each publication cycle in the 1990s. The relative sophistication of the literature also grew over time, with the earlier works focusing on advocacy of a feminist consciousness in nursing, to more complex analyses and well-conceived research and theoretical development.

Along with the growing sophistication of the literature, greater diversity in feminist perspective is reflected. The major limitation in this literature is that it draws on a limited scope of feminist theory and knowledge that has proliferated in recent years. Understandably, much of the feminist literature that forms the foundation for nursing scholarship is that related to women's health and women's social role as caregivers. There is yet to emerge work that draws significantly on debates that abound in the feminist literature and that brings those debates into nursing discourse. For example, feminist literature is inclusive of a substantive discourse concerning caring and women's roles in caring. The nursing literature tends to reflect either the assumption that feminist perspectives eschew women's caring roles, or draws on literature that valorizes women's caring roles.

Factors, such as class, race, age, or sexual preference, as significant contextual factors are not adequately accounted for in feminist nursing scholarship. The perspective remains predominantly that of white, middle class, young or midlife heterosexual women. To their credit, nurse authors reflect awareness of the need for diversity, often integrate other perspectives than their own, and insist on accounting for social, cultural, and political variables. Actualizing this awareness seems much more difficult to accomplish and will probably emerge only when the authors themselves represent the same diversity that is advocated in principle.

Changes in social and cultural environments, and in the health care system, demand focused attention on the issues that are addressed in feminist nursing literature. The trends that are already evident in this literature are important to sustain in future feminist nursing scholarship, which include increased focus on substance, depth, and breadth of analysis grounded in deeper and more diverse feminist perspectives, and the development of approaches to scholarship that more fully achieve the ideals reflected in this literature. The most pressing need for the future remains in making the critical connection between the insights of scholarship and the realities of nursing practice. Only then will the visions and ideals of feminist scholars begin to be tested and actualized.

REFERENCES

Allan, J. D. (1988). Knowing what to weigh: Women's self-care activities related to weight. *Advances in Nursing Science, 11*(1), 47–60.

Allen, D. G. (1987). Professionalism, occupational segregation by gender and control of nursing. *Women and Politics, 6*(3), 1-24.

Allen, D. G., Allman, K. K., & Powers, P. A. (1991). Feminist nursing research without gender. *Advances in Nursing Science, 13*(3), 49–58.

Anderson, J. M. (1985). Perspectives on the health of immigrant women: A feminist analysis. *Advances in Nursing Science, 8*(1), 61–76.

Anderson, J. M. (1991a). Current directions in nursing research: Toward a poststructuralist and feminist epistemology. *The Canadian Journal of Nursing Research, 23*(3), 1-3.

Anderson, J. M. (1991b). Reflexivity in fieldwork: Toward a feminist epistemology. *Image: The Journal of Nursing Scholarship, 23*, 115–118.

Ashley, J. (1975). Nurses in American history: Nursing and early feminism. *American Journal of Nursing, 75*, 1465–1467.

Ashley, J. (1976). *Hospitals, paternalism, and the role of the nurse*. New York: Teachers College Press.

Ashley, J. (1980). Power in structured misogyny: Implications for the politics of care. *Advances in Nursing Science, 2*(3), 3-22.

Baer, E. D. (1991). Even her feminist friends see her as "only" a nurse. *International Nursing Review, 38*, 121.

Baer, E. D. (1992). American nursing: 100 years of conflicting ideas and ideals. *Journal of the New York State Nurses Association, 23*(3), 16–21.

Beeber, L. S. (1990). To be one of the boys: Aftershocks of the World War I nursing experience. *Advances in Nursing Science, 12*(4), 32–43.

Bent, K. N. (1993). Perspectives on critical and feminist theory in developing nursing praxis. *Journal of Professional Nursing, 9*, 296–303.

Bevis, E. O. (1993). A symphony of caring: Shared visions and eloquent futures for nursing education and practice. In M. Burke & S. Sherman (Eds.), *Gerontological nursing: Issues and opportunities for the twenty-first century* (Publication No. 14-2510, pp. 81-97). New York: National League for Nursing.

Bunting, S., & Campbell, J. C. (1990). Feminism and nursing: Historical perspectives. *Advances in Nursing Science, 12*(4), 11–24.

Campbell, J. (1980). The relationship of nursing and self-awareness. *Advances in Nursing Science, 2*(4), 15–25.

Campbell, J. (1981). Misogyny and homicide of women. *Advances in Nursing Science, 3*(2), 67–85.

Campbell, J. C., & Bunting, S. (1991). Voices and paradigms: Perspectives on critical and feminist theory in nursing. *Advances in Nursing Science, 13*(3), 1–15.

Carnegie, M. E. (1986). *The path we tread: Blacks in nursing, 1854–1984*. Philadelphia: Lippincott.

Carryer, J. (1992). A critical reconceptualization of the environment in nursing: Developing a new model. *Nursing Praxis in New Zealand, 7*(2), 9–14.

Chinn, P. L. (1985a). Debunking myths in nursing theory and research. *Image: The Journal of Nursing Scholarship, 17*, 45–49.

Chinn, P. L. (1985b). Historical roots: Female nurses and political action. *Journal of the New York State Nurses Association, 16*(2), 29–36.

Chinn, P. L. (1987). Response: Revision and passion. *Scholarly Inquiry for Nursing Practice, 1*, 21–24.

Chinn, P. L. (1989). Nursing patterns of knowing and feminist thought. *Nursing & Health Care, 10*, 71–75.

Chinn, P. L., & Wheeler, C. E. (1985). Feminism and nursing. *Nursing Outlook, 33*, 74–77.

Chinn, P. L., Wheeler, C. E., Roy, A., Berrey, E., & Madsen, C. (1988). Friends on friendship. *American Journal of Nursing, 88*, 1094–1096.

Chinn, P. L., Wheeler, C. E., Roy, A., & Wheeler, E. M. (1987). Just between friends. *American Journal of Nursing, 87*, 1456–1458.

Cohen, J. A. (1993). Caring perspectives in nursing education: Liberation, transformation and meaning. *Journal of Advanced Nursing, 18*, 621–626.

Connors, D. D. (1980). Sickness unto death: Medicine as mythic, necrophilic and iatrogenic. *Advances in Nursing Science, 2*(3), 39–51.

Connors, D. D. (1985). Women's "sickness": A case of secondary gains or primary losses. *Advances in Nursing Science, 7*(3), 1–17.

Connors, D. D. (1988). A continuum or researcher-participant relationships: An analysis and critique. *Advances in Nursing Science, 10*(4), 32–42.

DeMarco, R. (1993). Mentorship: A feminist critique of current research. *Journal of Advanced Nursing, 18*, 1242–1250.

Dickson, G. L. (1990). A feminist poststructuralist analysis of the knowledge of menopause. *Advances in Nursing Science, 12*(3), 15–31.

Dickson, G. L. (1993). The unintended consequences of a male professional ideology for the development of nursing education. *Advances in Nursing Science, 15*(3), 67–83.

Doering, L. (1992). Power and knowledge in nursing: A feminist poststructuralist view. *Advances in Nursing Science, 14*(4), 24–33.

Donovan, J. (1985). *Feminist theory: The intellectual traditions of American feminism*. New York: Ungar.

Duffy, M. E. (1985). A critique of research: A feminist perspective. *Health Care for Women International, 6*, 341–352.

Glazer, N. Y. (1991). "Between a rock and a hard place": Women's professional organizations in nursing and class, racial and ethnic inequalities. *Gender and Society, 5*, 351–372.

Gordon, S. (1991). Fear of caring: The feminist paradox. *American Journal of Nursing, 91*, 45–48.

Greenleaf, N. P. (1980). Sex-segregated occupations: Relevance for nursing. *Advances in Nursing Science, 2*(3), 23–37.

Hagell, E. I. (1989). Nursing knowledge: Women's knowledge. A sociological perspective. *Journal of Advanced Nursing, 14*, 226–233.

Hagell, E. I. (1993). Reproductive technologies and court-ordered obstetrical interventions: The need for a feminist voice in nursing. *Health Care for Women International, 14*, 77–86.

Hall, J. M., & Stevens, P. E. (1991). Rigor in feminist research. *Advances in Nursing Science, 13*(3), 16–29.

Haney, E. H. (1985). *A feminist legacy: The ethics of Wilma Scott Heide and company*. Buffalo: Margaretdaughters.

Heide, W. S. (1973). Nursing and women's liberation. *American Journal of Nursing, 73*, 824–827.

Heide, W. S. (1985). *Feminism for the health of it*. Buffalo: Margaretdaughters.

Hine, D. C. (1989). *Black women in white*. Bloomington, IN: Indiana University Press.

Hoffman, F. L. (1991). Feminism and nursing. *National Women's Studies Association Journal, 3*, 53–69.

Huggins, E., & Scalzi, C. (1988). Limitations and alternatives: Ethical practice theory in nursing. *Advances in Nursing Science, 10*(4), 43–47.

Hughes, L. (1980). The public image of the nurse. *Advances in Nursing Science, 2*(3), 55–72.

Hughes, L. (1990). Professionalizing domesticity: A synthesis of selected nursing historiography. *Advances in Nursing Science, 12*(4), 25–31.

Keddy, B. A. (1993). Dis-ease between nursing and feminism: Nurses caring for one another within a feminist framework. *Issues in Mental Health Nursing, 14*, 237–292.

Kendall, J. (1992). Fighting back: Promoting emancipatory nursing actions. *Advances in Nursing Science, 15*(2), 1–15.

Kleffel, D. (1991). Rethinking the environment as a domain of nursing knowledge. *Advances in Nursing Science, 14*(1), 40–51.

Laing, M. (1993). Gossip: Does it play a role in the socialization of nurses? *Image: The Journal of Nursing Scholarship, 25*, 37–43.

Liaschenko, J. (1993). Feminist ethics and cultural ethos: Revisiting a nursing debate. *Advances in Nursing Science, 15*(4), 71–81.

Lovell, M. C. (1980). The politics of medical deception: Challenging the trajectory of history. *Advances in Nursing Science, 2*(3), 73–86.

Lovell, M. C. (1981). Silent but perfect "partners": Medicine's use and abuse of women. *Advances in Nursing Science, 3*(2), 25–40.

Lovell, M. C., & Fiorino, D. (1979). Combating myth: A conceptual framework for analyzing the stress of motherhood. *Advances in Nursing Science, 1*(4), 75–84.

Lucas, J. (1991, autumn). Sexual harassment, current models of occupational health and safety and women. *Australian Feminist Studies, 13*, 59–70.

MacPherson, K. I. (1981). Menopause as disease: The social construction of a metaphor. *Advances in Nursing Science, 3*(2), 95–113.

MacPherson, K. I. (1983). Feminist methods: A new paradigm for nursing research. *Advances in Nursing Science, 5*(2), 17–25.

MacPherson, K. I. (1985). Osteoporosis and menopause: A feminist analysis of the social construction of a syndrome. *Advances in Nursing Science, 7*(4), 11–22.

MacPherson, K. I. (1990). Nurse-researchers respond to the medicalization of menopause. *Annals of the New York Academy of Science, 592*, 180–184.

Malloy, G. B., & Berkery, A. C. (1993). Codependency: A feminist perspective. *Journal of Psychosocial Nursing, 31*(4), 15–19.

Mason, D. J., Backer, B. A., & Georges, A. (1991). Toward a feminist model for the political empowerment of nurses. *Image, The Journal of Nursing Scholarship, 23*, 72–77.

Meleis, A. I. (1987). ReVisions in knowledge development: A passion for substance. *Scholarly Inquiry for Nursing Practice, 1*, 5–19.

Melosh, B. (1982). *The physician's hand*. Philadelphia: Temple University Press.

Miller, J. B., & Mothner, I. (1978). Psychological consequences of sexual inequality. *Nursing Digest, 6*, 27–31.

Moccia, P. (1988). A critique of compromise: Beyond the methods debate. *Advances in Nursing Science, 10*(4), 1–9.

Moccia, P. (1993). About anger and power. In M. Burke & S. Sherman (Eds.), *Gerontological nursing: Issues and opportunities for the twenty-first century* (Publication No. 14-2510, pp. 69–79). New York: National League for Nursing.

Muff, J. (Ed.). (1982). *Socialization, sexism, and stereotyping*. St. Louis: Mosby.

Noel, N. L., & Yam, M. (1992). Domestic violence: The pregnant battered woman. *Nursing Clinics of North America, 27*, 871–885.

Parker, B., & McFarlane, J. (1991). Feminist theory and nursing: An empowerment model for research. *Advances in Nursing Science, 13*(3), 59–67.

Patterson, E. T., & Hale, E. S. (1985). Making sure: Integrating menstrual care practices into activities of daily living. *Advances in Nursing Science, 7*(3), 18–31.

Pohl, J. M., & Boyd, C. J. (1993). Ageism within feminism. *Image: The Journal of Nursing Scholarship, 25*, 199–203.

Poslusny, C. M. (1989). Feminist friendship: Isabel Hampton Robb, Lavinia Lloyd Dock, and Mary Adelaide Nutting. *Image: The Journal of Nursing Scholarship, 21*, 64–68.

Raymond, J. (1986). *A passion for friends: Toward a philosophy of female affection*. Boston: Beacon Press.

Reverby, S. (1987a). A caring dilemma: Womanhood and nursing in historical perspective. *Nursing Research, 36*, 5–11.

Reverby, S. M. (1987b). *Ordered to care: The dilemma of American nursing, 1850–1945*. New York: Cambridge University Press.

Reverby, S. M. (1993). Other tales of the nursing-feminism connection. *Nursing & Health Care, 14*, 296–301.

Roberts, S. J. (1983). Oppressed group behavior: Implications for nursing. *Advances in Nursing Science, 5*(4), 21–30.

Rose, J. F. (1990). Psychologic health of women: A phenomenologic study of women's inner strength. *Advances in Nursing Science, 12*(2), 56–70.

Rutnam, R. (1991, summer). Is equity enough? Feminist perspectives on health technology assessment policy. *Australian Feminist Studies, 14*, 47–56.

Sampselle, C. M. (1990). The influence of feminist philosophy on nursing practice. *Image: The Journal of Nursing Scholarship, 22*, 243–247.

Sandelowski, M. (1981). *Women, health, and choice*. Englewood Cliffs, NJ: Prentice Hall.

Sandelowski, M. (1988). A case of conflicting paradigms: Nursing and reproductive technology. *Advances in Nursing Science, 10*(3), 35–45.

Sarnecky, M. T. (1993). Julia Catherine Stimson: Nurse and feminist. *Image: The Journal of Nursing Scholarship, 25*, 113–119.

Sexton, P. C. (1981). *The new Nightingales: Hospital workers, unions, new women's issues*. New York: Enquiry Press.

Shattuck, J. C., & Schwarz, K. K. (1991). Walking the line between feminism and infertility: Implications for nursing, medicine, and patient care. *Health Care for Women International, 12*, 331–339.

Sherwin, S. (1989). Ethics, feminism, and caring. *Queen's Quarterly, 96*(1), 3–13.

Smith, F. T. (1981). Florence Nightingale: Early feminist. *American Journal of Nursing, 81*, 1021–1024.

Sohier, R. (1992). Feminism and nursing knowledge: The power of the weak. *Nursing Outlook, 40*, 62–66, 93.

Stern, P. N. (1993). *Lesbian Health: What are the issues?* Bristol, PA: Taylor & Francis. (Reprinted from *Health Care for Women International, 1992, 13*.)

Stevens, P. E. (1989). A critical social reconceptualization of environment in nursing: Implications for methodology. *Advances in Nursing Science, 11*(4), 56–68.

Thompson, J. L. (1987). Critical scholarship: The critique of domination in nursing. *Advances in Nursing Science, 10*(1), 27–38.

Thompson, J. L. (1991). Exploring gender and culture with Khmer refugee women: Reflections on participatory feminist research. *Advances in Nursing Science, 13*(3), 30–48.

Tong, R. (1989). *Feminist thought: A comprehensive introduction*. Boulder: Westview Press.

Travis, C. B., Gressley, D. L., & Crumpler, C. A. (1991). Feminist contributions to health psychology. *Psychology of Women Quarterly, 15*, 557–566.

Valentine, P. (1992). Feminism: A four-letter word? *The Canadian Nurse, 88*(11), 20–23.

Watson, J. (1990). The moral failure of the patriarchy. *Nursing Outlook, 38*, 62–66.

Webb, C. (1993). Feminist research: Definitions, methodology, methods and evaluation. *Journal of Advanced Nursing, 18*, 416–423.

Wheeler, C. E. (1984). Viewpoint: Essay in response to republication of a biography. *Advances in Nursing Science, 6*(4), 74–79.

Wheeler, C. E. (1985). *The American Journal of Nursing* and the socialization of a profession, 1900–1920. *Advances in Nursing Science, 7*(2), 20–33.

Wheeler, C. E., & Chinn, P. L. (1991). *Peace and power: A handbook of feminist process* (3rd ed., Publication No. 15-2404). New York: National League for Nursing.

White, J. H., & Schroeder, M. A. (1986). Femininity, image, feminism and a decision to seek treatment in obese women. *Health Care for Women International, 7*, 455–467.

White, J. H. (1991). Feminism, eating, and mental health. *Advances in Nursing Science, 13*(3), 68–80.

Wiens, A. G. (1993). Patient autonomy in care: A theoretical framework for nursing. *Journal of Professional Nursing, 9*, 95–103.

Williams, D. M. (1989). Political theory and individualistic health promotion. *Advances in Nursing Science, 12*(1), 14–25.

Wuest, J. (1993). Removing the shackles: A feminist critique of noncompliance. *Nursing Outlook, 41*, 217–224.

PART V

Other Research

Chapter 12

Health Risk Behaviors for Hispanic Women

SARA TORRES
COLLEGE OF NURSING
UNIVERSITY OF NORTH CAROLINA AT CHARLOTTE

ANTONIA M. VILLARRUEL
SCHOOL OF NURSING
UNIVERSITY OF MICHIGAN

CONTENTS

This chapter contains an integrated review of health risk behavior research of Hispanic women. The goal is to synthesize the literature on selected health risk behaviors in Hispanic women and thus provide a knowledge base from which researchers and practitioners can draw to create strategies for improving health outcomes. The health risk behaviors addressed are adolescent pregnancy, sexually transmitted diseases (including AIDS), and substance abuse (alcohol, drugs, and cigarette smoking).

Research literature was abstracted by conducting on-line computer search of the CINAHL, AIDSLINE, MEDLINE, and PSYCHOLOGICAL ABSTRACTS databases. Each article was examined to determine if: (a) it was focused on risk behaviors related to adolescent pregnancy, sexually transmitted disease, or substance abuse; (b) it was a report of research; (c) Hispanic women were included in the sample; (d) results by gender and ethnicity were reported in the analysis; and (e) the research was conducted in the United States, or if conducted in Puerto Rico or Latin America, a comparable Hispanic sample in the United States was used. To ensure a review of current issues and problems on health risk behaviors in Hispanic women, research reports published prior to 1985 were excluded. From this examination, 83 research articles were determined appropriate for inclusion in this review.

A theoretical or conceptual base was reported in only 11% of the reviewed studies. Theories serving as conceptual frameworks included Kleinman's Explanatory Model (Flaskerud & Calvillo, 1991), Theory of Reasoned Action (Norris & Ford, 1992), stress and coping models (Nyamanthi, Leake, Flaskerud, Lewis, & Bennet, 1993), and acculturation models (Amaro, Whitaker, Coffman, & Heeren, 1990; Caetano, 1987; Cervantes, Gilbert, Snyder, & Padilla, 1990–1991; Hser, Anglin, & Liu, 1991; Markides, Ray, Stroup-Benham, & Trevino, 1990; Velez & Ungemack, 1989).

In most studies (90%) researchers employed descriptive, correlational, or nonexperimental comparative designs. Experimental designs (3%) and qualitative methodologies (7%), including focus groups and content analysis of open-ended interviews, were used less frequently. Secondary analyses of national surveys such as: the National Survey of Family Growth (NSFG), the National Center for Health Statistics (NCHS, 1990), the Hispanic Health and Nutrition Examination Survey (HHANES) (NCHS, 1985), the National Center for Health Statistics (NCHS, 1987) and the National Institute on Drug Abuse (NIDA, 1985) comprised 24% of studies reviewed.

Probability sampling was employed in only 24% of studies, with most (76%) using convenience samples. Schools, neighborhoods, and homes were the primary context for 63% of studies, whereas 37% were conducted in hospitals, treatment centers, and clinics. Excluding national surveys, most studies were conducted in the western states, primarily in California (47%); fewer studies were conducted in the Southwest (16%), Midwest (1%), Northeast (14%), or Southeast (2%).

Excluding national studies, sample sizes in the studies varied widely: 5% had fewer than 15 subjects; 8% had 16 to 29 subjects each; 18% had 30 to 59 subjects; 12% had 60 to 99 subjects; and 57% had over 100 subjects identified as Hispanic women. Descriptive statistics were used in 62% of studies and inferential statistics in 38% of studies. About 8% of the articles were published in nursing journals.

Since cultural relevance of study design is a critical component in determining the scientific merit of research on culturally diverse groups, conceptual and methodological issues critical to studying Hispanics (Marin & Marin, 1991; Porter & Villarruel, 1993) were assessed. Across the studies, the majority of subjects were Mexican-American (70%), whereas Puerto Rican (14%), Central and South American (17%), and Cuban (9%) subjects were studied less frequently. Hispanic subgroups were not identified in 25% of studies. The small and disproportionate numbers of different Hispanic subgroups and the failure to report specific subgroups precluded drawing conclusions for subgroups in most studies.

The level of acculturation of subjects, typically defined as the various degrees of changes in Hispanics' cultural orientation which result from adaptation to U.S. society, was reported in only 47% of studies. Social class was reported in 55% of the studies, of these, 52% were primarily low-income subjects, and 3% were middle-income subjects. No study included high-income-level Hispanic women. Interviews and instruments were available in English and Spanish in 57% of studies, whereas 10% of studies were conducted in English only. The language for the instruments and interview was not reported in the remaining studies. The unequal attention paid to the cultural relevancy of conceptual and methodological issues across studies suggests that biases may exist in the current state of knowledge development on risk behaviors of Hispanic women.

Findings on health risk behaviors, prevalence, and associated risk factors of adolescent pregnancy, sexually transmitted diseases, and substance abuse in Hispanic women cannot be generalized to all Hispanic subgroups. Thus, an effort has been made to identity specific Hispanic subgroups when possible. The words "Hispanic" and "Latina" are used interchangeably throughout this chapter. The review in each area begins with an overview of incidence and prevalence data. Major themes and patterns emerging from research on adolescent pregnancy, sexually transmitted diseases and substance abuse then are summarized. The state of knowledge development in these areas is presented and recommendations for future research efforts are suggested.

PREGNANCY AMONG HISPANIC ADOLESCENTS

Prevalence of Adolescent Pregnancy

The incidence of live births to Hispanic adolescents is greater than that of the general population. In 1988 live births to Hispanic women under the age of 20 were 16.4% compared to 9.7% among non-Hispanic white and 22.9% among non-Hispanic black women. Further analysis of birth rates by Hispanic subgroup indicated that the prevalence of births to adolescent mothers is highest among Puerto Rican (21.4%) and Mexican-American (17.3%) populations and lowest among Cuban (6.1%) and Central and South American (8.1%) populations (NCHS, 1990). It is important to note that in 1988 only 30 states and the District of Columbia included a Hispanic-origin item on birth certificates, and not all states required identification of Hispanic subgroups. Although it is estimated that approximately 95% of the Hispanic population resided in the areas that require identification, the limitations of this data set should be recognized.

Trends in adolescent pregnancy and age-specific birth rates among Hispanic subgroups were reported by Pletsch (1990) in a secondary analysis of the HHANES. In comparison with Puerto Rican adolescents ($n = 300$) in New York, and Cuban adolescents ($n = 85$) in Miami, Mexican-American adolescents ($n = 638$) had the shortest mean-person months of fertility (40.4 months), the highest use of oral contraceptives (14.5%), and the highest proportion (10%) of those ever married. Mexican-Americans were comparable with Puerto Rican adolescents in being reported as ever pregnant, 14.1% and 14.6%, respectively. Mexican-Americans had the lowest number of miscarriages (14/1000) and the highest number of live births (141/1000) among the three Hispanic subgroups, however, Cuban-Americans were the group least likely to use oral contraceptives (6.5%) but had the lowest reports of pregnancy (4.4%) and number of live births (37/1000). Although Puerto Rican adolescents had the highest percentage living in poverty (59.5%), and the longest mean-person months of fertility (46.1 months), they had the lowest percentage (4.1%) of adolescents who were ever married. Results from this study clearly depict intracultural variation among Hispanic adolescents in socioeconomic status, contraceptive behavior, and birth outcomes.

Studies conducted with Mexican-American adolescents provided additional support to the findings of the HHANES. In primarily regional studies conducted with nonprobability samples, Mexican-American adolescents were more likely to be married prior to conceiving or prior to delivery (Smith, McGill, & Wait, 1987; De Anda, Becerra, & Fielder, 1988), more likely to give birth (De Anda et al., 1988; Aneshensel, Becerra, Fielder, & Schuler, 1990) and more likely to use birth control measures after they were married or had given birth (Darabi & Ortiz, 1987; De Anda et al., 1988; Felice, Shragg, James, & Hollingsworth, 1987). Further, low and inconsistent rates of contraceptive use among Mexican-American adolescents have been reported (Padilla & Baird, 1991; Wiemann & Berenson, 1993). From these findings a pattern of Mexican-American adolescent fertility is suggested; however this pattern cannot be generalized to other Hispanic subgroups. No studies were found specifically related to the contraceptive use, pregnancy rates, or birth outcomes of Puerto Rican, Cuban, or Central and South American adolescents.

In addition to variation in fertility patterns between Hispanic adolescents, variation within Hispanic subgroups has been suggested. Acculturation and generational distance, for example, are variables that have been proposed as affecting the early initiation of sexual intercourse among Mexican-American adolescents (Reynoso, Felice, & Schragg, 1993) and the greater number of premarital births among Hispanic adolescents (Aneshensel et al. 1990; Darabi & Ortiz, 1987). Despite the importance of these indicators of Hispanic ethnicity, few studies, including national data sets, have adequately included these variables in research.

Knowledge and Attitudes About Sexuality, Contraceptive Use, Pregnancy, and Motherhood

Low levels of knowledge among Hispanic adolescents related to sexuality and contraceptive use consistently have been reported (Moore & Erickson, 1985; Scott, Shifman, Orr, Owen, & Fawcett, 1988; Smith et al., 1987; Padilla & Baird, 1991). In a study that examined sexual knowledge of primiparous, pregnant, and postpartum adolescents, Smith et al. (1987) reported that Hispanic subjects had lower scores on items related to knowledge of the menstrual cycle than African-American or white adolescents. In another study, sexual and contraceptive knowledge scores were lower among Hispanic adolescent males and females as compared with Euro-, African- and Asian-American adolescents (Moore & Erickson, 1985). Similarly, Mexican-American adolescents correctly answered an average of only 33% of items related to sexual knowledge (Padilla & Baird, 1991). While no differences in knowledge scores were reported in this study among gender, age, or whether sexual activity had been initiated, females reported they had more knowledge of specific birth control methods than did males.

Only a few researchers examined the sources of contraceptive or sexual knowledge and the relationship between knowledge and sexual behavior. In one study (Moore & Erickson, 1985) no differences were found among adolescent groups in regard to communication about sexual and contraceptive issues among same-sex parents and friends. However De Anda et al. (1988), reported that Mexican-American adolescents who were or had been pregnant indicated they had received no instruction from their mothers about sexual behavior or the use of birth control measures. Knowledge about birth control was reportedly learned during prenatal visits and nearly 100% of subjects indicated they intended to use some form of birth control following delivery. While these researchers used nonprobability samples, similar findings across studies point to the necessity of providing culturally relevant and accessible sex and contraceptive teaching programs. Further, the relationship between level of sexual and contraceptive knowledge and behaviors needs to be explored.

Attitudes about child bearing, motherhood, and contraceptive use have been explored by several researchers. Further, a number of cultural tenets often deemed as characteristic of Hispanic subgroups, such as the importance of religion, gender role differentiation, familism or familial obligation have been linked with attitudes, sexual behaviors, and fertility patterns of Hispanic adolescents. For example, the importance of religion as conceptualized by religious practice and belief, church attendance, and valuing religion has been associated with less permissive attitudes about sex, limited sexual experience, and exerting protective behaviors in contraceptive use and pregnancy prevention (DuRant, Pendergrast, & Seymore, 1990; Scott et al., 1988). Similarly, among Hispanic adolescents familism and gender-role differentiation, which are components of the cultural imperative to be a mother, have been associated with (a) positive views of pregnancy and childbearing (De Anda et al.,1988; Moore & Erickson, 1985; Padilla & Baird, 1991; Smith et al., 1987; Russell, Williams, Farr, Schwab, & Plattsmier, 1993; Speraw, 1987); (b) low contraceptive use (Hodges, Leavy, Swift, & Gold, 1992); (c) higher pregnancy, birth, and marriage rates (Smith et al., 1987), and (d) supportive relationships with the baby's father and mother's family of origin (De Anda et al., 1988). The importance of the family, a component of familism, has also been associated with an increased likelihood of contraceptive use (DuRant et al., 1990). Other factors included the limited influence of peers in relation to decisions about sexual behavior (Christopher, Johnson, & Roosa, 1993; Padilla & Baird, 1991); and support, specifically for Puerto Rican adolescents to carry or terminate pregnancies (Berger et al., 1991; Ortiz & Vazquez-Nutall, 1987). Although it has been postulated that these norms are more predominant in Mexican Americans, the inter- and intra-cultural values of Hispanic subgroups and their relationship with sexual behavior of adolescents have not been studied or compared.

These studies support the link between cultural tenets and sexual behaviors of adolescents. However, existing cultural stereotypes, including rigid gender-role differentiation and strict adherence to Catholicism (which were the basis for interpreting findings of many of these studies), have been challenged for their accuracy (Amaro, 1988; Comas-Diaz, 1988; Darabi, Dryfoos, & Schwartz, 1985; Vazquez-Nutall, Romero-Garcia, & DeLeon, 1987) and criticized for the prevalent androcentric biases (Andrade, 1982, Cromwell & Ruiz, 1979). Thus there is need to accurately and systematically identify and describe cultural beliefs and their relation to: sexual behaviors, contraceptive use, birth outcomes, and the influence of peer and group norms.

Sexual and Contraceptive Behavior

Although few studies were found in which sexual behavior or patterns of intimacy were examined, beginning descriptions of sexual behavior among Hispanic adolescents have been provided. Years of dating were different among the five Hispanic subgroups. Data obtained from Hispanic adolescents from the NSFG indicated that although longer periods of dating were associated with sexual intercourse, no significant differences were found among groups in percentage of females who had engaged in sexual intercourse (DuRant et al. 1990). In a study which compared Hispanic and non-Hispanic white women's sexual activity, Mexican-American female adolescents were found to delay sexual activity longer from the time of onset of dating than non-Hispanic white groups (De Anda et al., 1988). Similarly, findings from a study in which sexual behaviors of a primarily Mexican-American sample of sixth through eighth graders were examined, lower percentages of girls than boys had indicated ever engaging in intercourse (Christopher et al., 1993). Among girls, more pronounced engagement in precoital behaviors was evident between sixth and seventh grades with kissing as the most frequent activity reported, and petting or fondling as the least frequent activity reported. In a related study, the presence of a biological factor, low self-esteem, and increased religious attendance were factors identified as influencing decisions to engage in intercourse for young Hispanic girls (Day, 1992). Despite a beginning profile of sexual behaviors among Hispanic adolescents, more extensive studies that describe intimate sexual behaviors of Hispanic preadolescents and adolescents, and the cultural norms that affect these behaviors are needed.

Few investigators examined the relationship of attitudes, values, or sociodemographic characteristics on sexual or contraceptive behavior of Hispanic adolescents, however, low contraceptive use by Hispanic adolescents consistently has been reported. Norris and Ford (1992) reported that only 50% of sexually active Hispanic females reported thinking about using condoms, in comparison to 95% to 100% of Hispanic males and African-American adolescents. Further, similarities in the intention to use and actual use of condoms were reported in both ethnic groups. In another study, Hispanics were the group least likely to continue oral contraceptive use or to return for follow-up clinic counseling or follow-up (Wiemann & Berenson, 1993). Similarly, findings from a secondary analysis of the National Adolescent Student Health Survey (Hodges et al., 1992) suggested that eighth and tenth grade Hispanic females were less likely than Euro-, African-, or Asian-American adolescents to support condom use. However, it was not possible to discern, within the context of this study, factors that contributed to the difference in attitudes among the groups of adolescents. Finally, in a secondary analysis of the NSFG, DuRant, Seymore, Pendergrast, and Beckman (1990) found that 7 variables (e.g., lower frequency of intercourse, older postmenarchal age, fewer years of dating, low attendance at church, and never experiencing a pregnancy scare) accounted for 61.8% of the variance in low contraceptive use by sexually active Hispanic adolescents. A finding of interest in this study was the association of social stability (church attendance, good communication with parents, enrollment in school) with low contraceptive use. The researchers suggested that because sexual values were not consistent with sexual behaviors, Hispanic adolescents were less likely to use effective birth control. Although values related to childbearing were not measured in this study, additional studies to explore the relationship between attitudes, values, and sexual and contraceptive behavior are warranted. Similarly, the examination of correlates of sexual and contraceptive behavior, including self-esteem, pubertal and hormonal development, peer, family, school, and community influences, has not been adequately studied. Future research in these areas would be an important contribution to existing knowledge in the area of Hispanic adolescent pregnancy.

AIDS

Prevalence of AIDS Among Hispanic Women

The incidence of AIDS in the United States, except in the District of Columbia and states bordering Mexico, was higher among Hispanics than for non-Hispanic Whites, and highest among U.S. born Hispanics (Diaz, Buehler, Castro, & Ward, 1993) and Hispanics residing in the Northeast and Puerto Rico (Diaz et al., 1993). Regional and national studies have suggested that African American and Hispanic women are at greater risk than Whites for contracting AIDS and the investigators predict higher increases of AIDS among these groups of women (Capell et al., 1992; Gayle, Selik, & Chu, 1990; Smith, McGraw, Crawford, Costa, & McKinlay, 1993; Sabogal, Faigeles, & Catania, 1993). Intravenous (IV) drug use or heterosexual contact with intravenous drug users (IVDU) were the primary modes of transmission for the majority of AIDS cases (81%) among Hispanic women. Transmission by Hispanic women of AIDS to others occurs through heterosexual contact in 37% of cases (NCHS, 1990). The rate of AIDS by heterosexual contact is similar to the rate for African American women and is 11 times higher than for Euro-American women (Holmes, Karon, & Kreiss, 1990).

Diversity in AIDS trends among female Hispanic subgroups has been noted. For example, in a study that analyzed AIDS cases in the United States and Puerto Rico that were reported to the Center for Disease Control between 1988 and 1991, IVDU was the predominant mode of exposure for U.S. and Puerto Rican born women. Sexual intercourse with an IVDU was the predominant mode of exposure for women born in South America and Puerto-Rico. Sexual intercourse with an HIV positive man (whose mode of exposure was unknown) was the primary mode of exposure among Central American, Cuban and Mexican born women. Finally, blood transfusion was reported by 34% of Mexican born women who had contracted AIDS (Diaz et al., 1993). The diversity among Hispanic women in relation to the prevalence and primary modes of transmission of AIDS is an important consideration in the design of effective prevention and treatment efforts and planning future studies.

Knowledge and Attitudes about AIDS and Condom Use

Most studies about AIDS and Hispanic women focused on AIDS-related knowledge and the relationship between attitudes about AIDS and condom use. Investigators that examined AIDS knowledge among Hispanics have consistently reported that, while Hispanics have a basic knowledge about AIDS (i.e., AIDS is a virus; it can be acquired through sexual contact), Hispanics also are more likely to hold beliefs that AIDS can be transmitted through casual contact (Aruffo, Coverdale, & Valbona, 1991; Flaskerud & Calvillo, 1991; Flaskerud & Uman, 1993; Marin & Marin, 1992a; Nyamanthi, Bennett, Leake, Lewis, & Flaskerud, 1993). Although gender differences in AIDS knowledge were not significant (Aruffo et al., 1991; Marin & Marin, 1992a), low acculturation levels were found to be significant predictors of less and incorrect knowledge about transmission of AIDS for both Hispanic men and women (Nyamanthi, Bennett, et al., 1993, Marin & Marin, 1992a; Flaskerud & Uman, 1993). Further, beliefs about AIDS transmission, both true and erroneous, have been found to be congruent with professional and traditional beliefs about health and illness (Flaskerud & Calvillo, 1991). Traditional beliefs held by a sample of low-income Latina women were related to causes of AIDS and selected treatments including contact with impurities, imbalance, and religious beliefs. The relationship of traditional beliefs about health and illness to beliefs about AIDS did not distinguish between Spanish and indigenous beliefs and did not account for the diversity within Hispanic culture. Flaskerud and Calvillo's findings (1991) suggest a necessity to tailor health education programs to address both professional and lay beliefs about AIDS.

The relationship between knowledge of AIDS and attitudes and beliefs about condom usage has been explored. A consistent conclusion in the studies is that women who are only partially acculturated are at greater risk of contracting AIDS because they (a) have limited knowledge of AIDS (Berger, Rivera, Perez, & Fierman, 1993; Nyamanthi et al., 1993); (b) retain specific cultural values which adversely affect condom use (Marin & Marin, 1992a; Mikawa et al., 1992; Ortiz & Casas, 1990; Rapkin & Erickson, 1990) and (c) despite limited engagement in risky behavior, their partners' behavior places them at greater risk (Flaskerud & Nyamanthi, 1989; Rapkin & Erickson, 1990; Sabogal et al., 1993). From studies in which cultural values and condom usage have been explored, low condom usage has been associated with discomfort in talking about AIDS and embarrassment in buying or asking partners to use condoms (Flaskerud & Nyamanthi, 1989; Mikawa et al., 1992; Marin & Marin, 1992b; Ortiz & Casas, 1990). Findings from these studies suggested that low acculturated women maintain aspects of traditional male-female roles, therefore, they are less likely to have access to condoms and they have limited ability to negotiate condom use with their partners because the use of condoms is viewed as a male prerogative. On the other hand, an obligation to protect women is another part of the machismo or traditional male role. This aspect can be viewed as a factor that could be used to promote condom use.

Contrary to findings from other studies, Kline, Kline, and Oken (1992) reported that a lack of power in relationships and economic dependence on men was not a major factor that led to risk-taking behavior in a predominantly Puerto Rican sample of women. Decisions to use condoms were influenced by the women's HIV status, the intimacy of the relationship with the partner, and a personal sense of responsibility. Although Hispanic women had perceptions of their partners not wanting to use condoms, women used abstinence and incorporated cultural values to negotiate safer sexual practices. Clearly, the role of Hispanic cultural patterns in both supporting and deterring health-promoting behaviors has been demonstrated in these studies. More and better designed studies about the influence of cultural patterns on sexual behaviors are needed. Strategies for women that are independent of men's behavior and emphasize cultural values (to support safer sexual behaviors) are important factors in the development of culturally relevant health promoting strategies.

There are a few intervention studies related to AIDS prevention in Hispanic women. In one such study, the effects of a didactic AIDS education program on low income African American and Latina women were examined (Flaskerud & Nyamanthi, 1990). Significant improvements were found in knowledge and attitudes post intervention, but only knowledge scores remained at the higher level at retest. Differences in sexual and drug use practices were evident and approached significance in pretest to posttest, and retest scores. Nyamanthi et al. (1993) compared the effectiveness of two programs: the control condition consisted of a traditional teaching program focused on AIDS education and community resources alone and the experimental program focused on improving risk reduction skills and enhancing self-esteem and coping skills. While significant improvements on post test knowledge scores, risk-taking activities, and emotion-focused coping were found, problem-focused coping did not change over time. Both programs provided effective interventions for Latina women and it was postulated that the culturally sensitive components employed in both programs may have been sufficient to reduce high-risk activities. Further, the researchers suggested that women in the experimental group may have been able to more accurately evaluate risk for HIV, thus the group served more as a stressor. Additional studies that systematically examine interventions directed toward reducing the risk of AIDS in Hispanic women are in order.

OTHER SEXUALLY TRANSMITTED DISEASES

Only two studies were found on sexually transmitted diseases other than AIDS among female Hispanics. Schilling, El-Bassel, Gilbert, and Schinke (1991) conducted a study in New York City with a randomly selected sample of African-American and Hispanic women from methadone clinics. Puerto Rican women comprised 96.6% of the Hispanic segment of the sample. Hispanic respondents agreed more strongly than their African-American counterparts that getting AIDS depended on luck, felt that it was more embarrassing to talk about sex with their sexual partners, and believed more strongly that their sexual partners would become upset at any change in their sexual practices. Even though the sample size was small this study had the possibility of adding to the knowledge of sexually transmitted diseases in Hispanic women.

The extent and correlates of infection with herpes simples virus type 1 (HSV-1) and type 2 (HSV-2) in an inner-city community with a representative cross-sectional sample of unmarried Euro-, African-, and Hispanic American adults of which 119 were Hispanic women were examined by Siegel, Golden, Washington, Morse, Fullilove, Catania, Marin, and Hulley (1992). Hispanic women were at higher risk than were white women for HSV-1 (84% vs. 43%) and HSV-2 (39% vs. 35%) infection and Hispanic women born within the United States were more likely to be HSV-1 positive (91% vs. 68% for women) than immigrants. The limitation of this study is that the identity of the Hispanic subgroup is not given, therefore, applicability is limited.

These studies indicated that Hispanic women have a higher incidence of non-AIDS sexually transmitted diseases compared to white women. However, there are very few studies in this area where Hispanic women are included. Additional studies examining sexual behaviors and other sexually transmitted diseases other than AIDS on Hispanic women are essential in order to develop interventions and prevention strategies in this area.

ALCOHOL USE

Prevalence of Alcohol Use in Hispanic Women

The prevalence of alcohol use is lower among Hispanic females than among non-Hispanic females. The National Household Survey of Drug Abuse (NIDA, 1987) estimated that Hispanic females have lower lifetime alcohol use rates (62.9%) than Euro-American women (85.6%). This pattern of use was consistent with the reported current use of alcohol. A smaller percentage of Hispanic females (35.2%) reported drinking in the month prior to the survey compared to Euro-American (54.7%) or African-American females (39.2%). The HHANES (NCHS 1985), which surveyed Mexican Americans, Puerto Ricans and Cubans, found that the vast majority of Hispanic women who drank alcoholic beverages, regardless of ethnicity, reported being light drinkers, with 17% to 24% of women in each subgroup reporting light drinking, no more than 7% moderate drinking, and 2% or less heavy drinking. However, variation in drinking patterns exists across Hispanic subgroups. The highest rates of abstention were found among foreign-born Central and South American (75%), followed by Mexican (71%), Cuban (48%), and Puerto Rican (45%) women (Caetano, 1987). Less frequent (less than once a month) but heavier drinking (five or more drinks per occasion) was most prevalent among Puerto Rican females (29%).

These studies suggested that in general, Hispanic women drink less than their Anglo counterparts but that patterns of heavier drinking exist among certain subgroups of Hispanics with Puerto Ricans being the heaviest drinkers. However, the question can be raised if this variation in drinking actually exists between subgroups or rather can be attributed to the widely discrepant assessment measures used between different studies. Further studies using consistent measures of alcohol use are needed.

Research indicates that Hispanic adult males have a much greater tendency to drink and to drink more heavily than Hispanic females (Cervantes et al., 1990–1991; Corbett, Mora, & Ames, 1991; Gilbert, 1987). This has been demonstrated for Hispanics in general and the Mexican subgroup in particular. Cervantes et al. (1990–1991) found that immigrant and Mexican-U.S.-born women were less likely to be heavy drinkers than their male counterparts or to expect that alcohol consumption would enhance social acceptance, enhance relationships, make sex more enjoyable, and make it easier to talk with others.

The pattern of alcohol use in Hispanic women also has been found to differ by acculturation level and generational status. The acculturation model predicts that alcohol consumption patterns of Hispanics will reflect the extent to which the drinking norms and practices of the larger society have been adopted. The relationship between acculturation and drinking is stronger among women than men (Caetano, 1987; Markides et al., 1990). Support for the acculturation model has been found in several studies (Caetano, 1987; Markides et al., 1990). In studies by Caetano (1987), Cervantes et al. (1990–1991), and Fernandez-Pol, Bluestone, Missouri, Morales, Mizruchi (1986), the more acculturated Hispanic women were more likely than less acculturated Hispanic women to drink alcohol, hold more liberal drinking views, and endorse a greater number of acceptable reasons for drinking. In the generations following immigration, women have been found to move from abstention and infrequent drinking to moderate drinking levels (Cervantes et al., 1990–1991). Data obtained in a national survey showed that very infrequent drinking (less than once a month but at least once a year) still was common among the second-generation females born in the United States

(48%) as well as among Cuban females (35%). Women and older people were found to drink less frequently and consume less alcohol than men, middle-aged and younger people (Markides et al., 1990).

Studies on the relationship between acculturation and alcohol use by Hispanic women lend strong support for the acculturation model and provide a good foundation for further studies. However, all but one of the studies on acculturation and generational status were conducted on the Mexican population. Further research to explore the relationship between generational status, and acculturation on other Hispanic ethnic groups would be an important contribution to existing knowledge in this area.

Psychological Factors Related to Alcohol Use

Three studies were found that examined psychological factors and alcohol use by Hispanic women. One study examined the relationship of hostility to alcohol consumption in a convenience sample of Mexicans (Lee, Leon, & Markides, 1988). Results indicated that among females, hostility was moderately related to the frequency and volume of alcohol consumed. Two studies examined depressive symptoms and the use of alcohol in Mexican women. Golding, Burnam, and Wells (1990) found that Mexican women who drank in heavier quantities or those who abstained were both more likely to report depression. Also, depressed Mexican-American men reported drinking to forget worries, relieve tension, and have more confidence, while depressed Mexican-American women drank to reduce stress. In contrast, Cervantes et al. (1990–1991) found no correlation between depression and alcohol use among Mexican women. While depression was not predictive of drinking level among women, it was for men.

Thus, there are conflicting reports on the relationship between psychological factors and alcohol use by Hispanic women. However, strong conclusions cannot be drawn on the basis of three studies. A limitation of the studies is that all were conducted with a Mexican population and thus cannot be generalized to other Hispanic subgroups. Further studies on the psychological effects of alcohol on subgroups of Hispanic women are needed. These studies need to be correlated to the acculturation and generational status of the women.

ILLEGAL DRUG USE

Prevalence of Illegal Drug Use in Hispanic Women

An overview of the prevalence of illicit drug use among Hispanics from the 1987 National Household Survey on Drug Abuse (NIDA, 1987) indicated that Hispanic women were less likely than white women to ever have used marijuana, cocaine, hallucinogens, inhalants, and PCP. Similar to patterns of alcohol use, the use of drugs among Hispanic women was found to vary among Hispanic subgroups. The HHANES (NCHS, 1985), which surveyed Mexican Americans, Cubans, and Puerto Ricans on the use of marijuana, cocaine, and inhalants, indicated that, in general, Puerto Rican women had a greater drug problem than Mexican-American or Cuban-American women; Mexican-American women had a greater drug problem than Cuban-American women. Lifetime use of cocaine and marijuana was found to be higher for Puerto Rican (16.8% and 35.8%) than Mexican-American (5.6% and 27.9%), or Cuban-American (4.9% and 13.1%) women. Current use of cocaine and marijuana was also higher for Puerto Rican (6.4%) than for Mexican-American (0.9%) women (Amaro, Whitaker, Coffman, & Heeren, 1990). No difference was found in the lifetime use of inhalants among Puerto Rican and Mexican-American women (no analysis was done on Cuban women due to the small sample size). Several geographically localized studies conducted on the use of drugs by Mexican Americans and Puerto Ricans supported the results of the HHANES Survey (Amaro et al., 1990; Anglin, Booth, Ryan, & Hser, 1988; Berenson, Stiglich, Wilkinson, & Anderson, 1991; Hser, Anglin, & Liu, 1991; Zambrana, Hernandez, Dunkel-Schetter, & Scrimshaw, 1991). However, Anglin, Hser, and McGlothlin (1987) reported that the use of drugs in Mexican-American women is dominated by heroin use. Together, study findings suggested that illicit drug use by Hispanic women is a significant problem.

Gender differences in illicit drug use and death rates from drug dependence also have been reported among Hispanics. National studies on drug use found that Hispanic men were more likely to have used drugs or be current users of drugs than Hispanic women (NIDA, 1987; NCHS, 1985). By subgroup, Mexican-American, Puerto Rican, and Cuban men were found to use cocaine and marijuana at much higher rates than their female counterparts (Chavez, Edwards, & Oetting, 1989). A study of death rates from drug dependence in Puerto Ricans indicated that men had a risk of dying from drug dependence several times that of women with female rates being the smallest to those of males in the age group of 15 to 24. Thereafter, the female rate was one quarter of male rates (Shai, 1990).

The concepts of acculturation and generational status also have been investigated in relationship to drug use. Amaro et al. (1990) found that acculturation into U.S. society, as reflected by language use, was accompanied by a higher prevalence of illicit drug use. This relationship held true even when sociodemographic variables were taken into account. Acculturation was more strongly associated with drug use among Mexican American women than among Mexican American men; cocaine use was more strongly associated among Puerto Rican men than among Puerto Rican women. The use of marijuana and cocaine was reported more often by U.S.-born Hispanic men and women of all groups and was higher among English-speaking Hispanic men and women than among those who were bilingual, who in turn were generally more likely to report drug use than those who were primarily Spanish speakers (Velez & Ungemack, 1989). By subgroup, Puerto Rican men and women reported the highest use of marijuana and cocaine across language categories and birthplace. Moreover, Hispanic females from all Hispanic subgroups appear more vulnerable to acculturation than males (Amaro et al., 1990; Berenson et al., 1991; Hser, Anglin, & Liu, 1991; Velez & Ungemack, 1989; Zambrana et al., 1991). Female immigrants have demonstrated greater increases in drug use than male immigrants with each additional year spent in the United States.

Research findings in the area of acculturation, generational status and illicit drug use are similar to the findings related to alcohol. It may be that adjusting to the Anglo culture places stress on Hispanic women who turn to alcohol and drugs to cope. Further research on the relationship between degree of acculturation and alcohol and drug use is needed. In addition, it is important to develop preventive programs appropriate to the unique needs of Hispanic women.

Psychosocial and Psychological Factors in Drug Use

Few researchers have examined the relationship between psychological and psychosocial factors with illegal drug use by Hispanic women. An exception is a study by Nyamanthi and Flaskerud (1992) which found that Hispanic drug-abusing women tended to neglect their children, lacked financial security, and social support, and suffered racial discrimination. Personal effects of their drug use were: loss of control, low self-esteem, loneliness, and helplessness.

In a series of articles results were reported from a research study designed to examine the process of addiction among Mexican and Anglo men and women addicted to heroin (Anglin, Booth, Ryan, & Hser, 1988; Anglin, Hser, & Booth, 1987; Anglin, Hser, & McGlothlin, 1987; Cervantes et al., 1990–1991; Hser, Anglin, & Booth, 1987; Hser, Anglin, & McGlothlin, 1987). Addictive careers were divided into four distinct periods related to narcotics use: preexperimentation, experimentation, addiction, and first methadone treatment. Overall, there were more similarities than differences in the addictive careers of Mexican and Anglo women. Although the careers were similar, it is interesting to note that on the average Mexican women entered the process of addiction a year later in the first three phases, were 2 years older entering treatment, and three years older at discharge from treatment than Anglo women. Also, in contrast to Anglo women, Mexican women engaged in prostitution less often, had more arrests, were rearrested more quickly after discharge, and had lower employment rates. Mexican women had higher discharge and relapse rates than Anglo women.

Despite the prevalent drug abuse problem, only one intervention study focused on treating Hispanics was found (Malgady & Rogler, 1990). A hero/heroine intervention was developed using adult Puerto Rican role models to foster ethnic identity, self-concept, and adaptive coping behavior in adolescents. The intervention significantly increased adolescents' ethnic identity and self-concept and reduced anxiety. However, treatment for stopping drug abuse was not significantly effective for girls in father-absent families or for boys in father-present families; a strong treatment effect was found for girls in father-present families.

The majority of the research on Hispanic women and drug abuse has been descriptive. Most studies have used samples of convenience and lack generalizability across Hispanic subgroups. There is a dearth of research on treatments, interventions and drug abuse theories to account for the special circumstances of Hispanic women.

PRESCRIPTION DRUGS AND OVER-THE-COUNTER MEDICATIONS

Little is known about the use of prescription drugs and over-the-counter (OTC) medications by Hispanic women. Studies that have investigated nonprescription and prescriptions drug use in Hispanic women have focused solely on prevalence. Two national studies found no differences between Mexican-American and Puerto Rican women in the use of sedatives (NIDA, 1987). Other studies have found the incidence of prescription drug use to differ among women in Hispanic subgroups. In a Florida, community-based, nonprobability sample of Cuban born women, all subjects reported using benzodiazepines, 22.9% reported using phenothiazines, and 13.1% reported using propanediols (Kirby, 1989). In contrast, a California study examined the patterns of substance use before and during pregnancy in a sample of low-income, primiparous African-American, Mexican-American and Mexican immigrant women. Twenty-four percent of the recent Mexican immigrant respondents reported prescription drug use, whereas the U.S.-born Mexicans reported no use of prescription drugs. Use of OTC medications was reported by 31% of recent Mexican immigrants and 21% of U.S.-born Mexican women (Zambrana et al., 1991).

These findings suggest that there are intra- and intergroup differences in the use of prescription and OTC medications by Hispanic women. Results suggest that some Hispanic women may overly depend on the use of prescription drugs and OTC medications. However, strong conclusions cannot be drawn because of methodological limitations, such as nonprobability sampling and small sample size. Again, the need for additional systematic studies on Hispanic subgroups with attention to acculturation and generation status is emphasized.

SMOKING

Prevalence of Smoking Among Hispanic Women

The rate of cigarette smoking among Hispanic women varies according to age, Hispanic subgroup, generational status, and acculturation level (Samet, Coultas, Howard, & Skipper, 1988). In the HHANES (Haynes, Harvey, Montes, Nickens, & Cohen, 1990; NCHS, 1985) the prevalence of cigarette smoking among Mexican Americans, Puerto Ricans, and Cuban Americans was examined. The age-adjusted rates were 23.8, 30.3, and 24.4 percent respectively. Puerto Ricans and Cuban-American women were more likely to be heavy smokers than Mexican-American women. Some studies have shown that Hispanic women have a higher prevalance of smoking than Anglo women. Puerto Rican women under the age of 40, Mexican-American women in their 40s, and Cuban American women in their 30s were found to have a smoking prevalence higher than the national average for women (Escobedo, Anda, Smith, Remington, & Mast, 1990; Escobedo, Remington, & Anda, 1989a; Pletsch, 1991). Interestingly, other studies have found that Hispanic women smoke less than Anglo women (Humble, Samet, Pathak, & Skipper, 1985; Marin, Perez-Stable, Marin, Sabogal & Otero-Sabogal, 1990).

As with alcohol and drug use, the prevalence of cigarette smoking has been found to be higher in Hispanic men than women (Escobedo, Anda, Smith, Remington, & Mast, 1990; Lee & Markides, 1991). Some findings indicate that cigarette smoking among Hispanic males has decreased but the same is not true for Hispanic women (Escobedo & Remington, 1989; Escobedo, Remington, & Anda, 1989a, 1989b). The age at which cigarette smoking is initiated greatly influences smoking prevalence. Among subgroups, Puerto Rican women have been found to start smoking earlier and have higher smoking initiation rates than Mexican American, Cuban or Anglo women (Escobedo, Anda, Smith, Remington, & Mast, 1990). This could be one explanation for the higher prevalence of smoking in Puerto Rican women. Authors of one study indicated that Mexican Americans may underreport the quantity of cigarette smoking and those reporting light smoking may truly by moderate or heavy smokers (Perez-Stable, Marin, Brody, & Benowitz, 1990).

Cigarette smoking in relationship to acculturation and generational status of Hispanic women also has been studied. Several studies have shown that smoking rates for Hispanic women increases with greater acculturation (Coreil, Ray, & Markides, 1991; Haynes, Harvey, Montes, Nickens, & Cohen, 1990; Dusenbury et al., 1992; Marin, Perez-Stable, & Marin, 1989; Marin, Perez-Stable, Marin, Sabogal, & Otero-Sabogal,1990; Smith & McGraw, 1993; Zambrana et al., 1991). Interestingly, the relationship between acculturation and smoking seems independent of gender (Lee & Markides, 1991; Marin et al., 1989). Positive associations between smoking status and heavy coffee consumption have been found across gender and age groups (Lee, Leon, & Markides, 1988).

Psychosocial and Psychological Factors in Smoking

Studies have attempted to link psychosocial and health behaviors with cigarette smoking by Hispanic women. Major social predictors of experimental smoking have been found to be the proportion of friends who smoke, number of siblings who smoke, presence of other smokers in the immediate social environment (home and workplace), and maternal smoking (Coreil et al., 1991; Dusenbury et al., 1992). Also educational attainment, religious affiliation, and marital status have been found to influence the probability of smoking. High school graduates were one half as likely to be smokers than those who had not graduated, those who attended Catholic or fundamentalist churches were much less likely to smoke than those who did not attend, and respondents with spouses or partners who did not smoke were also less likely to do so.

Lower systolic and diastolic blood pressures in middle-aged smokers, and higher level of depressive symptomatology have been found among smoking women (Samet, Coultas, Howard, & Skipper, 1988). Interestingly, Hispanic women have been found less likely to smoke during pregnancy than their non-Hispanic counterparts (Marin, Perez-Stable, Marin, Sabogal, & Otero-Sabogal, 1990; Wolff, Portis, & Wolff, 1993). Hostility as measured by an irritability scale has been shown to have little relationship to smoking (Lee, Leon, & Markides, 1988).

One survey (Marin, Perez-Stable, Marin, Sabogal, & Otero-Sabogal, 1990) has been conducted to evaluate the effectiveness of a smoking cessation program for Hispanics. Nearly 50% of respondents were Central Americans and nearly one third were of Mexican ancestry. Results indicated that an increased awareness of cessation services occurred after implementation of the intervention with the change occurring primarily among the less acculturated Spanish-speaking Hispanics. The Hispanic subjects considered willpower and knowing the negative effects of smoking to be the most helpful techniques for quitting.

In summary, many clinicians and researchers have conjectured that a combination of one or more of the following factors have contributed to the substance abuse problem currently experienced by U.S. Hispanics: (a) the poverty-striken conditions in which many Hispanics live; (b) the limited school and employment opportunities available to them; (c) the discrimination they experience; (d) stress related to adapting to a new culture and loss of cultural identity by many young Hispanic immigrants; and (e) the disintegration of the extended family system that in the past provided emotional and financial help during times of crises and served as a positive socialization mechanism against the adoption of deviant behavior, such as substance abuse. However, these hypotheses have not been substantiated with research.

Furthermore, a major limitation to the studies reviewed in the area of substance abuse among Hispanic women has been the lack of standard means to measure acculturation and the use of alcohol, drugs, and smoking. Nonetheless, an important finding is that similar results have been obtained across studies and across samples regarding the relevance of the acculturation model to substance abuse in Hispanic women; the increased acculturation among Hispanics has been associated with higher incidence of alcohol, drug, and smoking use. Thus, strategies need to be developed to intervene with Hispanic women, helping them to cope with the stress of acculturation.

RECOMMENDATIONS

The authors of this chapter have attempted to give some clarity to the incidence, prevalence, and characteristics associated with adolescent pregnancy, sexually transmitted diseases, and substance abuse in Hispanic women. The review has shown that a fuller understanding of these health risk behaviors and their implications for the Hispanic population is needed. Conceptual and methodological problems plague much of this body of research making it difficult to gain a lucid picture of the phenomena of adolescent pregnancy, sexually transmitted diseases, and substance abuse as they occur in this population.

Most of the research conducted with Hispanics has been with the largest Hispanic subgroup, Mexicans (70%) which make up 60% of the Hispanic population in the United States. Only 34% of the Hispanic population lives in California; however, 47% of the studies reviewed were conducted in California. Over one half of the studies were conducted with lower socioeconomic class Hispanics (social class was not reported in 45% of studies); thus, it appears that most of the body of literature available describes lower socioeconomic Hispanic women living in California.

The research reviewed suggests that there is considerable variation across localities in terms of the incidence and prevalence of adolescent pregnancy, sexually transmitted diseases and substance use in Hispanics. However, much of this variation could be due to the widely discrepant assessment measures used in the different studies. We cannot conclude that systematic differences across Hispanic subgroups exist without further research which examines large samples of Hispanics from different regions of the country, across socioeconomic classes, and using comparable measures. Other methodological issues that have implications for future research include the following:

- "Hispanic" has been used as a "catch-all" term. Hispanic subgroups need to be distinguished when conducting research with Hispanics.
- Most studies on the health risk behavior on Hispanic women have been conducted at the local level. More large-scale studies with consistent measures are needed to understand the phenomena fully.
- Research on adolescent pregnancy, sexually transmitted diseases and substance abuse has mostly been restricted to descriptive studies. Consequently, more experimental and intervention studies in the Hispanic population are needed in all areas.
- Theory development attempting to account for the special circumstances of Hispanic women is in its infancy. Consequently, there is only a limited body of empirical literature to guide the design and selection and treatment and prevention interventions specific to health risk behaviors among Hispanic women.
- More research on the health risk behaviors of Puerto Rican women is warranted. Puerto Rican women have higher incidence of adolescent pregnancy, sexually transmitted diseases, and substance abuse

- Research by nurses related to adolescent pregnancy, sexually transmitted diseases and substance abuse problems of Hispanics women is also almost nonexistent. There is a need for nursing research in health risk behaviors of Hispanic women.

In conclusion, limitations in treatment and prevention programs reflect limitations in the existing body of literature on health risk behaviors among Hispanic women as a population and among the subpopulations. Without basic information regarding etiological factors in the development of health risk behaviors, treatment and prevention programs targeted at the subgroups of this population may be misguided.

REFERENCES

Amaro, H. (1988). Women in the Mexican-American community: Religion, culture, and reproductive attitudes and experiences. *Journal of Community Psychology, 16*, 6-20.

Amaro, H., Whitaker, R., Coffman, G., & Heeren, T. (1990). Acculturation and marijuana and cocaine use: Findings from HHANES, 1982-1984. *American Journal of Public Health, 80*(Suppl.), 54-60.

Andrade, S. J. (1982). Social science stereotypes of the Mexican-American woman: Policy implications for research. *Hispanic Journal of Behavioral Sciences, 4*, 223-244.

Aneshensel, C. S., Becerra, R. M., Fielder, E. P., & Schuler, R. H. (1990). Onset of fertility-related events during adolescence: A prospective comparison of Mexican-American and non-Hispanic White females. *American Journal of Public Health, 80*, 959-963.

Anglin, M. D., Booth, M. W., Ryan, T. M., & Hser, Y. (1988). Ethnic differences in narcotics addiction: 2. Chicano and Anglo addiction career patterns. *The International Journal of the Addictions, 23*, 1011-1027.

Anglin, M. D., Hser, Y., & Booth, M. W. (1987). Sex differences in addict careers: 4. Treatment. *American Journal of Drug and Alcohol Abuse, 13*, 253-280.

Anglin, M. D., Hser, Y., & McGlothlin, W. H. (1987). Sex differences in addict careers: 2. Becoming addicted. *American Journal of Drug and Alcohol Abuse, 13*, 59-71.

Aruffo, J. F., Coverdale, J. H., & Valbona, C. (1991). AIDS knowledge in low-income and minority populations. *Public Health Reports, 106*, 115-119.

Berenson, A., Stiglich, N. J., Wilkinson, G. S., & Anderson, G. D. (1991). Drug abuse and other risk factors for physical abuse in pregnancy among white non-Hispanic, black, and Hispanic women. *American Journal of Obstetrics and Gynecology, 164*, 1491-1499.

Berger, D. K., Kyman, W., Perez, G., Menendez, M., Bistritz, J. F., & Goon, J. M. (1991). Hispanic adolescent pregnancy testers: A comparative analysis of negative testers, childbearers, and aborters. *Adolescence, 26*, 951-962.

Berger, D. K., Rivera, M., Perez, G., & Fierman, A. (1993). Risk assessment for human immunodeficiency virus among pregnant Hispanic adolescents. *Adolescence, 28*, 598–607.

Caetano, R. (1987). Acculturation, drinking and social settings among U.S. Hispanics. *Drug and Alcohol Dependence, 19*, 215-228.

Cervantes, R. C., Gilbert, M. J., Snyder, N. S., & Padilla, A. M. (1990–1991). Psychosocial and cognitive correlates of alcohol use in younger adult immigrant and U.S.-born Hispanics. *The International Journal of the Addictions, 25*, 687–708.

Chavez, E. L., Edwards, R., & Oetting, E. R. (1989). Mexican American and white American school dropouts' drug use, health status, and involvement in violence. *Public Health Reports, 104*, 594–604.

Christopher, F. S., Johnson, D. C., & Roosa, M. W. (1993). Family, individual, and social correlates of early Hispanic adolescent sexual expression. *Journal of Sex Research, 30*, 54–61.

Comas-Diaz, L. (1988). Mainland Puerto Rican women: A sociocultural approach. *Journal of Community Psychology, 16*, 21–31.

Corbett, K., Mora, J., & Ames, G. (1991). Drinking patterns and drinking-related problems of Mexican-American husbands and wives. *Journal of Studies on Alcohol, 52*, 215–223.

Coreil, J., Ray, L. A., Markides, K. S. (1991). Predictors of smoking among Mexican-Americans: Findings from the Hispanic HANES. *Preventive Medicine, 20*, 508–517.

Cromwell, R., & Ruiz, R. (1979). The myth of macho dominance in decision making within Mexican and Chicano families. *Hispanic Journal of Behavioral Sciences, 1*, 355–373.

Darabi, K. F., Dryfoos, J., & Schwartz, D. (1985). Hispanic adolescent fertility. *Hispanic Journal of Behavioral Sciences, 8*, 157–171.

Darabl, K. F., & Ortiz, V. (1987). Childbearing among young Latino women in the United States. *American Journal of Public Health, 77*, 25–28.

Day, R. D. (1992). The transition to first intercourse among racially and culturally diverse youth. *Journal of Marriage and the Family, 54*, 749–762.

De Anda, D., Becerra, R. M., & Fielder, P. (1988). Sexuality, pregnancy, and motherhood among Mexican-American adolescents. *Journal of Adolescent Research, 3*, 403–411.

Diaz, T., Buehler, J. W., Castro, K. G., & Ward, J. W. (1993). AIDS trends among Hispanics in the United States. *American Journal of Public Health, 83*, 504–509.

DuRant, R. H., Pendergrast, R., & Seymore, C. (1990). Sexual behavior among Hispanic female adolescents in the United States. *Pediatrics, 85*, 257–261.

DuRant, R. H., Seymore, C., Pendergrast, R., & Beckman, R. (1990). Contraceptive behavior among sexually active Hispanic adolescents. *Journal of Adolescent Healthcare, 11*, 490–496.

Dusenbury, L., Kerner, J. F., Baker, E., Botvin, G., James-Ortiz, S., & Zauber, A. (1992). Predictors of smoking prevalence among New York Latino youth. *American Journal of Public Health, 82*, 55–58.

Escobedo, L. G., Anda, R. F., Smith, P., Remington, P. L., & Mast, E. E. (1990). Sociodemographic characteristics of cigarette smoking initiation in the United States: Implications for smoking prevention policy. *Journal of American Medicine Association, 264*, 1550–1555.

Escobedo, L. G., Remington, P. L., & Anda, R. F. (1989a). Long-term age-specific prevalence of cigarette smoking among Hispanics in the United States. *Journal of Psychoactive Drugs, 21*, 307–318.

Escobedo, L. G., Remington, P. L., & Anda, R. F. (1989b). Long-term secular trends in initiation of cigarette smoking among Hispanics in the United States. *Public Health Reports, 104*, 583–587.

Escobedo, L. G., & Remington, P. L. (1989). Birth cohort analysis of prevalence of cigarette smoking among Hispanics in the United States. *Journal of American Medical Association, 261*, 66–69.

Felice, M. E., Shragg, G. P., James, M., & Hollingsworth, D. R. (1987). Psychosocial aspects of Mexican-American, white, and black pregnant teenagers. *Journal of Adolescent Health Care, 8*, 330–334.

Fernandez-Pol, B., Bluestone, H., Missouri, C., Morales, G., & Mizruchi, M. S. (1986). Drinking patterns of inner-city black Americans and Puerto Ricans. *Journal of Studies on Alcohol, 47*, 156–160.

Flaskerud, J. H., & Calvillo, E. R. (1991). Beliefs about AIDS, health, and illness among low-income Latina women. *Research in Nursing & Health, 14*, 431–438.

Flaskerud, J. H., & Nyamanthi, A. M. (1989). Black and Latina women's AIDS related knowledge, attitudes, and practices. *Research in Nursing & Health, 12*, 339–346.

Flaskerud, J. H., & Nyamanthi, A. M. (1990). Effects of AIDS education program on the knowledge, attitudes, and practices of low income black and Latina women. *Journal of Community Health, 15*, 343–355.

Flaskerud, J. H., & Uman, G. (1993). Directions for AIDS education for Hispanic women based on analyses of survey findings. *Public Health Reports, 108*, 298–304.

Gayle, J. A., Selik, R. M., & Chu, S. Y. (1990). Surveillance for AIDS and HIV infection among black and Hispanic children and women of childbearing age: 1981–1989. *MMWR Surveillance Summaries, 39*(3), 23–30.

Gilbert, M. (1987). Alcohol consumption patterns on immigrant and later generation Mexican-American women. *Hispanic Journal of Behavioral Sciences, 9*, 299–313.

Golding, J. M., Burnam, M. A., & Wells, K. B. (1990). Alcohol use and depressive symptoms among Mexican Americans and Non-Hispanic whites. *Alcohol & Alcoholism, 25*, 421–432.

Haynes, S. G., Harvey, C., Montes, H., Nickens, H., & Cohen, B. H. (1990). Patterns of cigarette smoking among Hispanics in the United States: Results from HHANES, 1982–1984. *American Journal of Public Health, 80*, 47–53.

Hodges, B. C., Leavy, J., Swift, R., & Gold, R. S. (1992). Gender and ethnic differences in adolescents' attitudes toward condom use. *Journal of School Health, 62*, 103–106.

Holmes, K. G., Karon, J. M., & Kreiss, J. (1990). The increasing frequency of heterosexually acquired AIDS in the United States, 1983–1988. *American Journal of Public Health, 80*, 858–863.

Hser, Y., Anglin, M. D., & Booth, M. A. (1987). Sex differences in addict careers: 3. Addiction. *American Journal of Drug and Alcohol Abuse, 13*, 231–251.

Hser, Y., Anglin, M. D., & Liu, Y. (1991). A survival analysis of gender and ethnic differences in responsiveness to methadone maintenance treatment. *The International Journal of Addictions, 25*, 1295–1315.

Hser, Y., Anglin, M. D., & McGlothlin, W. (1987). Sex differences in addict careers: 1. Initiation of use. *American Journal of Drug and Alcohol Abuse, 13*, 33–57.

Humble, C. G., Samet, J. M., Pathak, D. R., & Skipper, B. J. (1985). Cigarette smoking and lung cancer in Hispanic whites and other whites in New Mexico. *American Journal of Public Health, 75*, 145–148.

Kirby, G. K. (1989). Immigration, stress and prescription drug use among Cuban women in South Florida. *Medical Anthropology, 10*, 287–295.

Kline, A., Kline, E., & Oken, E. (1992). Minority women and sexual choice in the age of AIDS. *Social Science and Medicine, 34*, 447–457.

Lee, D. J., & Markides, K. S. (1991). Health behaviors, risk factors and health indicators associated with cigarette use in Mexican Americans: Result from the Hispanic HANES. *American Journal of Public Health, 81*, 859–864.

Lee, D. J., Mendes de Leon, C. F., & Markides, K. S. (1988). The relationship between hostility, smoking, and alcohol consumption in Mexican Americans. *The International Journal of Addictions, 23*, 887–896.

Malgady, R. G., & Rogler, L. H. (1990). Hero/heroine modeling for Puerto Rican adolescents: A preventive mental health intervention. *Journal of Consulting and Clinical Psychology, 58*, 469–474.

Marin, B. V., & Marin, G. (1992a). Effects of acculturation on knowledge of AIDS and HIV among Hispanics. *Hispanic Journal of Behavioral Sciences, 12*, 110–121.

Marin, B. V., & Marin, G. (1992b). Predictors of condom accessibility among Hispanics in San Francisco. *American Journal of Public Health, 82*, 592–595.

Marin, B. V., Perez-Stable E. J., Marin, G., Sabogal, F., & Otero-Sabogal, R. (1990). Attitudes and behaviors of Hispanic smokers: Implications for cessation interventions. *Health Education Quarterly, 17*, 287–297.

Marin, G., & Marin, B. V. (1991). *Research with Hispanic Populations*. Newbury Park, CA: Sage.

Marin, G., Marin, B. V., Perez-Stable, E. J., Sabogal, F., & Otero-Sabogal, R. (1990). Changes in information as a function of a culturally appropriate smoking cessation community intervention for Hispanics. *American Journal of Community Psychology, 18*, 847–864.

Marin, G., Perez-Stable, E. J., & Marin, B. V. (1989). Cigarette smoking among San Francisco Hispanics: The role of acculturation and gender. *American Journal of Public Health, 79*, 196–198.

Markides, K. S., Ray, L. A., Stroup-Benham, C. A., & Trevino, F. (1990). Acculturation and alcohol consumption in the Mexican-American population of the southwestern United States: Finding from HHANES 1982–1984. *American Journal of Public Health, 80*, 42–46.

Mikawa, J., Morones, P. A., Gomez, A., Case, H. L., Olsen, D., & Gonzales-Huss, M. J. (1992). Cultural practices of Hispanics: Implications for the prevention of AIDS. *Hispanic Journal of Behavioral Sciences, 14*, 421–433.

Moore, D. S., & Erickson, P. I. (1985). Age, gender, and ethnic differences in sexual and contraceptive knowledge, attitudes, and behaviors. *Family and Community Health, 8*, 38–51.

National Center for Health Statistics. (1984). *Public use data tape documentation: National survey of family growth, cycle III, 1982*. Hyattsville, MD: Department of Health and Human Services.

National Center for Health Statistics. (1985). *Plan and operation of the Hispanic Health and Nutrition Examination Survey, 1982–1984*. (DHHS Publication No. PHS 85-1321). Washington, DC: Government Printing Office.

National Center for Health Statistics. (1990). *Health, United States, 1990*. Hyattsville, MD: Department of Health and Human Services.

National Institute of Drug Abuse. (1987). *1985 National household survey on drug abuse: Population estimates* (DHHS Publication No. ADM 87-1539). Rockville, MD: U.S. Government Printing Office.

Norris, A. E., & Ford, K. (1992). Beliefs about condoms and accessibility of condom intentions in Hispanic and African American youth. *Hispanic Journal of Behavioral Sciences, 14*, 373–382.

Nyamanthi, A., Bennett, C., Leake, B., Lewis, C., & Flaskerud, J. (1993). AIDS-related knowledge, perceptions, and behaviors among impoverished minority women. *American Journal of Public Health, 83*, 65–71.

Nyamanthi, A. M., & Flaskerud, J. (1992). A community-based inventory of current concerns of impoverished homeless and drug-addicted minority women. *Research in Nursing & Health, 15*, 121–129.

Nyamanthi, A. M., Leake, B., Flaskerud, J., Lewis, C., & Bennett, C. (1993). Outcomes of specialized and traditional AIDS counseling programs for impoverished women of color. *Research in Nursing & Health, 16*, 11–21.

Ortiz, C. G., & Vazquez-Nutall, E. (1987). Adolescent pregnancy: Effects of family support, education, and religion on the decision to carry or terminate among Puerto Rican teenagers. *Adolescence, 22*, 897–916.

Ortiz, S., & Casas, J. M. (1990). Birth control and low income Mexican-American women: The impact of three values. *Hispanic Journal of Behavioral Sciences, 12*, 83–92.

Padilla, A. M., & Baird, T. L. (1991). Mexican-American sexuality and sexual knowledge: An exploratory study. *Hispanic Journal of Behavioral Sciences, 13*, 95–104.

Perez-Stable, E. J., Marin, B. V., Marin, G., Brody, D. J., & Benowitz, N. L. (1990). Apparent underreporting of cigarette consumption among Mexican American smokers. *American Journal of Public Health, 80*, 1057–1061.

Pletsch, P. K. (1991). Prevalence of cigarette smoking in Hispanic women of childbearing age *Nursing Research, 40*, 103–106.

Pletsch, P. K. (1990). Hispanics: At risk for adolescent pregnancy? *Public Health Nursing, 7*, 105–110.

Porter, C. P., & Villarruel, A. M. (1993). Nursing research with African American and Hispanic people. *Nursing Outlook, 41*, 59–67.

Rapkin, A. J., & Erickson, P. I. (1990). Differences in knowledge of and risk factors for AIDS between Hispanic and non-Hispanic women attending an urban family planning clinic. *AIDS, 4*, 889–899.

Reynoso, T. C., Felice, M. E., Schragg, G. P. (1993). Does American acculturation affect outcome of Mexican-American teenager pregnancy? *Journal of Adolescent Health, 14*, 257–261.

Russell, A. Y., Williams, M. S., Farr, P. A., Schwab, A. J., & Plattsmier, S. (1993). Patterns of contraceptive use and pregnancy among young Hispanic women on the Texas-Mexico Border. *Journal of Adolescent Health, 14*, 373–379.

Sabogal, F., Faigeles, B., & Catania, J. A. (1993). Multiple sexual partners among Hispanics in high-risk cities. *Family Planning Perspectives, 25*, 257–262.

Samet, J. M., Coultas, D. B., Howard, C. A., & Skipper, B. J. (1988). Respiratory diseases and cigarette smoking in a Hispanic population in New Mexico. *American Review of Respiratory Disease, 137*, 815–819.

Schilling, R. F., El-Bassel, N., Gilbert, L., & Schinke, S. P. (1991). Correlates of drug use, sexual behavior, and attitudes toward safer sex among African-American and Hispanic women in methadone maintenance. *The Journal of Drug Issues, 21*, 685–698.

Scott, C. S., Shifman, L., Orr, L., Owen, R. G., & Fawcett, N. (1988). Hispanic and black American adolescents' beliefs relating to sexuality and contraception. *Adolescence, 23*, 667–687.

Shai, D., & Apteker, L. (1990). Factors in mortality by drug dependence among Puerto Ricans in New York City. *American Journal of Drug and Alcohol Abuse, 16*, 97–107.

Siegel, D., Golden, E., Washington, A. E., Morse, S. A., Fullilove, M. T., Catania, J. A., Marin, B., & Hulley, S. B. (1992). Prevalence and correlates of herpes simplex infections: The population-based AIDS in multiethnic neighborhoods study. *Journal of American Medical Association, 268*, 1702–1708.

Smith, K. W., & McGraw, S. A. (1993). Smoking behavior of Puerto Rican women: Evidence from caretakers of adolescents in two urban areas. *Hispanic Journal of Behavioral Sciences, 15*, 140–149.

Smith, K. W., McGraw, S. A., Crawford, S. L., Costa, L. A., & McKinlay, J. B. (1993). HIV risk among Latino adolescents in two New England Cities. *American Journal of Public Health, 83*, 1395–1399.

Smith, P. B., McGill, L., Wait, R. B. (1987). Hispanic adolescent conception and contraception profiles: A comparison. *Journal of Adolescent Health Care, 8*, 352–355.

Speraw, S. (1987). Adolescents' perceptions of pregnancy: A cross-cultural perspective. *Western Journal of Nursing Research 9*, 180–197.

Vazquez-Nutall, E., Romero-Garcia, I., & DeLeon, B. (1987). Sex roles and perceptions of femininity and masculinity of Hispanic women. *Psychology of Women Quarterly, 11*, 409–425.

Velez, C. N., & Ungemack, J. A (1989). Drug use among Puerto Rican youth: An exploration of generational status differences. *Social Science Medicine, 29*, 779–789.

Wiemann, C. M., & Berenson, A. B. (1993). Contraceptive discontinuation among white, black, and Hispanic adolescents. *Adolescent Pediatric Gynecology, 6*, 75–82.

Wolff, C. B., Portis, M., & Wolff, H. (1993). Birth weight and smoking practices during pregnancy among Mexican-American women. *Health for Women International, 14*, 271–279.

Zambrana, R. E., Hernandez, M., Dunkel-Schetter, C., & Scrimshaw, S. (1991). Ethnic differences in the substance use patterns of low-income pregnant women. *Family and Community Health, 13*, 1–11.

Index

A

Q

R

Contents of Previous Volumes

VOLUME II

VOLUME III

VOLUME IV

VOLUME X

Springer Publishing Company

SCHOLARLY INQUIRY FOR NURSING PRACTICE

JOURNAL

An International Journal

Harriet R. Feldman, PhD, RN,
Ruth Bernstein Hyman, PhD,
Barbara Kos-Munson, PhD, RN, and
Pierre Woog, PhD, Editors

Scholarly Inquiry for Nursing Practice applies the spirit of inquiry to every aspect of nursing practice. Articles often cross disciplinary and international borders to bring readers up-to-date, thought-provoking, and penetrating analyses of nursing practice, research, and theory. Each article is accompanied by commentary by a noted expert on the topic, so that readers can get an immediate sense of the material's significance in the field.

Sample Contents:

- ❑ The Common Sense Model: An Organizing Framework for Knowledge Development in Nursing, *S.E. Ward*
- ❑ Response by *B.J. Lowery*
- ❑ Development and Validation of the Perinatal Nursing Self-Efficacy Scale, *C.A. Murphy and L.A. Kraft*
- ❑ Response by *R. Froman*
- ❑ Unwritten Knowledge in Nursing: Consider the Spoken as well as the Written Word, *B. O'Brien and A. Pearson*
- ❑ Response by *C.A. Tanner*
- ❑ Patient Advocacy – An Important Part of the Daily Work of the Expert Nurse, *K. Segesten*
- ❑ Response by *L.A. Copp*

4 issues annually • ISSN 0889-7182

536 Broadway, New York, NY 10012-3955 • (212) 431-4370 • Fax (212) 941-7842

Springer Publishing Company

WRITING AND GETTING PUBLISHED

A Primer for Nurses

Barbara Stevens Barnum, RN, PhD, FAAN

This book, by one of nursing's most accomplished authors, is a step-by-step guide to developing professional writing skills and navigating the publication process. It includes pointers on structuring one's writing, avoiding common mistakes, making a term paper or dissertation publishable, writing query letters and book proposals, and finding and working with a publisher. The ability to communicate effectively in writing is an important tool for sharing knowledge and expertise, and for advancing a career. This concise guide demystifies the skills and procedures necessary to make this happen.

Contents:

Part I. Writing the Article • Finding the Right Topic • Writing the Article • Avoiding Common Mistakes • It's a Great Term Paper: Why Don't You Get it Published • Publication Options: Sending Your Article to the Right Journal • What about a Query Letter? • Submitting Articles: Getting the Procedure Right • When Your Article Reaches the Journal

Part II. Writing the Book • How Book Writing Differs from Article Writing • The Edited or Co-authored Book • It's a Great Dissertation, but is it a Book? • Producing the Book Prospectus • Finding and Working with a Publisher

Part III. Special Issues • Writing with Colleagues • Writing from Research • Writing about Work Instruments

Appendices • Appendix A. List of Nursing Journals. • Appendix B. List of Nursing Book Publishers • Appendix C. Additional Writing Resources

1995 216pp 0-8261-8690-4 hardcover

536 Broadway, New York, NY 10012-3955 • (212) 431-4370 • Fax (212) 941-7842

SP ***Springer Publishing Company***

ADVANCING NURSING EDUCATION WORLDWIDE

Doris Modly, RN, PhD,
Renzo Zanotti, IP, AFD, PhD (C),
Dott. **Piera Poletti**, & **Joyce J. Fitzpatrick**, RN, PhD, FAAN, Editors

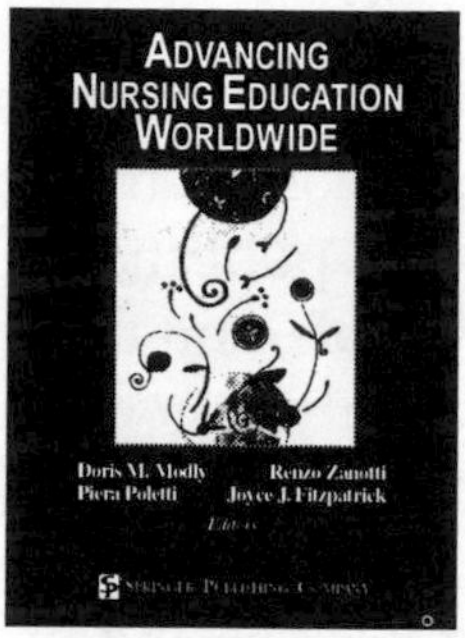

The purpose of the book is to describe global trends in nursing education, share innovative approaches to it, report and develop cross-cultural and collaborative research, and provide a model for future international collaborations in nursing. The book concludes with a blueprint for action that nurses can apply to improve the status of nursing education.

Partial Contents:

Part I: Nursing Education Requirements Worldwide. Global Trends in Nursing Education: A World Health Organization Perspective, *J. Salvage* • Broadening Nursing Boundaries Through Nursing Education and Nursing Education Research, *R. Zanotti*

Part II: Teaching Practices Worldwide. Designing Curriculum to Advance Nursing Science and Professional Practice, *D.M. Modly*

Part III: Issues Important to Nurse Educators Worldwide. Management Education for Nurses in the United States, *S.A. Ryan & C. Conway-Welch* • Computers in Nursing Education, *M. Tallberg* • Re-entry of Students, *D. McGivern*

Part IV: Advancing Research in Nursing Education. Pathways to Implementing Nursing Education Research Globally, *J.J. Fitzpatrick* • A Blueprint for Advancing Nursing Education Research Globally, *Scientific Committee Members*

1995 200pp 0-8261-8650-5 hardcover

536 Broadway, New York, NY 10012-3955 • (212) 431-4370 • Fax (212) 941-7842

Springer Publishing Company

NURSING RESEARCH AND ITS UTILIZATION

BOOK WINNER AWARD

International State of the Science

Joyce J. Fitzpatrick, PhD,
Nikki S. Polis, PhD, and
Joanne S. Stevenson, PhD, Editors

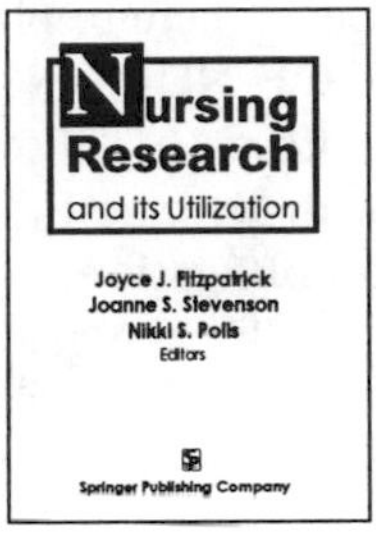

Leading experts in various areas of nursing research discuss the current state and future of the field. Specific topics in nursing practice, care delivery, and professional training are examined. Contributors include Nancy Fugate Woods, Kathleen A. McCormick, Ada Sue Hinshaw, Ada Jacox, and May Wykle.

Partial Contents:

I: Nursing Practice. Prevention and Primary Health Care Delivery, *D.L. Powell* • Classification of Nursing Interventions: Implications for Nursing Research, *J.C. McCloskey & G. Bulechek*

II: Nursing Care Delivery. The Effects of Practice Model Implementation, *J.A. Verrano* • Research on Nursing Case Management, *G.S. Lamb*

III: Research Training and Career Development. Developing a Research Career: A Trajectory for Career Development, *A.S. Hinshaw* • Nursing Research Training and Career Development Around the World, *T. Oguisso*

IV: International Perspectives. Nursing Research in the Western Pacific Region and Future Directions, *M.I. Kim* • Challenges in Conducting Cross-National Nursing Research, *L.F. Degner & M.E. Williams*

1994 256pp 0-8261-8090-6 hardcover

536 Broadway, New York, NY 10012-3955 • (212) 431-4370 • Fax (212) 941-7842

ORDER FORM

Save 10% on Volume 14 with this coupon.

____ Check here to order the ANNUAL REVIEW OF NURSING RESEARCH, Volume 14, 1996 at a 10% discount. You will receive an invoice requesting prepayment.

Save 10% on all futures volumes with a continuation order.

____ Check here to place your continuation order for the ANNUAL REVIEW OF NURSING RESEARCH. You will receive a prepayment invoice with a 10% discount upon publication of each new volume, beginning with Volume 14, 1996. You may pay for prompt shipment or cancel with no obligation.

Name ____

Institution ____

Address ____

City/State/Zip _____________________________________

Examination copies for possible adoption are available to instructors "on approval" only. Write on institutional letterhead, noting course, level, present text, and expected enrollment (include $3.50 for postage and handling). Prices slightly higher overseas. Prices subject to change.

Mail this coupon to:
SPRINGER PUBLISHING COMPANY
536 Broadway, New York, N.Y. 10012